H. Breuer · B. J. Smit
Proton Therapy and Radiosurgery

This book is dedicated to our teachers
Rossal Sealy and Peter Brix

Springer

Berlin
Heidelberg
New York
Barcelona
Hong Kong
London
Milan
Paris
Singapore
Tokyo

Hans Breuer
Berend J. Smit

Proton Therapy and Radiosurgery

With 88 Figures in 112 Separate Illustrations and 60 Tables

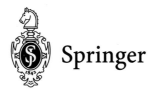 Springer

Hans Breuer, Dr.
18, Constantia Avenue
7600 Stellenbosch
Rep. of South Africa

Berend J. Smit, Professor
Tygerberg Hospital
Department of Radiation Oncology
Gene Louw Buillding
7505 Tygerberg
Rep. of South Africa

ISBN 3-540-64100-9 Springer-Verlag Berlin Heidelberg New York

CIP data applied for

Die Deutsche Bibliothek - CIP-Einheitsaufnahme
Breuer, Hans: Proton therapy and radiosurgery / H. Breuer; B. J. Smit. – Berlin; Heidelberg;
New York; Barcelona; Hongkong; London; Mailand; Paris; Singapur; Tokio: Springer, 2000
ISBN 3-540-64100-9 DBN: 95.644007.X

© Springer-Verlag Berlin Heidelberg 2000
Printed in Germany

Cover design: Erich Kirchner, Heidelberg

Typesetting: Verlagsservice Teichmann, Mauer

SPIN: 10559166 21/3135 - 5 4 3 2 1 0 – Printed on acid-free paper

Preface

The book is divided into two parts: Part I deals with the relevant physics and planning algorithms of protons (H Breuer) and Part II with the radiobiology, radiopathology and clinical outcomes of proton therapy and a comparison of proton therapy *versus* photon therapy (BJ Smit). Protons can be used for radiosurgery and general radiotherapy.

Since proton therapy was first proposed in 1946 by Wilson, about sixteen facilities have been built globally. Only a very few of these have isocentric beam delivery systems so that proton therapy is really only now in a position to be compared directly by means of randomised clinical trials, with modern photon radiotherapy therapy systems, both for radiosurgery and for general fractionated radiotherapy.

Three-dimensional proton planning computer systems with image fusion (image registration) capabilities of computerised tomography (CT), magnetic resonance imaging (MRI), stereotactic angiograms and perhaps positron emission tomography (PET) are essential for accurate proton therapy planning. New planning systems for spot scanning are under development.

Many of the older comparisons of the advantageous dose distributions for protons were made with parallel opposing or multiple co-planar field arrangements, which are now largely obsolete. New comparative plans are necessary once more because of the very rapid progress in 3-D conformal planning with photons. New cost-benefit analyses may be needed.

Low energy (about 70 MeV) proton therapy is eminently suitable for the treatment of eye tumours and has firmly established itself as very useful in this regard.

Medium to high-energy proton therapy by means of horizontal beams has produced very good results for chondromas, chordomas and chondrosarcomas near the spinal cord and brain stem.

Protons seem to have an advantage for the larger intra-cranial (and large lesions at other body sites) lesions like arteriovenous malformations, relative to photons, but for the smaller lesions alternatives like the Gamma Knife and linear accelerator appear to be equally effective and may be less costly.

The relative biological effectiveness (RBE) of protons in the distal dose fall-off zone may be 1.5 or higher than the generally quoted 1.1, and this may have important implications, especially for fractionated therapy, where fractionation may cause greater than expected damage in the penumbral zone of treatment plans.

Reliability of beam availability is an extremely important clinical consideration. Pre-therapy delays of up to 10 days for the preparation of collimator, immobilisation device and planning should be avoided for new facilities which should have isocentric beam delivery with reliable accelerators and beam lines equipped with spot scanning systems or multileaf collimators and motorised compensator cutters.

The prospect of superconducting magnets may make new facilities compact enough to fit into hospital environments, and spot scanning techniques may obviate all the "slow" hardware in the beam line.

The cost of constructing proton therapy centres remains a major stumbling block to the wider implementation of proton facilities.

Exciting new concepts like ECRIPAC (Electron Cyclotron Resonance Ion Plasma Accelerator) may eventually deliver proton therapy facilities, which can be compact, cheap and hospital-based.

This book may be of use to all involved in proton therapy: radiation oncologists, neurosurgeons, medical physicists, radiobiologists, the relevant specialists-in-training, and the radiographer/technician or student.

The text, especially Part I, is kept short. The cited literature contains more detailed information.

Acknowledgements
The hard work of Mrs Roswitha Mouton in preparing the manuscript and drawings is gratefully acknowledged. The valuable editorial advice of Dr RF Mould and the contributions of Dr Wilhelm Groenewald and the encouragement of colleagues is appreciated. Dr WA Groenewald (PhD) made all the calculations for the chapter on dose-volume relationships in Part II (BJS)

HB is grateful to Dr Sinclair Wynchank for patient discussions and valuable advice. Rosie deflected my stress into harmless channels, thank you.

BS and HB 1999

Table of Contents

Part I Radiation Physics

PART II Proton Therapy and Radiotherapy

Radiation Physics

A General Aspects

A.1
A Brief History of Charged Particle Radiotherapy

About half a century after Röntgen (1896) discovered X-rays, another physicist – this time from Harvard University – suggested utilising high energy protons for radiotherapy (Wilson 1946). He described in detail the very favourable depth-dose distribution of fast protons inside the body, now called the Bragg distribution (named after W.H.Bragg, 1862–1942). However, the medical profession had to wait another four years until the cyclotron could accelerate protons, deuterons and alpha particles to a sufficiently high energy. In contrast, the first therapeutic application of X-rays began merely a few months after its discovery.

Following a then medical trend, the first irradiation target for protons was the pituitary gland. The aim was, to suppress its function in order to influence favourably the metastatic development of breast carcinoma. Apparently the therapists did not trust in the development of a Bragg peak deep inside the tissue but utilised a "cross fire" irradiation technique. The first publication (Tobias et al. 1954) dealt with the effectiveness of fast deuterons on rats. A medical application of protons was published three years later from Berkeley, USA, by Lawrence (1957), reporting the first patient treatment. After that only a He^{++}-beam remained available for medical investigations, high energy protons were exclusively reserved for physics experiments.

The new synchrocyclotron in Uppsala, Sweden, extended the work of Berkeley in 1954 by refining the functional radiosurgery of the brain. Among other methods, the Uppsala group pioneered radiotherapy utilising a Spread Out Bragg Peak (SOBP) for the treatment of large tumours. In the early sixties, the Harvard Cyclotron Group in Cambridge, USA, took over an obsolete physics accelerator and developed most of the proton irradiation techniques currently in use. A few years later, scientists at Dubna, Russia, prepared a high energy proton beam for medical treatment on a large scale. At present, a large fraction of all patients treated with fast protons have received their treatment at this accelerator north of Moscow.

The use of fast protons for treatment of the eye – predominantly the irradiation of uveal melanoma – was started in the early seventies at the Massachusetts Eye and Ear Infirmary (Constable et al. 1976), using the proton beam of the Harvard Cyclotron. The Japanese proton machines in Chiba and – a few years later – Tsukuba introduced in 1979 sophisticated beam scanning techniques to cover large and irregularly shaped targets. Hand in hand with those developments three-dimensional irradiation planning techniques of rapidly growing complexity appeared.

Realising that heavy charged particles, especially fast protons, are a superior medical irradiation modality, more and more physics accelerators were – at least part-time

– utilised for medical treatment. At present there are, world-wide, more than twenty heavy charged particle sources available to the medical profession. By the end of 1998 about 23 000 patients had been treated, 90% with protons.

Proton accelerators cost at least an order of magnitude more than betatrons and electron linear accelerators (linacs). Small wonder, that during the first fifty years only old and mainly obsolete physics machines carried the main burden. However, cost-effectiveness can be achieved with single purpose proton accelerators. The first medically dedicated proton treatment facilities have been built. Leading this path was Loma Linda, California, opening for treatment in 1991 (Slater et al. 1988). Massachusetts General Hospital in Boston, USA, followed in 1998. Two dozen further institutions are either under construction or at the planning stage, for a listing see Sect. A.2.

To accelerate heavy ions, i.e. positively charged particles having a mass exceeding that of He^{++}, into an energy range suitable for medical treatment is even more expensive than producing appropriate protons. However, heavy particles combine the sharp delineation of the dose distribution achieved by protons with a radiobiologically desirable high Linear Energy Transfer (LET). Berkeley combined in 1974 its heavy ion accelerator HILAC with its circular accelerator BEVATRON to form the new machine BEVALAC. Mainly He- and Ne-ions were employed for medical treatment. The results are at least as promising as those for protons. Nevertheless, all treatment ceased in 1992. This very promising work is now continued at the heavy ion facilities in Darmstadt, Germany and Chiba, Japan.

A.2
Heavy Charged Particle Radiotherapy Facilities

The folowing tables are based on the regularly updated information in PARTICLES, Newsletter of the Proton Therapy Co-operative Group (PTCOG), edited by Janet Sisterson (Sisterson 1999).

A.2.1
Proton Radiotherapy Facilities in Operation

Table A2.1

Location		Patients	Max. energy (in MeV)
North America			
Berkeley CA, USA	1954-1957	30	910
Harvard MA, USA	1961	8160	160
IUCF IN, USA	1993	9	
Loma Linda CA, USA	1990	4330	250
UCSF CA, USA	1994	214	
Vancouver, CAN	1995	47	

Table A2.1 Continue

Location		Patients	Max. energy (in MeV)
Europe			
Berlin, D	1998	30	72
Clatterbridge, GB	1989	817	172
Dubna, RU	1967, 1987	150	660
Louvain-la-Neuve, B	1991	30	85
Moscow, RU	1969	3000	200
Nice, F	1991	1350	65
Orsay, F	1991	1219	200
St.Petersburg, RU	1975	1029	1000
Uppsala, S	1957, 1989	200	185
Villingen, CH	1984, 1996	2773	72, 250
Other			
Chiba, JP	1979	100	70
Faure, ZA	1993	310	200
Kashiwa, JP	1998	8	235
Tsukuba, JP	1983	606	250

A.2.2
Other Heavy Charged Particle Facilities

Table A2.2

Location	Particles		Patients
Berkeley CA, USA	$>d^+$	1957-1992	2000
Berkeley CA, USA	Ne^+	1975-1992	450
Chiba, JP	$>d^+$	1994	473
Darmstadt, D	$>d^+$	1997	20
Los Alamos NM, USA	π^-	1974-1982	290
PSI, CH	π^-	1980-1993	500
Vancouver, CAN	π^-	1979-1994	400
Villingen, CH	π^-	1980-1993	500

A.2.3
Facilities under Construction or at the Planning Stage

Table A2.3

Location	Particles	Opening	Max. energy (in MeV)
AUSTRON, A	p, $>d^+$		
Beijing, China	p		250
Bratislava, SK	p	2003	
Erlangen, D	p		
Hyogo, JP	$>d^+$	2001	
ISS, I	p		200
ITEP, RU	p		320
Krakow, PL	p		60
Kyoto, JP	p	2002	230
NC Star, USA	p	1999	300
NPTC, USA	p	2000	235
PROTOX, GB	p	2001	250
TERA, I	p, $>d^+$	2002	250

B Basics

B.1
Protons

B.1.1
Physical Properties

Protons, symbol p or H^+, are positively charged elementary particles, the nuclei of light hydrogen atoms. Protons are members of the baryon-group and were discovered in 1920 by Ernest Rutherford. They are a basic component of all atomic nuclei, consisting of two up-quarks and one down-quark.

The proton carries one positive elementary electric charge and has a rest mass of 1.67×10^{-27} kg (= 938 MeV), i.e. it is 1836 times more massive than the electron. Most likely the proton is a stable particle, for the latest measurements assign it a lifetime of $> 10^{30}$ a.

A free proton is obtained by stripping a hydrogen atom of its electron. To achieve this a minimum energy of 13.5 eV is needed. The proton reverts rapidly to hydrogen by capturing an electron from its surroundings.

High energy protons occur naturally in cosmic radiation. Protons are released in nuclear reactions, during the decay of neutrons and by stripping hydrogen of its electron. Protons are accelerated in Van de Graaff generators, various types of cyclotrons, linear accelerators, etc.

B.1.2
The Proton's Position in the Hierarchy of Particles

The proton is just one member in the very involved hierarchy of relatively stable particles, partly listed below. For comparison the positions of the electron (e^-) and of the neutron (n) are emphasised.

B.1.3
Proton Radiotherapy

The radiation dose deposited by X-rays entering a body drops off exponentially with penetration depth. Consequently, the entrance dose is much greater than the dose at the position of any target deep inside. The exit dose produced by X-rays cannot be neglected. Although the depth dose distribution of high energy bremsstrahlung displays a maximum, its descending part drops slowly.

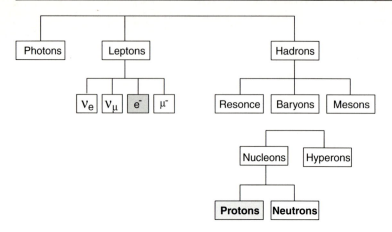

Fig. B1.1. Hierarchy of relatively stable particles.

The dose distribution produced by electrons, a light and negatively charged particle, is more favourable for radiotherapy. The shape of the dose distribution inside a body presents a broad maximum at a few centimetres depth, about 20% higher than the entrance dose. The distal fall-off of the dose distribution is moderately steep, the exit dose low. See Fig. B1.2.

The main advantage of the proton radiation – as compared with X-rays and electron beams – is its finite range and the shape of its depth dose distribution. If a proton beam enters a body, its locally deposited dose increases very slowly for about 3/4 of the beam's range. While passing through the last quarter of its path length, the radiation dose deposited by the protons rises steeply, reaches a maximum value and then drops off rapidly to zero. If the diameter of the proton beam exceeds approximately 15 mm, its entrance dose is only about 25% of the dose value at its maximum. If the proton energy is selected properly, i.e. its range is shorter than the body's diameter, the exit dose is virtually zero.

The cost of radiotherapy using protons is significantly higher than the expenses incurred utilising X-rays, bremsstrahlung or electrons. Nevertheless, the superior depth dose distribution of a proton beam justifies, in many instances, its application.

Beams of other heavy charged particles like deuterons, Helium ions, Carbon ions, etc. display a depth dose distribution as superior to that of X-rays as that of protons. However, there is always an unavoidable exit dose of about 1/10 of the peak dose value. In addition, the costs to produce those particles for radiotherapy is even higher than the costs for proton therapy.

The following table compares some irradiation modalities used in radiotherapy.

The following figure presents the depth dose distributions (deposited relative radiation dose versus penetration depth) of various types of radiation used in radiotherapy. The curve shapes are are approximations and merely illustrate the general behaviour of the various modalities.

Table B1. Properties relevant to radiotherapy of various types of radiation. The values for relative costs are very approximate. The depth dose types refer to Fig. B1.2.

Radiation	Rel.mass	Rel. costs	RBE	Depth dose type
Bremsstrahlung (linac)	-	0.1	1.0	A
Electron	5.4×10^{-4}	0.2	1.0	B
Proton	1.0	1	1.1	C
Neutron	1.0	0.3-1.5	2-4	B
π^-	0.15	3	2-3	D
d-Ion	2.0	3	1.1	C
He^{++}-Ion	4.0	3	1.2-1.6	C
C^{+6}-Ion	12.0	3	2-3	D
Ne-Ion	20.2	3	2.5-3.5	D
Si-Ion	28.1	3	3-4	D

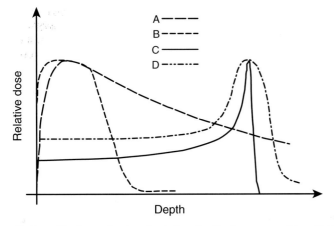

Fig. B1.2. The shape of various depth dose distribution types used in radiotherapy. A. Bremsstrahlung: With increasing bremsstrahlung energy the position of the maximum shifts slowly to the right. The distribution width remains about the same. B. High-energy electrons: With increasing energy the dose maximum shifts toward the right. C. Protons: The peak's position (Bragg peak) is proportional to the particle energy. The distal fall-off is very steep and the particle range is well defined. D. Pions: The dose distribution displays a 'tail' beyond the distal part of the peak.

B.2
Sources of Protons

Radiotherapy proton beams must fulfil two basic requirements. Their energy has to be high enough to reach the target volume inside the patient's body. Their intensity must be sufficient to deliver the required radiation dose within a reasonable treatment time.

Natural sources of protons are rare and unsuitable: In cosmic rays their energy is much too high, from radioactive decay their intensity is too low. Only accelerators can produce protons of sufficient energy and intensity.

Table B2.1. General require-ments at the target site (1 litre volume) for charged particle radiotherapy.	Particle beam	Maximum beam energy in MeV	Minimum beam intensity for 10 Gy/min
	Protons	250	4×10^9
	α-particles	1000	1×10^9
	C^{+6}-ions	4800	2×10^8
	π^--mesons	100	6×10^9

B.2.1
Proton Accelerators

Protons injected into accelerators are produced by stripping hydrogen atoms of their electrons. These free protons are accelerated by electric fields to the desired energy.

The same process applies (except for pions) for the production of therapeutic beams of other heavy charged particles, i.e. electrons are removed from the appropriate atoms and the remaining nuclei are accelerated.

B.2.1a
General Requirements

Until very recently accelerators used in radiotherapy were machines originally designed for experimental physics. They were either given up as being outdated, or produced therapeutic beams as a sideline. A dedicated medical accelerator should fulfil the following requirements:

Energy. The maximum beam energy must be sufficient to penetrate about 30 cm of inhomogeneous tissue. This requires a maximum proton energy of approximately 250 MeV. To tailor the beam energy to the depth of the irradiation site, the beam energy should be continuously adjustable. With modern accelerators this is either impossible to do directly (due to the accelerating principle) or impracticable (due to the time needed for an energy change). Consequently, in general, the energy change takes place close to the irradiation site by employing energy reduction devices. This unavoidably leads to an increase in background radiation, mainly neutrons. To utilise the well defined particle range, the energy precision should be 0.2%.

Energy width. The energy spectrum of the proton beam reaching the patient site should be as narrow as possible in order to exploit fully the steep distal fall-off of the Bragg distribution. Since this requirement coincides with the needs of an efficient beam transport system, it is always fulfilled.

Intensity. A proton current of about 1 nA delivers a dose-rate of (2 to 4) Gy/min at the required site into a volume of approximately 1 litre of tissue. The resulting treatment time would be a few minutes. Since the efficiency of a beam transport and beam handling system is about 5%, a proton current of approximately 20 nA must exit from the accelerator.

In general the particle extraction efficiency is low, requiring a proton current inside the accelerator of the order of some μA.

Time structure. Due to saturation effects in monitors and possible biological dose-rate effects, a continuous proton beam is desirable. However, except for cyclotrons, all proton accelerators of practical interest emit pulsed beams.

Compactness. In contrast to accelerators used in experimental physics, compact and light accelerator designs are at a premium for radiotherapy. Ideally the machine would be hospital-based, where space for it and its shielding is extremely limited. In addition, the irradiation techniques often require a changing proton beam direction. Consequently, a dedicated medical proton accelerator should be compact and light enough to fit directly into a gantry, to facilitate varying the incident beam direction. Most likely this condition can only be met by a new type of accelerator, possibly by the Electron Cyclotron-Resonance Ion Plasma Accelerator (ECRIPAC).

Other requirements. Ease of operation and reliability are outstanding factors. It should be a push button operation. After setting a series of green knobs, the red and final one should produce the desired proton beam. Some accelerators achieve this and a 95% overall beam availability is not unheard off. This will help to make the treatment system cost-effective. However, the overall system should remain flexible enough to allow the introduction of new treatment concepts.

B.2.1b
Proton Accelerators Suitable for Radiotherapy

Cyclotron. In 1929 E.O.Lawrence invented the classical cyclotron and developed it further during the thirties. It produced free protons (or other ions) by stripping the electrons from hydrogen (or other elements). The protons are injected at the center of the cyclotron to move between the poles of an electrically powered dipole magnet having a constant (guiding) magnetic field. This circular magnet is separated vertically into two halves, called 'dees'. The acceleration occurs within the relatively narrow gap between the two half-magnets employing a correctly phased alternating electric field. The protons gain energy, twice for each revolution, the magnetic field remaining constant. Consequently, the accelerated particles travel outward in a spiral trajectory. Accelerated proton currents of up to 1 mA or more can be achieved. A continuous proton beam is extracted by various means and fed into a beam transport system.

Due to the relativistic mass increase of the accelerated protons, the maximum energy attainable by such a very simple classical cyclotron is about 20 MeV.

Synchro-cyclotron. This is a cyclotron where the frequency of the accelerating electric field is modulated to compensate for the relativistic mass increase of the protons. Due to the spiral trajectory of the particles inside, the necessary size of the (very expensive) magnets increases rapidly with energy.

Isochronuous or sector-focusing cyclotron. Here the pole faces of the magnets are specially shaped, so that the average magnetic field strength increases toward the outside in such a way, that the accelerated particles need the same time for each revolution. In addition, the particles are focused onto a stable orbit. This configuration is called Fixed Focus Alternating Gradient (FFAG). It requires – besides the specially shaped pole faces – high magnetic field strength. In general, the magnets are split along the radius into separated sectors.

Table B2.2. Typical data for two medically dedicated FFAG-cyclotrons. IBA: Cyclotron magnets at ambient temperature. CAL/Siemens: Superconducting magnets.

	IBA	CAL/Siemens
Number of sectors	4	3/6
Diameter	4.30 m	3.10 m
Total weight	220 t	80 t
Power consumption	200 kW	53 kW

Superconducting cyclotrons achieve higher magnetic field strength by employing superconducting magnets (and possibly also superconducting electric power coils). Advantage: For the same physical dimensions they can achieve significantly higher particle energies (and higher beam currents).

Linear accelerator (Linac). This type of machine was developed parallel to the cyclotron and at the same time. Initially designed for electrons, it has now been modified to accelerate also positively charged particles into an energy range of interest for radiotherapy. The protons are injected as short bunches (of milli- or microsecond duration) into a straight vacuum tube subdivided into many sections. The protons are accelerated by a succession of alternating electromagnetic fields applied to the individual sections and appropriately timed. Since the protons gain a constant amount of energy in each section and the number of sections is constant, the linac is an accelerator emitting particles with a fixed energy only. At best, the maximum energy may be varied in large steps, e.g. 10 MeV. Advantages: Very high and stable proton current output (1 mA is readily achieved), no magnets. Disadvantages: Length (to produce 250 MeV protons the linac is at least 8 m long), output of a pulsed particle beam.

B.2.2
Comparison of Existing Proton Accelerator Types

Table B2.3. Comparison of proton accelerators.

	Trajectory	Current	Size	Max. energy	Time structure
Cyclotron	Spiral	High	Compact	< 20 MeV	Continuous
Synchro-cyclotron	Spiral	Low	Large	< 1 GeV	Pulsed
FFAG-cyclotron	Circular	Low	Medium	< 1 GeV	Pulsed
Linac	Linear	Very high	Very long	> 1 GeV	Pulsed

B.3
The Proton Beam Line

B.3.1
Beam Transport System

The beam transport system carries the protons (or light ions) exiting the accelerator inside an evacuated tube to the patient site. In most cases, the proton beam is transported horizontally. The main transport elements are focusing quadrupoles, horizontally beam bending magnets, beam switching, shaping and monitoring devices, and possibly one or more gantries. Since the length of a beam line may easily exceed 20 m, all its elements must be extremely stable – mechanically and electrically – so that the beam at the patient site moves less than about 1 mm laterally during the entire treatment time. In general the beam transport system must accommodate a beam diameter of up to a few centimetres until the beam shaping site is reached.

It is desirable that the patients are treated in the supine position, the same position used for diagnostic procedures. This requires at least two additional bending magnets, moving the proton beam upward and downward through about 180 degrees. Such a beam line was achieved for the first time 1991 in Loma Linda, USA.

A gantry is formed, if the last bending magnets are designed to move orthogonally around the horizontal beam axis.

Gantry. This device moves the proton beam axis around a supine patient in order to apply the proton beam from many directions without changing the patient's position with respect to his support. There are a number of possible arrangements, e.g. the patient's support could move through a restricted arc in order to minimise the gentry's movement. It is important, that the beam entering the gantry is symmetrical in phase space and has a very narrow energy spectrum; otherwise the beam transfer efficiency through the gantry will depend on the gantry angle.

In general beam shaping elements are placed at the gantry's exit.

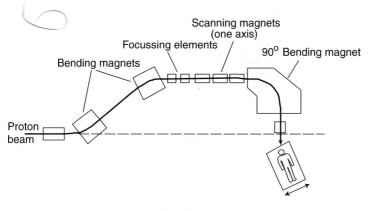

Fig. B3.1. Cross section of the compact PSI gantry in Villingen, Switzerland. The entire arrangement can move around the beam axis. This gantry is specifically designed for a spot scanning system. Redrawn after Pedroni et al. 1995.

At ambient temperatures the maximum achievable bending radius for 200 MeV protons is about 1.3 m. Superconducting coils or magnets or both will reduce this value considerably. Since light ion beams are 2 to 3 times more magnetically rigid than proton beams, an appropriate gantry can become very large and heavy. A gantry is a complex device and easily the most expensive element of the entire particle beam transport system.

B.3.2
Shielding of the Beam Transport System

For a hospital based proton accelerator adequate shielding is of the utmost importance. The main problems here are not the protons escaping from the beam transport system, but neutrons produced by protons striking material in their flight path. e.g. vacuum tube walls, slits, scattering devices, monitors, etc. This is called neutron leakage. In addition, materials struck by protons are activated and can remain radioactive for hours after the beam is switched off (residual activity).

Neutron leakage. To estimate the need for shielding, it can be assumed, that the neutrons are emitted from point sources along the proton beam line. The neutrons produced cover a wide energy range. The following will consider only fast neutrons, i.e. those in the MeV energy range. The water content within the shielding concrete will reduce the flux of low energy neutrons sufficiently.

At a distance d from the point source and behind a thickness x of shielding material, the equivalent dose D (measured in Sv/m^2) caused by fast neutrons is

$$D = (D_0/d^2) \exp(-x/\lambda)$$

where

D_0: equivalent dose at the radiation source
λ: attenuation length of the shielding material for fast neutrons.

The first term of the equation indicates the influence of the distance, the second term describes the effect of the absorbing material.

Unfortunately, the values for D_0 and λ are rather uncertain. They depend on the proton energy, the direction of the neutrons with respect to the proton beam, the RBE of the fast neutrons, the type of shielding material, etc. Experience demonstrates, that D is predominated by the bulk density of the shielding material. The type of material struck by the proton beam is of secondary importance.

The most widely used shielding material is concrete, sometimes loaded with special neutron absorbing substances.

A first order estimate for the attenuation length yields $\lambda = 850$ kg/m^2 for neutrons emitted into the forward direction and $\lambda = 530$ kg/m^2 for laterally emitted neutrons.

When designing shielding at the patient site, it must be realised that access has to be safe and easy. This prevents the usage of massive sliding doors, as encountered in physics installations. Instead, mazes with at least two 90 degree bends are utilised.

Residual activity. This activity is produced wherever the proton beam strikes matter, including the patient himself. The activity has a typical half-life of about 3 h. However, most parts of the beam line struck are rarely accessed and then only by trained personnel. Due to low proton radiation intensities received and short exposure times, the residual activity of patients is insignificant.

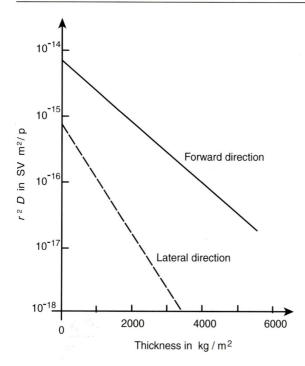

Fig. B3.2. Reduction of the fast neutron dose behind various thicknesses of concrete. The neutrons are produced by 230 MeV protons totally absorbed in Al. Redrawn after Siebers (1995a).

B.4
A Future Proton Source for Medical Applications

Currently, proton radiotherapy depends on large accelerators and complex beam transport systems housed in big buildings. This is a very expensive set-up. Even using liquid helium cooled superconducting facilities will not reduce the overall costs involved substantially. Consequently, proton treatment is more often than not financially out of reach even for large treatment centres.

A radically new accelerator design based on plasma physics is being developed in France, see Geller et al. 1996. This Electron Cyclotron-Resonance Ion Plasma Accelerator (**ECRIPAC**) produces an overall electrically neutral plasma disk consisting of electrons, protons and ions. The electron plasma is accelerated by a diamagnetic force to 4 MeV. The trapped protons cannot escape but obtain the same velocity as the electrons and thus reach energies of up to 400 MeV. The electrons are stripped away by guiding them onto a ring-shaped absorber and the remaining protons leave the accelerator in the forward direction.

There is no need for a complex beam transport system, for ECRIPAC could be mounted directly into a gantry. Consequently, this would lead to a very compact, and thus relatively inexpensive proton radiotherapy source.

The components of ECRIPAC have been tested successfully and a prototype is expected to be ready at the beginning of the millennium.

Table B4. Some design features of ECRIPAC.

Maximum proton energy: 400 MeV	This energy can be varied between radiation pulses.
Proton beam current: > 1 nA at 200 MeV	The beam current increases with decreasing proton energy.

Beam pulse rate: 1 Hz

Beam pulse length: < 10 μs

Total accelerator length: 1 m

Total weight: 300 kg

Cost: about the same as medically dedicated electron linacs

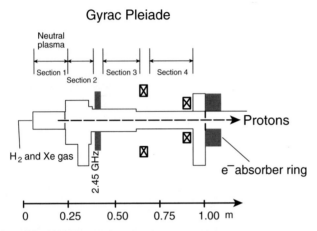

Fig. B4. Sketch of ECRIPAC. Section 1 transforms a gas mixture into a neutral plasma. This plasma diffuses into section 3 (GYRAC), where it is transformed into a dense, highly magnetised plasma disc of electrons, protons and Xe-ions. After accelerating the plasma (PLEIADE), an inhomogenuous magnetic field shakes out the Xe-ions. A fraction of the magnetic energy of the plasma disc is imparted as kinetic energy to the protons. The last coil separates away the electrons. The protons leave through a 1 cm diameter central opening. Modified after Geller et al. 1996.

B.5
Summary: Design Criteria for Radiotherapy Proton Beams

The following considerations could be the basis for the design of a medically dedicated proton beam. In general, those criteria also apply to beams of charged particles like D-, He-, C-, and Ne-Ions.

The overwhelming criterion is to deliver a therapeutic dose to an irregularly shaped target volume. At the same time the unavoidable irradiation of healthy tissue, especially of radio-sensitive structures, should be minimised.

B.5.1
Clinical Requirements

B.5.1a
Beam Penetration and Precision

A **maximum penetration depth** of 30 cm to 35 cm of tissue will easily handle more than 95% of all patients. The setting of this depth should ideally be reproducible within 0.1 cm, an easy task for a well designed proton transport system. However, it must be realised that this precision is quite illusionary for actual treatments, due to the accumulating uncertainties in pixel size of the CT images, extent of inhomogeneities penetrated, treatment planning algorithms, etc. (see section E3.2).

A **minimum penetration depth** is set by the proton energy degrader. Since during energy-downgrading the width of the original Bragg peak is essentially preserved, its full width at half maximum (FWHM) value of about 1.5 cm is the minimum penetration depth.

The **minimum proton penetration step width** is determined by the distal fall-off of the Bragg distribution. About 0.5 cm appear to be a reasonable value.

The **maximum available field size** for a fixed beam should be 30 cm × 30 cm. If a gantry is available, this condition can be relaxed due to the possibility of overlapping smaller field sizes. Mechanically shifting the patient in at least one direction during treatment also relaxes the above requirement. In this case an additional dose uncertainty is unavoidable. The maximum available field size itself determines the dimensions of beam spreaders, collimators, monitors, distance between the beam exit and the patient surface, etc.

The **minimum available field size** is about 1.5 cm diameter. Below this size the height of the Bragg peak relative to the entry dose is not fully developed and so the skin saving property of proton irradiation diminishes.

The **distal dose fall-off** is dominated by the distal decrease of the Bragg distribution for the maximum proton energy of the accelerator. Range straggling due to the energy width of the original proton beam increases the value of the distal dose fall-off.

The **lateral dose fall-off** is influenced by many factors but dominated in general by edge scattering and by the penetration of the therapeutic beam into the patient's tissue.

B.5.1b
Radiation Dose and Dose Rate

The **dose rate** should be about 2 Gy/min resulting in a treatment time of up to 5 min for one large field and maximum penetration depth.

A **dose accuracy and uniformity** of 2% are the most widely quoted requirements. Taking into account inhomogeneities, edge effects, range uncertainties, pixel sizes and irradiation planning algorithms, this requirement currently remains a target to be aimed for. A week-to-week dose reproducibility of about 2% is desirable and can be achieved.

The **time structure of the delivered radiation dose** depends on the accelerator type employed. Little is known about the consequences of a dose delivered by a train of microsecond radiation bursts, as e.g. by a linac, as compared with a proton beam from a cyclotron having a pulse length more than three orders of magnitude longer. Most likely there is little difference in biological effect.

B.5.2
Patient Set-up

For many reasons the irradiation of a patient should take place in the supine position. Immobilisation of the patient is essential. Ensuring that the uncertainty of the local dose delivered is well below the uncertainty of the treatment planning system, requires a target immobilisation within 1 mm. This means, that during the course of a treatment session, which will last some minutes, no target structure should shift by more than 1 mm. Since such immobilisation is usually accompanied by patient discomfort, the setting-up room should be close to the treatment area.

For a last minute check of the patient set-up, an X-ray system is needed which can move easily in and out of a beam's-eye position.

B.5.3
Accelerator

To fulfil the clinical requirements as stated above, a proton accelerator must meet the following requirements:

The **proton energy** to achieve the required penetration depth is 200 MeV to 250 Mev at the patient site. Since the proton beam loses energy within the beam handling system, e.g. in scattering facilities, monitors, beam shaping devices, dosimeters, etc., the design proton exit energy of the accelerator should be about 10% larger. There is no need for a high precision calibration of the proton beam energy because the measured beam equivalent range is utilised.

Proton energy changes in steps of about 0.4 MeV are desirable. This cannot be achieved by the accelerator itself, nor could it be handled by the proton beam transport system within a suitable time period. Consequently, energy degraders – essentially material layers in the proton beam line – are utilised. Nevertheless, since those degraders are a strong source of neutrons, large energy changes should be achieved by the accelerator itself, if at all feasible. Placing the energy degrader as far upstream as possible, e.g. in front of the last bending magnet, will substantially reduce the neutron leakage at the patient site.

The **proton beam energy spread** at the accelerator exit is normally about 0.1%, i.e. ≤ 0.25 MeV. This spread is increased by many devices within the beam line, especially by the energy degrader. The energy spread reduces the steepness of the distal dose fall-off inside the patient. For all practical purposes, the energy spread of the exiting proton beam dominates.

The **proton radiation intensity** is determined by the desirable dose rate. To achieve about 2 Gy/min at the patient site requires a proton current of a few nA. Many protons are scattered out of the beam direction, e.g. in beam spreading devices, the energy degrader, dosimeters, etc. Consequently, the proton intensity at the accelerator exit must be about 2 orders of magnitude larger than at the patient site.

Interestingly, scattering and scanning beam spreading devices require about the same proton radiation intensity.

The required output of about 4×10^{11} protons/min is met by all modern circular accelerators. Linacs exceed this output intensityby orders of magnitude.

The beam emittance determines the diameter of the vacuum lines for the beam transport system and the pole face separation of magnets and quadrupoles. Since the costs increase proportionally with the square of the beam emittance, the emittance should be as small as possible.

C Interaction of Protons with Matter

C.1
Energy Loss

Protons and other light ions having kinetic energy E will interact with atoms and molecules of matter that they penetrate.

The following refers mainly to protons, but may easily be extended to low Z light ions.

Every interaction results in a change in flight direction (scattering) and/or a partial (or even total) loss of energy. The energy loss per unit distance is called **differential energy loss** or **linear stopping power,** abbreviated dE/dx. By definition, the proton (or low Z ion) is presumed to have lost all its kinetic energy if $E \leq 10$ eV. Energy loss also means a reduction in the speed for the penetrating particle, a slowing down.

Example: A 200 MeV proton moves with about 2×10^6 m/s (about 65% of the speed of light). After a very large energy loss of 99%, i.e. down to $E_p = 2$ MeV, its speed is reduced to about 2×10^5 cm/s.

For the energy range of interest, i.e. $E \leq 300$ MeV, the energy loss process is dominated by interaction of the proton with the bound outer-shell electrons of atoms or molecules in the matter penetrated. This leads to an excitation of the atom as a whole, or to its ionization and consequently to the removal of an electron. Since the energy loss per interaction is $\ll E$, the slowing down process can be considered as continuous and uniform. It may be treated as a transport phenomenon.

Interaction with the atomic nucleus contributes significantly to the energy loss, only for a relatively high particle energy, i.e. for about $E \geq 100$ MeV. Exotic processes like proton bremsstrahlung production begin to contribute significantly only in the GeV energy region.

In general, the energy loss is computed for interactions with atoms only. To extend it to compounds (i.e. molecules), the losses due to the individual components of a molecule are simply added. This is justified, because the intramolecular binding energy is very small compared to the ionization potentials of the individual atoms, and the value of these ionization potentials dominates the size of the energy loss. The uncertainty introduced due to this simplification is negligible for $E \geq 1$ MeV.

The differential energy loss for $E \geq 0.1$ MeV declines steeply with increasing E. However, after reaching a minimum value at a few GeV the differential energy loss slowly begins to increase.

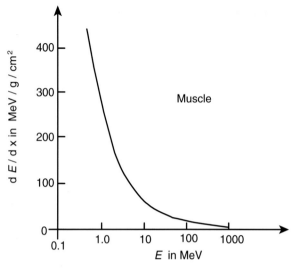

Fig. C1.1. Proton linear stopping power (dE/dx) in muscle tissue for the energy range 0.1 MeV to 1000 MeV. Semi-log plot. Numerical values after Janni (1982).

C.1.1
Energy Loss by Excitation and Ionization

Assuming differential energy loss due only to excitation and ionization and E $\geq$ 0.5 MeV, the following Bethe-Bloch relation(Bethe 1930, Bloch 1933) describes the total mass stopping power for protons.

$$\frac{dE}{\rho dx} = \frac{2\pi N_A z_p^2 e^4 Z}{m_e c_0^2 \beta^2 A_r} \left[\ln \frac{2m_e c_0^2 \beta^2 W}{I_{adj}^2 (1 - \beta^2)} - 2\beta^2 - \frac{2}{Z} \sum_i C_i - \Delta \right.$$
$$\left. + \pi \alpha Z_p \beta + \frac{2z_p Z \alpha^3 F(\beta, Z)}{\beta^3} \right]$$

(C1.1)

where

dE/dx : linear stopping power, in MeV/cm
ρ : density of stopping material, in g/cm^3
$dE/(\rho\, dx)$: total mass stopping power, in MeV/(g/cm^2)
N_A : Avogadro's number
z_p : atomic number of the proton (= 1)
A_r : relative atomic mass
e : elementary charge
Z : atomic number of penetrated material
m_e : rest mass of the electron
c_0 : speed of light in vacuum
β : speed of proton / speed of light
W : maximum energy transfer from the proton to a free electron
I_{adj} : adjusted ionisation potential

ΣC_i : sum of effects of the shell corrections
Δ : polarization effect
α : fine-structure constant = 1/137
$F(\beta,Z)$: correction term due to the Second Born Approximation.

The first term of equation C1.1 dominates the differential energy loss, the other factors represent corrections of a few percent.

The differential energy loss for a low Z ion is larger than that of a proton. Example: For a 200 MeV totally stripped carbon ion it follows that $(dE/dx)_{C^{6+}}$ is approximately $1.6 \times (dE/dx)_p$.

Figure C1.2 presents (dE/dx) in the energy region of interest for proton radiotherapy.

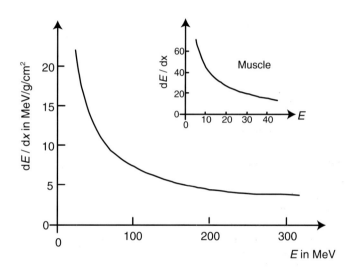

Fig. C1.2. Linear stopping power of protons in muscle tissue in the energy range 5 MeV $\leq$ E $\leq$ 300 MeV. Linear diagram.

Because of the transfer of energy from the proton (mass m_p) to an outer atomic electron, the proton is scattered, i.e. it changes its flight direction. The maximum proton scattering angle (expressed in radian) accompanying dE/dx is $\sin \theta \approx m_e/m_p$.

Example: The maximum scattering angle for a 200 MeV proton is approximately 8.2×10^{-4} rad and about 0.68×10^{-4} rad for 200 MeV Carbon ions.

While penetrating matter a parallel beam of protons in the energy range of interest, spreads insignificantly sideways due to excitation and ionisation; the spreading is dominated by scattering. The lateral spread of the radiation dose is negligible, considering that the maximum range of the secondary electrons ejected by protons is ≤ 0.1 cm in solid organic substances.

C.1.2
Energy Loss by Nuclear Interactions

C.1.2a
Elastic Nuclear Interactions

The elastic interaction of incoming protons with the atomic nucleus leads to an energy transfer to the nucleus and a change in flight direction of the protons. Since the interacting partners in the collision have masses of the same order of magnitude, the energy transferred to the recoil nucleus is comparatively large. For a 1 MeV proton scattered off a carbon nucleus, the maximum energy loss is 0.09 MeV. The associated maximum scattering angle of the proton is approximately 5 degree. However, the interaction probability is very low, only about 0.1% and it further decreases with increasing energy. Consequently, elastic nuclear interactions can be neglected for E $\geq$ 1 MeV, i.e. they only play a small role toward the very end of the proton path.

C.1.2b
Inelastic Nuclear Interactions

This type of interaction of the proton with the atomic nucleus leads to the excitation of the nucleus, to the formation of a compound nucleus or to a direct interaction between the incoming proton and individual components of the nucleus. The result is an energy loss of many MeV per collision, in general accompanied by the emission of secondary protons, neutrons and/or other low Z particles, and by a significant change in the flight direction of the proton.

The probability for inelastic nuclear reactions increases rapidly with increasing proton energy; it dominates the energy loss of protons for E exceeding a few hundred MeV. Janni (1982) calculated the probability for an inelastic nuclear interaction and thus the reduction of the initial proton fluence in the central proton beam. Bortfeld (1997) presents a relationship for the relative proton fluence ϕ (x) at the depth x:

$$\phi (x) \approx 1 + 0.018 \, (R_0 - x)^{0.87} \tag{C1.2}$$

R_0 is the mean range of the proton.

Example: The relative probability for an inelastic nuclear interaction in solid organic materials for a 25 MeV proton is about 1%, rises to 25% for 200 MeV and dominates the energy loss for $E \geq$ 500 MeV.

Inelastic nuclear interactions are localised predominantly in the region proximal to the Bragg peak, thus affecting mainly the entrance dose.

The range of secondary particles produced by inelastic nuclear interactions can exceed the range of the primary particles. This is because for the same particle velocity the range is inversely proportional to the square of the charge of the charged particle and the secondary particle may be completely ionized. This leads to a 'tail' distal to the Bragg peak, a feature well developed for low Z ions other then protons.

The energy deposited by neutrons is insignificant, because the number of neutrons $\ll$ number of protons, see Sandison et al. 1997.

C.1.3
Energy Losses for E ≤ 0.5 MeV

Since the Bethe-Bloch formula (C1.1) applied for $E \leq 0.5$ MeV leads to unreliable results, the differential energy loss in this energy range is determined experimentally. Its numerical value continues to increase rapidly with decreasing energy until it reaches about 1 GeV/(g/cm^2) for E approximately 0.1 MeV. For lower proton energies the differential energy loss declines steeply.

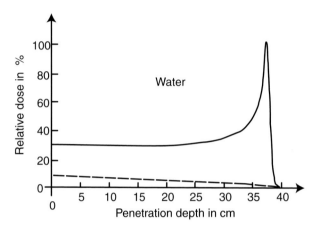

Fig. C1.3. Broad-beam central axis depth-dose distribution for 250 MeV protons. The dashed curve indicates thecontributions due to inelastic nuclear interactions. Adapted from Carlsson et al 1997.

C.1.4
Summary

Figure C1.4 summarises the dominating processes for the interaction of protons with matter.

C.2
Proton Scattering

Scattering theory calculates the shape and the width of the angular distribution of the scattered protons (p). The elastic interaction of the proton with the Coulomb fields of the nucleus and the orbiting electrons (e) dominates the scattering process in the region of interest (proton energy ≤ 300 MeV). The main contribution results from Coulomb interaction of the proton with the nucleus; the p-e interaction is taken into account as a correction factor.

The influence of inelastic nuclear interactions of the proton is treated separately because:
1. The interaction probability decreases rapidly with increasing proton energy, consequently it has little influence on the region of main interest, the Bragg peak.

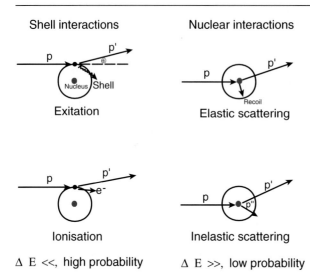

Fig. C1.4. Simplified schematics of the energy loss processes encountered by protons in the energy range of interest for radiotherapy.

2. The scattering angles and the energy losses involved are so large, that very few, inelastically scattered protons will reach the region of interest, the target volume.

C.2.1
Elastic Coulomb Scattering

C.2.1a
Introduction

Elastic Coulomb scattering dominates the proton-nucleus interaction. It results in numerous very small angular deflections. It is called elastic scattering, because:
1. The incident particle is also the exiting particle.
2. The energy loss of the incident proton during each single scattering event is very small.
3. The total kinetic energy of all participants is conserved.

Elastic scattering results in an angular spread of an initially parallel proton beam. The shape of the distribution is Gaussian only if a very thin layer of material is penetrated. After traversing thicker layers, the shape of the angular distribution deviates significantly from a Gaussian. The relative contributions to its 'tail' are especially enhanced.

The theory of elastic Coulomb scattering covers penetration depths up to the full proton range. For practical applications convenient approximations are available. The treatment includes penetration of composite materials.

It is worthwhile to note that the dominant paper (Molière 1948) was published over fifty years ago. Gottschalk et al. 1993 summed up its relevance: "At present one can conclude that Molière theory, carefully evaluated, has an average error no more than 1% and a maximum error no more than ± 5% for protons."

Vavilov (1957) treats the ionization energy loss as a compound Poisson process. Sandison et al. 1997 demonstrate the excellent agreement between the approaches of Molière and Vavilov. (Contrary to a remark by Sandison, Molière theory does not include a small angle approximation).

The following summarises Molière theory. For details see Molière (1948) or Bethe (1953) (a mathematically more lucid publication including all previous theoretical treatments) or Gottschalk et al. 1993 (a condensed version which includes a critical comparison with all previous experiments).

C.2.1b
Molière Theory

Molière (1948) expanded his theory of single scattering (Molière 1947) of charged particles to cover multiple scattering. In this case, the number of scattering events for each proton is ≤ 20. As long as the value of $\sin \theta$ is about θ (in radian, i.e. the scattering angle $\theta \leq 20$ degrees) the scattering is equivalent to the diffusion of protons in the plane of θ.

As a first step Molière derived the probability function for the scattered particle distribution for small scattering angles and very small energy losses. He presents this function, the Molière distribution (MD), as the sum of analytical terms. The following expression for the MD for protons is normalised to a peak value of 1.

$$f(\theta, d) = \frac{1}{4\pi\theta_M^2} \left[f^{(0)}(\theta') + \frac{f^{(1)}(\theta')}{B} + \frac{f^{(2)}(\theta')}{B^2} \cdots \right] \qquad (C2.1)$$

where

θ : proton angle with respect to the forward direction, in radian
d : penetrated thickness, in g/cm^2
θ_M : characteristic multiple scattering angle, in radian

$$\theta_M^2 = 1.56 \, d \, B \, Z^2/(2A \, (pv)^2) \qquad (C2.2)$$

where

B : a quantity depending on the number of collisions for the proton
Z, A : atomic number, relative atomic weight of scatterer
p, v : momentum, speed of proton
θ' : reduced angle, introduced for convenience, $= \theta/(\theta_M\sqrt{2})$

For incident particles other than protons, (C.2.1) must be multiplied by z^2, the square of the relative charge of this particle. Note, the equation C2.1 is almost independent of the (normalised) thickness of the scatterer.

The first term $f^{(0)}$ of (C.2.1) is a Gaussian:

$$f^{(0)}(\theta') = 2\exp[(-\theta')^2] = 2\exp(-\theta^2/2\theta_M^2) \qquad (C2.3)$$

If (C2.3) is used as a zero order approximation for (C2.1), the resulting Gaussian is too wide and its lateral distribution (the 'tails') is orders of magnitude too low. This deviation becomes significant for $\theta \leq \theta_M$.

The second term $f^{(1)}$ of (C2.1) is presented by Molière as an analytical expression. Tabulated values can be found in Molière (1948) and Bethe (1953). For small angles the contribution of $f^{(1)}$ to the Gaussian of (C2.3) is only about 10%, Bethe (1953).

The third term $f^{(2)}$ (again tabulated by Molière (1948) and Bethe (1953)) transforms for large scattering angles into the formula for single scattering.

The following higher terms $f^{(n)}, n > 2$ are correction terms that practically cancel each other out.

Influence of proton-electron scattering. Molière theory neglects the proton scattering caused by the electrons orbiting the nucleus. Fano's (Fano 1954) correction takes care of those contributions for thin layers, while Scott (1963) extends the correction toward large values of d. The results deviate only by a few percent from Molière theory.

Bethe took account of p-e scattering by replacing Z^2 in (C2.2) by $Z(Z-1)$. For low values of Z Fano's (respectively Scott's) correction yields better agreement with experiments than Bethe's, see; below.

Thick scatterer. Equation C2.1 is valid for a relatively thin scatterer only. To extend it to large values of d, i.e. large energy losses, Molière generalised the characteristic single scattering angle for all thicknesses and redefined the screening angle used in the Born approximation. This extension pre-supposes that the energy of the proton at any position inside the scatterer is known. After those changes, the general shape of the MD, as presented by (C2.1), remains unchanged.

To compute actual characteristic scattering angles, Gottschalk et al. 1993 introduced a polynomial best-fit for Janni's (Janni 1982) range-energy values which presents (in

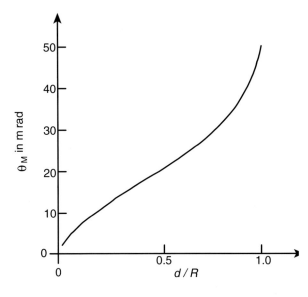

Fig. C2.1. The characteristic multiple scattering angle θ_M as a function of penetration depth (measured as normalised depth, i.e. penetration depth d/proton range R). Drawn for Be after Table 1 in Gottschalk et al. 1993.

tabular form) values for the characteristic multiple scattering angle θ_M for a proton energy of 158.6 MeV.

Gottschalk et al. 1993 points out that Molière theory is invalid for a very thick scatterer, e.g. for a thickness where the proton range straggling becomes significant. Experiments indicate that this is correct as soon as the proton reaches about 97% of its range.

Figure C2.1 presents an example of θ_M as a function of penetration depth.

The following figure compares experiment with the Molière theory and its corrections.

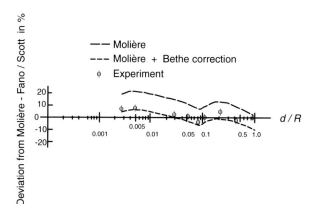

Fig. C2.2. Percentage deviation of the characteristic multiple scattering angle θ_M from Molière theory (incl. Fano/Scott correction) as a function of the normalised scatterer thickness. Scattering material Be. Redrawn after Gottschalk (1993).

Compound scatterer. Molière theory remains valid for compounds and mixtures of elements. In this case the weighted contributions due to the individual constituents i are summed. For example: The square of the characteristic multiple scattering angle θ_M (see (C2.2) becomes

$$\theta_M^2 = 1.56 \sum_i \frac{k_i Z_i^2}{A_i \int_0^d B_1 d' \, dd'} \tag{C2.4}$$

where

k_i : weighted contributions of constituents Z_i, A_i and B_i.

C.2.1c
Approximations for Molière's Distribution

Thin scatterer. Highland (1975/79) derived the following relation for the characteristic scattering width θ_{approx} of a Gauss distribution approximating (C2.1) (incl. Bethe correction):

$$\theta_{approx} = \frac{14.1}{pv} \left(\frac{d}{L_R} \right)^{-1/2} (1 + \epsilon) \tag{C2.5}$$

where

L_R : radiation length of scattering material, in g/cm^2
(L_R enters the equation only because it is convenient for the computation).

The correction term ε (expressed in radian) is

$$\epsilon = \frac{1}{9} \lg \left(\frac{L}{L_R} \right) \tag{C2.6}$$

The accuracy of (C2.5) is better than 5% for d ≥ 0.001 R.

Table C2 presents some relevant values for L_R.

Table C2. Radiation length L_R for some scattering materials. Numerical values adopted from Atomic and Nuclear Properties of Materials (1986).	Material	L_R in (g/cm^2)
	Lead	6.37
	Silicium	21.8
	Aluminium	24.0
	Shielding concrete	26.7
	Silica Aerogel	29.9
	Water	36.1
	Lucite, Plexiglas	40.6
	Carbon	42.7
	Polyethylene	44.8

Very thick scatterer. Hong et al. 1996 generalised Highland's approximation for a infinitely thick scatterer. Accordingly, the rms scattering radius y_{rms} as a function of depth d' is

$$y_{rms}(d') = 14.1(1 + (1/9) \log(d'/L_R))[\int ((d'- z)/pv)^2 \, (\rho/L^R) \, dz]^{1/2} \tag{C2.7}$$

where the integral extends from 0 to d';

p,v : proton momentum, speed at depth z inside the scatterer
ρ : density of scattering material.

The normalised rms scattering radius as a function of the normalised value for d' is a function independent of the material, see Figure C2.3 .
    Hong et al. 1996 show that the relation between rms scattering radius at the full proton range $y(R)$ and the proton range in water R_w is almost linear and can be represented by

$$y(R) = 0.0275 \, R_w + 1.2085 \times 10^{-5} \, R_w^2 \tag{C2.8}$$

C.2.1d
Comparison with Experiments

Precise measurements and a detailed survey of the literature by Gottschalk et al. 1993 show, that Molière theory (extended by taking e-p interactions into account) presents

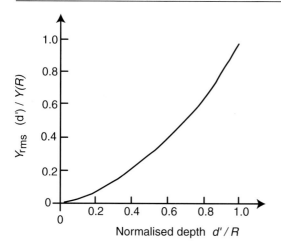

Fig. C2.3. The rms scattering radius $y_{rms} (d')$ divided by the rms scattering radius at the full proton range $y(R)$, as a function of depth d' divided by proton range R. After Hong et al. 1996.

the angular proton scattering distribution with an average accuracy of about 1% and the maximum deviations from theory do not exceed 5%. See Fig. C2.2

C.2.2
Inelastic Scattering

Inelastic proton scattering is characterised by very few scattering events for individual particles, but large directional changes. This is in contrast to elastic scattering, where individual protons are scattered very often but the directional change during each event is tiny.

During inelastic proton scattering, energy is transferred from the proton to the nucleus. A compound nucleus is formed which emits its excitation energy in the form of gamma rays or a secondary particle, e.g. a proton. The interaction takes place only when incident protons have an energy exceeding a few MeV, because the proton must

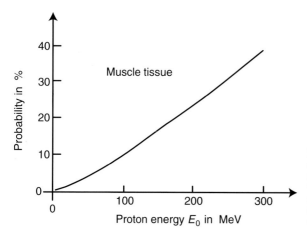

Fig. C2.4. Probability (in %) of a proton with initial energy E_0 undergoing inelastic scattering while penetrating muscle tissue. The values for bone are about 7% larger. Numerical values adopted from Janni (1982).

be able to penetrate the nuclear Coulomb barrier. The resulting angular distribution contributes mainly to the 'tail' of the MD, far outside the characteristic scattering angle.

Note, that a significant number of protons is inelastically scattered.

Example: 24% of 200 MeV protons undergo an inelastic scattering process penetrating through muscle. However, this value drops to 3.6% once the proton's energy is reduced (predominantly by elastic scattering) to 50 MeV.

The influence of inelastic scattering is noticeable only in the slowly rising portion of the Bragg distribution. The inelastically scattered protons are either scattered out of the forward direction and/or lose a significant percentage of their energy. In either event very few of those protons will reach the Bragg region.

For planning purposes the influence of this numerical loss of protons is neglected. Since the input to the proton radiation planning algorithm inevitably includes a measured depth dose distribution, it automatically adjusts for inelastic proton scattering. Nevertheless, inelastic proton scattering can be taken into account numerically, see Sandison et al. 1997.

C.3
Energy-Range Relation

Penetrating into matter, only charged particle radiation displays a pathlength. This is because these particles do not disappear while moving through the material, they merely lose energy due to interactions with the encountered atoms and molecules. The instant the energy of a charged particle has been reduced to thermal energy – about 10 eV – it is deemed to have attained its pathlength.

Contrary to the above, electromagnetic radiation while penetrating through matter will be absorbed, following an exponential relation. The process is characterised by an absorption or attenuation coefficient α. Sometimes a mean range $\bar{I}$ for electromagnetic radiation is defined as: $\bar{I} := \bar{I}_0/e$, where $\bar{I}_0$ is its intensity at zero penetration depth and $e = 2.718...$.

The pathlength of a charged particle inside a given substance depends on its mass, electrical charge and initial energy.

C.3.1
Pathlength, Mean Range and Water Equivalent Ratio

The **pathlength** P of a charged particle, e.g. a proton, is determined by its differential energy loss during penetration. Its pathlength along the x-axis is the integral over the energy-dependent differential energy loss until the particle energy is reduced to thermal energy:

$$P_x = \int_{E_f}^{E_o} \left(\frac{dE}{\rho dx} \right)^{-1} dE \tag{C3.1}$$

where

P_x : pathlength along the x-axis, in g/cm^2
E_0 : initial particle energy, in MeV

E_f: final particle energy ($\leq$ 10 eV)
ρ : density of material penetrated, in g/cm^3
dE/dx : differential energy loss, in MeV/cm.

The particle follows a zigzag path due to multiple scattering. Consequently, it is difficult to measure the pathlength directly.

Mean range R_0 is defined as the orthogonal projection of the entire path onto the forward direction:

$$R_o = \int_{E_f}^{E_o} \overline{\cos\theta} \left(\frac{dE}{\rho dx}\right)^{-1} dE \qquad (C3.2)$$

where

$\overline{\cos\theta}$: average cosine of incident and exit angle of the charged particle.

The difference between pathlength and mean range for protons in the energy range of interest, is about 0.1% for low Z materials and increases to about 0.2% for high Z materials.

Numerical values for P_x and R_0 have been tabulated, e.g. by Janni (1982) and in ICRU (1993). In general, particle range refers to mean particle range.

Figure C3.1 presents the range-energy relation for protons penetrating muscle.

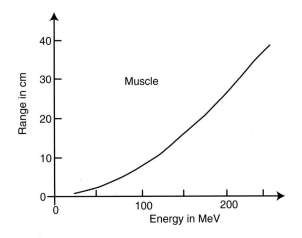

Fig. C3.1. Range-energy relation for protons in muscle-tissue. Drawn after Janni (1982).

A convenient formula for the mean range R_0 (measured in cm) for protons in water is given by Bortfeld (1997)

$$R_0 = \alpha \, E_0^{\,P} \qquad (C3.3)$$

where $\alpha \approx 0.0022$ and p ≈ 1.77

The formula presents R_0 with an accuracy of about 1.5 mm in the energy range from 1 MeV to 200 MeV.

Geiger-Nutall originally discovered this power function in 1911 (Segré 1965).

The presented value for α was extracted from a fit of the range-energy data tabulated in ICRU (1993).

The above power function holds well for many substances, keeping in mind that

$$\alpha \sim \sqrt{\overline{A}}/\rho \tag{C3.4}$$

where

$\overline{A}$: effective relative atomic mass.

If the number of charged particles N penetrating a substance is measured as a function of the depth x, the following curve results:

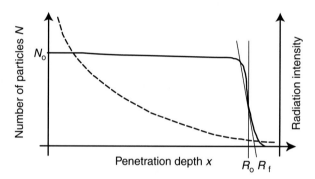

Fig. C3.2. Typical penetration curve for charged particles (solid line). The penetration depth x is in general presented in g/cm^2, i.e. length × density. N_0: initial number of particles. R_0 : mean range, R_f : extrapolated range. For comparison a typical attenuation curve for electromagnetic radiation is added (dotted line).

The above (solid) curve with its steep fall-off is typical for heavy charged particles characterised by an energy loss per interaction that is very small compared to the particle's energy. For electrons, losing more energy per collision, the distal fall-off is much more gentle.

The following notations are convenient (but not generally agreed upon):

R_0 : mean range of particle radiation, the position where $N = N_0/2$
R_f : extrapolated range, the intersection of the tangent at the point of steepest descent with the x-axis

As a rule (Berger 1993) R_0 equals the depth at which the absorbed radiation dose has dropped to 80% of its maximum value distal to the Bragg peak (see section C.4).

The **Water Equivalent Ratio** (WER) of a substance (sub) is a useful quantity. It is defined as:

$$\text{WER} = (dE/dx)_{\text{sub}} / (dE/dx)_{\text{water}} \tag{C3.5}$$

WER is useful in computations because it depends only slightly on the proton energy within the energy range of interest in radiotherapy.

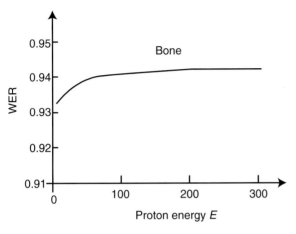

Fig. C3.3. The Water Equivalent Ratio (WER) for bone as a function of proton energy E. The value WER = 0.94 appears to be a good approximation within the energy range of interest. Numerical values from Janni (1982)

C.3.2
Range Straggling

If all protons would lose the same amount of energy per scattering event, all would display the same range, i.e. the penetration curve would be horizontal with a perpendicular drop at its end, see Figure C3.4. However, the interaction of charged particles with atoms and molecules is a statistical process. Consequently the energy loss for each individual particle varies to some degree, so particle path length and range are characterised by straggling.

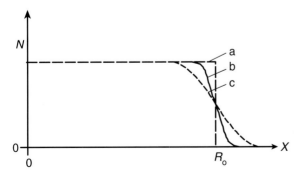

Fig. C3.4. Penetration curves. a: No energy loss fluctuations, b: Elastic electron-proton interactions, c: Curve b + inelastic interactions.

If energy loss is dominated by the heavy particle-electron interaction the distal fall-off is very steep (occurring within about 2% of the range for protons) and centred around R_0. With increasing mass of the heavy particle, the curve's steepness increases but its tail becomes more pronounced.

Range straggling is a measure of the uncertainty of the particle range. Under the reasonable assumption, that the difference $R_0 - R_f$ is approximately half the width of the Gaussian describing the range straggling, straggling can be calculated for p-e energy losses alone, Segré (1965), or in addition including multiple and nuclear scattering, Janni (1982). Inelastic nuclear scattering does not contribute, due to the large energy loss per interaction.

Figure C3.5 presents the range straggling in the energy range of interest.

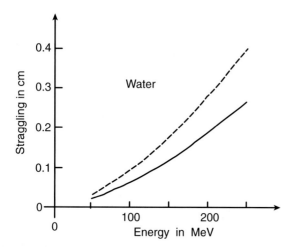

Fig. C3.5. Straggling ($R_f - R_0$) of protons in water, due to (p-e) interactions only (solid line), in addition including multiple and nuclear scattering (dotted line), after Janni (1982).

The range straggling for 200 MeV protons in water is 2 mm – 3 mm, i.e. about 1% of R_0.

C.3.3
Range Uncertainty

In radiotherapy the uncertainty in the range of charged particles is of vital interest because the main advantage of a charged heavy particle beam is its steep distal dose fall-off. To approach a radio-sensitive structure closely, but safely, when depositing a radiation dose, the uncertainty in the range calculation must be taken into account. The factors dominating range uncertainty are the energy-range relation, range straggling and the density of the matter penetrated.

Energy-range relation: The most thorough analysis of this factor was performed by Janni (1982). Although the uncertainties vary slightly with energy and substance penetrated, their mean values lead to an uncertainty of about 1% of the particle range. Taking this into account, the tabulated values of Janni (1982) agree well with the more recent calculations presented in ICRU (1993).

The energy of a proton beam leaving the beam transport system is known to hard-ly better than 1%.

Range straggling: This contributes another 1% uncertainty.

Electron density of the material penetrated: This is an important factor since the range is inversely proportional to it. For example, to use the density of water for calcu-lating the penetration into muscle introduces an uncertainty of the order of 1%. Although it is difficult to determine bone density, the beam path includes rarely more than 10% bone. However, an uncertainty of 10% in the bone density still causes an uncertainty of about 1% in the range.

Passing through a long inhomogeneity in the presence of a steep density step par-allel to the beam direction, Coulomb scattering will increase the range uncertainty. Goitin and Sisterson 1987 calculated this influence using a Monte Carlo technique, Schneider et al. 1998 present the same results analytically.

Summarising all those unavoidable uncertainties it is obvious, that the cumulative uncertainty R_0 is of the order of 2% to 3%. For a 200 MeV proton beam this leads to a range uncertainty of 5 mm to 7 mm!

C.4
Bragg Distribution

C.4.1
Shape of the Bragg Distribution

When a beam of protons passes into homogeneous matter, the differential energy loss increases rapidly with decreasing proton energy. Consequently, the differential dose deposited by protons slowing down rises steeply towards the end of the proton's path. Plotting the absorbed radiation dose versus the penetration depth of the protons, a dis-tribution emerges called the Bragg distribution or Bragg curve, see Wilson (1946).

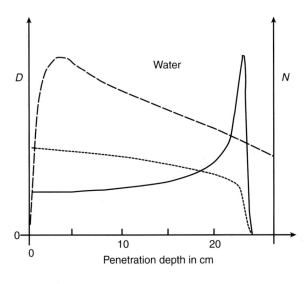

Fig. C4.1. Dose D deposited by secondary electrons resulting from the energy loss of protons (solid line). For comparison the relative particle fluence N (right hand scale, dotted line) and a bremsstrahlung depth-dose distribution (dashed line) are indicated.

The Bragg curve comprises different parts: A linear, slowly rising section, called the plateau. This is caused predominantly by the slowly increasing differential energy loss with decreasing proton energy. A rapid rise in the deposited dose follows, culminating in a maximum, reflecting a corresponding increase in the differential energy loss. The relative height of this 'Bragg peak' is about 3 to 4 times the entrance dose (the deposited dose at the beam's entrance). The distal fall-off is very steep: For a 200 MeV proton beam the fall from 90% of the peak dose to 10% occurs within about 7 mm. The corresponding full width at half maximum (FWHM) of this Bragg peak is approximately 22 mm.

In zero order approximation FWHM is independent of the initial energy of the charged particles, because it depends mainly on the shape of the ionisation differential energy loss curve. However, since inelastic energy losses and straggling increase with proton energy, the FWHM increases correspondingly. In addition, the energy spread of the incident proton beam widens the Bragg distribution.

Taking into account that the Relative Biological Effectiveness (RBE) increases with increasing ionisation density, the 'effective' Bragg peak is even more pronounced.

The **shape of the Bragg distribution,** i.e. the depth-dose along the centre line of the particle beam, is determined by two terms: Reduction of the particle energy E during its penetration and the removal of a number of particles out of the centre beam path. Consequently, the Bragg distribution can be described by:

$$D(x) = 1/\rho \ (N \ (x)(dE(x)/dx) + \gamma \ (dN \ (x)/dx)E(x))$$

where

N : particle fluence at depth x, in particles/cm^2
γ : in the centre beam path absorbed fraction of energy released by inelastic nuclear reactions.

The first term covers the differential energy loss, i.e. the Bethe-Bloch relation (equation C1.1). The second term encompasses the influences of nuclear interactions, of range straggling, and of the finite width of the particle energy spectrum.

Bortfeld (1997) presents a lengthy analytical expression, a combination of Gaussians and parabolic cylinder functions. For protons penetrating through water, this analytical expression is well represented by (Bortfeld 1997):

$$D(x) = \phi_0/(1 + 0.012 \ R_0)[17.93 \ (R_0 - x)^{-0.435} + (0.444 + 31.7 \ \varepsilon/R_0)(R_0 - x)^{0.565}] \quad \text{(C 3.6)}$$

where

ε : Non-Gaussian fraction contributing to the incident proton energy spectrum
R_0 : Mean proton range in cm.

The calculated shape of Bragg distributions in the energy range of interest for radiotherapy agree very well (deviations < 1%) with measurements.

Bortfeld and Schlegel (1996) approximate the shape of the Bragg distribution assuming that a power law describes the energy-range relation for protons. The influence of inelastic scattering is excluded. The authors derive a relatively simple expression for the Bragg distribution proximal to its end of range:

$$D(x) = \frac{1}{\rho p \alpha^{1/p} (R_0 - x)^{1-(1/p)}} \qquad (C3.7)$$

where $p = 1.8$ and $\alpha = 1.9 \times 10^{-3}$.

Due to the singularity at $x = R_0$ equation C3.7 can only be utilised for the design of a Spread Out Bragg Peak (SOPB) dose distribution. This approximation excludes the influence of inelastic nuclear scattering. It is interesting to note, that Bortfeld and Schlegel 1996 had to change the value of p (see Eq.C3.3) to 1.5 in order to design SOPB distributions which agree with measurements.

Employing the theory of Vavilov (1957), Sandison et al. 1997 computed the Bragg distribution including the influence of inelastic proton scattering (taken into account as an exponential extinction function). Using a Monte Carlo algorithm, the authors achieved a Bragg distribution in good agreement with experiment.

Other heavy charged particles also display a Bragg distribution favourable for radiotherapy. The higher the charge of the particles, the steeper the distal dose fall-off. However, there is a disadvantage: While the Bragg distribution for protons falls-off steeply to zero, for heavier particles a "tail" develops beyond the steep fall-off due to the production of secondary particles. The corresponding radiation dose may reach up to 10% of the peak dose.

C.4.2
Deviations from the Bragg Distribution

C.4.2a
Particle Beam Diameter and the Bragg Peak

Multiple scattering accompanies the energy reduction of a penetrating beam of charged particles. This, together with the very short range – maximal about 1.5 mm – of the secondary electrons, widens the lateral penumbra of an initially well defined particle beam. The numerical value of the penumbra width due to multiple scattering just before end of range is about 5% of the particle range. Since the particles are scattered out of the center beam line, the dose distribution of a very narrow proton beam does not display a Bragg peak. If the beam diameter increases, scattering toward the beam's centre line starts to cancel the out-scattering. E.g: Within a proton beam of 150 MeV and a diameter ≥ 9 mm in- and out-scattering cancel, the Bragg peak height is fully developed. In contrast, the same beam with a diameter ≤ 3 mm displays no position where there is a dose $\geq$ entrance dose, see figure C4.2.

C.4.2b
Influence of Inhomogeneous Media

Biological structures are rarely homogeneous. Bones of different densities, fatty tissues, air cavities, small fatty enclosures, etc. will be in the radiotherapy beam path.

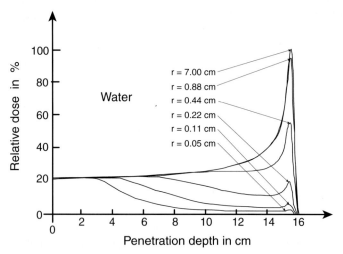

Fig. C4.2. Bragg distributions along central beam line for 150 MeV proton beams of various diameters. Modified after Carlsson et al. 1997.

Consequently, the specific energy losses within the beam path will vary with locality and the FWHM, and especially the distal fall-off of the Bragg distribution, will increase, possibly impairing the arguments in favour of charged particle radiotherapy.

As long as the density distribution along and across the beam path is known, the Bragg distributions for each sub-beam path can be calculated and the individual contributions combined to present a 3D Bragg distribution. This procedure is relatively simple for known and statistically distributed inhomogeneities, see e.g. Hiraoka et al. 1994. Otherwise the specific energy loss for each locality inside the 3D absorber must be taken into account.

C.5
Protons Penetrating Tissue

It is not straightforward to apply results gained from measurements in a water tank or a simple phantom to radiotherapy of patients. The reason is, that tissues are made up of different types of molecules and contain inhomogeneities of various sizes and shapes. It is not only that those structures influence the range of the protons, but non-uniform multiple scattering takes on an important role. Neglecting this could result in local under- or overdosage and in deformation of the distal end of the proton dose distribution, causing perhaps unintended irradiation of radiosensitive structures distal to the target volume.

C.5.1
Taking Account of Tissue Densities

The density ρ of the tissues penetrated by the particle beam is of utmost importance, because the particle range R is inversely proportional to ρ. It must be remembered, that this density is the relative electron density ρ_e.

For a composite substance it is

$$\rho_e = \frac{\rho N_g}{\rho_w N_w} \qquad (C3.8)$$

and

$$N_g = N_A \sum_i \frac{\omega_i Z_i}{A_i} \qquad (C3.9)$$

where

ρ : density of substance in g/cm^3
ρ_w : density of water in g/cm^3
N_w : number of water molecules per mol
N_A : Avogadro's number = 6.02×10^{23} per mol
ω_i : proportion of component by weight
Z_i : atomic number of the ith element
A_i : relative atomic mass.

Calculated and measured (indirectly measured via proton stopping powers) values for ρ_e agree within 1.6% (Schneider et al. 1996), however, even this excellent agreement implies a range uncertainty of about 3 mm for 200 MeV protons.

There is only one practical way to determine the 3D electron density distribution $\rho_e(x,y,z)$ inside the body, so essential for proton radiotherapy planning. This is by converting the absorption coefficient matrix extracted from Computed Tomography (CT) measurements into a corresponding ρ_e matrix.

Table C5 presents some measured values for ρ and ρ_e.

Table C5. Selected density values for organic tissues relative to water. The value of $K = \rho/\rho_e$ indicates the relation between bulk density and relative electron density. For later reference the CT numbers are also given. Extracted from Schneider et al. 1996.

Substance	ρ	ρ_e	K	CT no
Blood	1.06	1.050	1.01	1055
Bone, cranium	1.61	1.517	1.06	1903
Bone, femur	1.33	1.278	1.04	1499
Bone, sacrum	1.29	1.244	1.04	1413
Bone, C4 vertebra	1.42	1.355	1.05	1609
Bone, D6 vertebra	1.33	1.278	1.04	1477
Brain	1.04	1.035	1.00	1037
Breast	1.02	1.014	1.01	1003
Cartilage	1.10	1.083	1.02	1098
Lens	1.07	1.055	1.01	1050
Heart	1.06	1.051	1.01	1055
Liver	1.06	1.050	1.01	1053
Lung (inflated)	0.26	0.258	1.01	259
Lung (deflated)	1.05	1.041	1.01	1044
Muscle	1.05	1.040	1.01	1042
Skin	1.09	1.078	1.01	1075
Water (Def.)	1.00	1.000	1.00	1000

C.5.2
Tissue Density and CT Number

C.5.2a
Definitions

Hounsfield Unit (HU) $= 1000 \times (\mu_n - \mu_{water}) / \mu_{water}$
CT number (CT no.) $= HU + 1000$

Consequently

water: HU = 0,   CT no. = 1000
air: HU = -1000,   CT no. = 0

where

μ_n: total linear attenuation coefficient for X-rays emitted by the employed CT scanner

The subscripts indicate the substances penetrated by the X-rays.

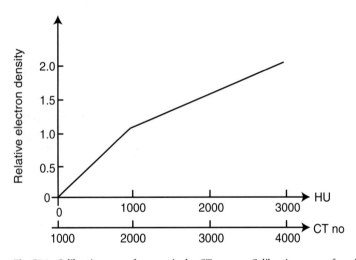

Fig. C5.1. Calibration curve for a particular CT scanner. Calibration curves for other CT scanners will differ.

C.5.2b
Accuracy of the CT Numbers

X-ray energy. The total attenuation coefficient is dominated by the photoelectric effect, although Compton scattering cannot be neglected for low Z materials. Since cross sections due to Compton scattering are proportional to Z and those of the photoelectric effect cross section increase with Z^3, the relative contribution of Compton scattering decreases for relatively high Z materials like bone. Consequently the CT numbers vary according to the mean energy emitted by the X-ray tube inside the CT scanner employed. Ideal solution: determination of ρ_e with a dual-energy CT scanner.

Ageing of the X-ray tube inside the CT scanner will change the X-ray spectrum and its mean energy. To a first approximation this will not affect the measured values for μ because the changes in the cross section for the Compton and photoelectric effects will cancel. This in turn means that the CT numbers are unaffected. This also holds for high Z tissues like bone.

Calibration. According to Schneider et al. 1996, calibrating a CT scanner using tissue substitutes could result in an error of 2% to 3%, with corresponding uncertainties in the proton range.

Influence of depth. An additional problem is the change of observed CT numbers with distance penetrated, e.g. in the head and in the pelvis the same tissue type will display different CT numbers.

Conclusion: Due to the above mentioned uncertainties, the conversion of measured CT numbers into values for ρ_e will lead to uncertainties in the particle range. This must be taken into account if proton radiotherapy is to fulfil its promise.

Table C5 and figure C5.1 allow the conversion of CT numbers into corresponding ρ_e values.

C.5.3
Influence of Edges and Inhomogeneities

If a proton beam passes through an inhomogeneity (density ρ_d) inside a homogeneous substance (density ρ) the dose distribution will depend on the inhomogeneity's spatial dimension and its relative density. To take full account of the influence of edges and small inhomogeneities, Monte Carlo calculations are called for. However, these influences may be evaluated qualitatively to try to avoid the creation of hot and cold dose spots inside the total dose distribution.

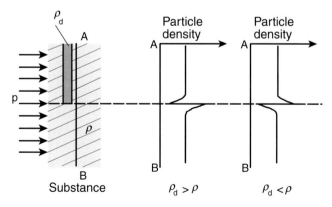

Fig. C5.2. Development of hot and cold spots in the dose distribution at the edge of a density step inside a homogeneous substance. For a beam not orthogonal to the density step, the edge effect will be partly washed out.

C.5.3a
Edge Effects

A density step inside a homogeneous substance and arranged orthogonal to the proton beam direction will create a disturbance around its edge, see Fig C5.2 on previous page. Multiple scattering at the edge will scatter more protons out of the direct shadow

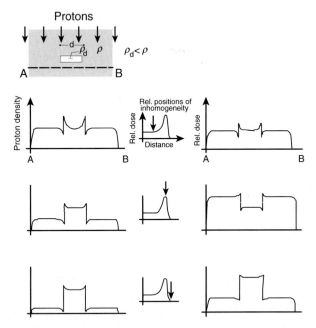

Fig. C5.3. Protons passing an inhomogeneous region inside a homogeneous substance. The reverse case of $\rho_d \geq \rho$ can be easily deduced. The effect is enhanced for emphasis.

of the denser material than into it, resulting in a cold spot with an immediate rise in absorbed dose to create a neighbouring hot spot. Inverting the densities will also invert the relative positions of the cold and hot spots.

C.5.3b
Small Inhomogeneities

If the size d of an inhomogeneity is smaller or equal than the width of the beam and $\rho_d \leq \rho$ (e.g. low density region inside bone), then more protons are scattered into the region directly behind the inhomogeneity than out of it. Its relative dose distribution will depend on the position of the inhomogeneity with respect to the Bragg peak. The effect diminishes for $d \leq$ FWHM and/or as $\rho_d \to \rho$.

The isodose lines are shaped according to the inhomogeneities encountered by the proton beam while penetrating a substance. Density and position of the inhomogeneities influence the curvature of the isodose lines, see figure C5.4.

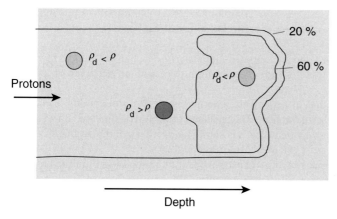

Fig. C5.4. Isodose lines (20%, 60%) for a proton beam penetrating a substance containing small inhomogeneities. The shape of the isodose lines is idealised.

C.5.3c
Narrow but Long (Thick) Inhomogeneities

If the width of a proton beam is larger than the width of a long and narrow inhomogeneity in the beam's path, only the shape of the distal fall-off will be affected, see figure C5.5.

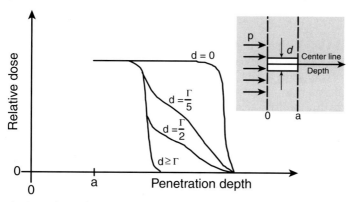

Fig. C5.5. Shape of SOBP along the centre beam line for various, relatively narrow inhomogeneities in the beam's path. d : width of inhomogeneity, γ : width of proton beam at position 0. In the presented case, the density of the inhomogeneity is higher than the density of its surroundings.

C.6
Proton Dosimetry and Proton Dose Measurement

The damaging effect of tissue irradiation with protons is caused by the energy loss of secondary electrons (also called delta rays) released by the penetrating protons. The energy of these photoelectrons and Compton-electrons is limited to a few hundred keV, consequently their influence is restricted to the direct beam path and a few mm around it.

Radiation dose is the energy dissipated and absorbed in a given volume. In radiotherapy it is desirable to determine the radiation dose with an accuracy of 2%–3% (Chu et al. 1993).

It must be realised that in general the energy loss of the protons due to nuclear interactions (non-elastic interactions), is neglected in proton dosimetry. However, the initial section of the proton's beam path is significantly affected: the probability for a non-elastic interaction for a 200 MeV proton is about 25%.

A protocol for proton dosimetry and proton beam calibration was published recently, ICRU (1998) and will most likely be internationally adopted.

C.6.1
Dosimetry Units

C.6.1a
Absorbed radiation Dose

Absorbed radiation dose (D) is a measure of the energy deposited by radiation in a given mass of tissue or other material.

Definition: 1 gray (Gy) = 1 joule (J) per kg

An obsolete (but still encountered) unit is the Rad (rad).
Conversion: 1 rad = 0.01 Gy

D can be calculated in principle if the proton energy, the number of secondary electrons released and the electron density of the substance traversed are known. D can be measured directly by employing a calorimeter. Since both methods are either of poor accuracy or cumbersome to use, the absorbed dose is in general calculated from the ion dose measured by an ionization chamber.

Radiotherapy clinics also employ the (unofficial) radiation unit cobalt-equivalent-dose, expressed in gray. See Part II.

C.6.1b
Ion Dose

The ion dose (J) is a measure of the number of ion pairs produced by radiation in a given mass. There is no special unit for J, it is expressed in coulomb (C) per kg (originally air).

An obsolete unit is the röntgen (R).
Conversion: 1 R = 0.258 mC per kg air

J is measured directly by employing an ionization chamber.

C.6.1c
Conversion of Ion Dose into Absorbed Radiation Dose

The average energy needed to remove 1 electron from an air molecule (and consequently to create an ion pair) is 34.3 eV = 5.49×10^{-18} J. If the proton beam produces n ion pairs in 1 kg of air, then the absorbed dose in air is:

$$D = 34.3 \text{ n eV/kg} = 5.49 \times 10^{-18} \text{ n Gy}$$

To calculate the absorbed dose for a 'standard' tissue, D must be multiplied by the factor 1.09.

C.6.2
Dose Display

The dose distribution inside irradiated tissue must be calculated for each spatial position (pixel). If tissue inhomogeneities and beam scattering are to be taken into account, the individual electron density for each pixel must be known, e.g. determined from a set of CT images. From the resulting density distribution the three-dimensional dose distribution is determined.

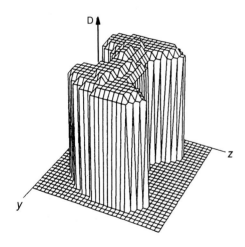

Fig. C6.1. Dose distribution through the y-z plane. The original distribution is shaped for optimal treatment of a complex target. After Brahme et al. 1995.

To assist visualisation of the computed dose distribution inside a 3D object various types of display are employed. The following presents only a few examples.

C.6.2a
Isodose Lines

Lines of equal dose are superimposed upon the CT plane of interest. It is helpful to display in addition the depth dose distributions along selected directions, see figure C6.2.

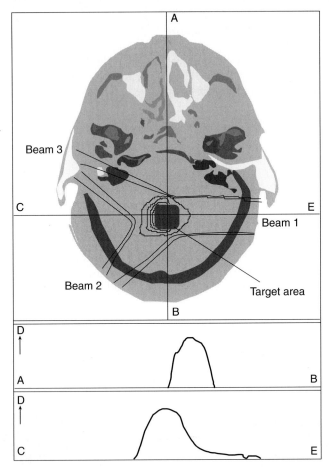

Fig. C6.2. Isodose lines in a selected CT slice. The isodose lines of three beams are overlapping at the target. Beam 1 enters in the plane of the CT, beams 2 and 3 are entering from below. The depth dose distributions along the (movable) lines A-B and C-D are presented.

In general, the CT images produced by the CT scanner are directly utilised for display. However, for special purposes the isodose lines in a series of parallel planes inclined at a fixed angle to the image plane of the CT, could be of value.

C.6.2b
3D and Beam's-Eye View

The 3D view presents a series of outlined CTs stacked in the proper succession. Target and other areas of interest are emphasised and can be observed in their 3D surroundings.

The beam's eye view presents the volume to be irradiated as seen along the centre line of the proton beam entering the object, see figure C6.3.

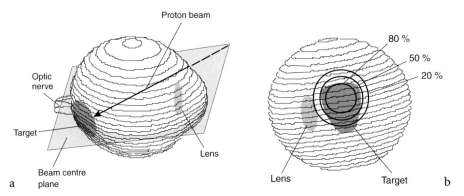

Fig. C6.3. 3D display of the eye, including optic nerve, target and lens. **a.** Display including a proton beam and the beam plane. **b.** Beam's eye view of display a. The projection onto the retina of 3 isodose lines is indicated. The 20% isodose line barely misses the lens.

An oxonometric display presents isodose lines simultaneously in three mutually orthogonal planes. By shifting those planes parallel to themselves an impression of the dose distribution in 3D is created.

C.6.2c
Dose-Volume Histogram (DVH)

In order to optimise the dose distribution inside the body and to compare alternative irradiation plans rapidly, the dose accumulated in the target volume, but also – inevitably – received by adjacent and possibly radiation sensitive structures, must be evaluated. This is difficult to quantify using the above mentioned displays. The problem can be partly overcome by a DVH.

There are various types of DVHs. Here a only 'differential DVH' is presented because the 'integral DVHs' are difficult to interpret and evaluate. Relatively small changes in the integral DVH could hide large local dose variations, see Fig. C6.4.

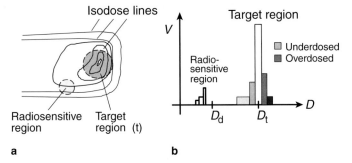

Fig. C6.4. a: Isodose distribution in a plane including an outlined target and a radiosensitive region. **b:** Calculated differential DVH (from a) for the target region (D_t = target dose) and for the radiosensitive region. A radiation dose exceeding D_d would cause irreversible damage. Over- and under-dosed regions are indicated.

In the differential DVH the displayed volume V is the fraction of the total target (or radiosensitive) volume irradiated up to a maximum dose D. Ideally, the differential DVH for the target is a vertical line at the required dose D_t. However, since the dose distribution over the entire target volume is rarely uniform, the DVH also displays over- and under-dosed regions, see figure C6.4.

The DVH of the radiosensitive volume helps to decide whether or not it receives a damaging radiation dose.

Every modern treatment planning computer program should present DVHs for any outlined structure of interest.

C.6.3
Instrumentation

Dosimeters for clinical use should measure the radiation dose with an accuracy of better than 5%.

International dose intercomparisons (e.g. Vatnitzky et al. 1999) demonstrate that, using ionization chambers, it is possible to achieve an agreement in dosimetry between various treatment centers of about 2.9%.

Descriptions and drawings of dosimeters suitable for proton-radiotherapy are described in many textbooks and reviews, e.g. in Chu (1995).

C.6.3a
Ionization Chamber

This is the most widely used instrument to monitor and measure ionising radiation. The charge of secondary electrons produced in the chamber walls and inside the chamber volume is collected by an electric field and measured at an electrode. The most popular version is the transmission parallel plate ionization chamber, with plates either metallised or made from tissue equivalent compounds. The edges of the cylindrical chamber volume are defined by borders of grounded electrodes and the chamber thickness is the separation between the measuring electrodes. Effective volumes down to a few mm^3 are achievable. In general the chamber volume is filled with air, N_2 or a noble gas. The secondary electrons set free by the protons passing through the measuring volume are all fully stopped within it.

The following relation holds:

$$D = n \, W_{gas} / \rho \, V$$

where

D : absorbed radiation dose, expressed in Gy
n : collected number of electrons (= measured electrical charges/elementary charge)
W_{gas} : energy needed to produce one ion pair of the gas filling the chamber, in J
ρ : density of chamber gas, in kg/m^3
V : chamber volume, in m^3.

For protons $W_{air} = 34.3$ eV is generally accepted, more recent measurements (Siebers et al. 1995b) indicate $W_{air} = 34.2 \pm 0.5$ eV

The following quantities determine the accuracy of D:

a. Amount of energy needed to form one ion pair in the chamber gas.

b. Recombination probability for the produced ions. This is especially difficult to evaluate if the proton beam is pulsed.

c. Relation of the mass stopping power in tissue to that in the gas filling the ionization chamber (if the absorbed radiation dose in tissue is to be determined).

Although D can be calculated directly from a measurement, due to the uncertainty in W ionization chambers in general are calibrated against calorimeters or Faraday cups. The absorbed dose received by tissue can be deduced from the ratio W_{gas}/W_{tissue}.

Besides monitoring and measuring radiation dose, segmented ionization chambers are useful instruments for aligning a proton beam.

C.6.3b
Faraday Cup

If a proton beam is totally absorbed inside an electrically isolated block of material contained within a vacuum, the charge collected is a measure of the number of incident protons. This methods yields a collection efficiency very close to one. From the computed beam fluence and the proton energy the absorbed dose can be calculated. This measurement is independent of proton fluence, thus it provides reliable results for both continuous and pulsed proton beams.

The Faraday cup is mainly employed to calibrate ionization chambers. A calibration accuracy of 1.6% may be achieved (Grusell et al. 1995). However, Faraday cup and ionization chamber measurements can differ by 6% (Cambria et al. 1997).

C.6.3c
Silicon Diode

Due to the much greater density of their measuring volumes, diodes – e.g. constructed of Si-Li – are about 3 orders of magnitude more sensitive to radiation than equally sized ionization chambers. This allows for detector sizes of ≤ 1 mm^3, suitable for mapping radiation fields as well as for measurements in vivo. However, diodes suffer radiation damage which will influence their sensitivity (exception: diodes made of diamond).

C.6.3d
Calorimeter

Calorimeters measure the temperature increase due to the energy deposited within them by a totally absored incident particle beam. Consequently, they directly measure the absorbed dose. Such measurements are cumbersome and thus unsuitable for routine use. Consequently calorimeters are mainly employed as calibration standards.

Calorimeters undervalue the dose by about 2.6% as compared with ionization chambers (Palmans et al. 1996). This difference is caused by wall effects in the ionization chamber, uncertainties in W and in the differential energy loss of protons in air and in the calorimeter substance.

For special purposes other dosimetry methods are employed: thermoluminescence, darkening of photographic emulsions, nuclear activation, oxidation from Fe^{++} to $Fe^{3}+$, etc.

C.7
Summary and Comparison with Photon Radiotherapy

Although protons and X-rays are very different radiation modalities, both act on tissue via secondary electrons. However, there is a fundamental difference: The radiation intensity of X-rays penetrating matter decreases exponentially, while a proton beam has a finite range.

A good approximation for the relation between the initial proton energy E_0 and its mean range R_0 in a substance with density ρ is presented by Bortfeld (1997):

$$R_0 \approx 0.0022 \, E_0^{1.77} \, / \, \rho$$

The radiation dose deposited by X-rays decreases exponentially with depth while the dose deposited by the penetrating protons remains almost constant for the initial 70% of the protons' path. After that, a surprising feature is observed: toward the end of the proton range, the absorbed dose rises steeply about threefold, culminates in the Bragg peak and then drops rapidly to zero. The depth position of this dose maximum within the irradiated material is proportional to the primary proton energy, indicating that the dose maximum may be shifted by merely varying the incident proton energy.

The decrease of the X-ray intensity with penetration depth is not very sensitive to density differences encountered. Consequently, irradiation planning for X-rays pays scarce attention to the structures encountered. On the other hand, the proton range is inversely proportional to any encountered density. It must therefore be taken into account to avoid severe over- or under-dosage of the target volume. For this reason, CT images of the region of interest are essential to evaluate quantitatively the tissue density via the Hounsfield numbers of each pixel.

Protons experience little elastic scattering, consequently the penumbra is only a few mm wide. This calls for different displays of the dose distributions to utilise fully the proton beam's favourable dose distribution. The standard planar isodose presentations for X-rays are still used for proton beams. However, 3D displays are essential in proton radiotherapy planning because of the significant range changes due to any inhomogeneity along the proton beam path. Isodose lines presented in an oxonometric display are very useful.

Dose-Volume histograms allow a quantitative evaluation of the dose fraction received by the target volume or any other (e.g. a radiosensitive) volume in the beam path. This is essential for choosing between competing treatment plans.

The instrumentation to monitor and measure radiation dose is similar for both protons and X-rays. It is easier to calibrate a proton dosimeter because protons have a finite range. This allows a direct absolute dose measurement using a calorimeter and indirect dose measurements employing a Faraday cups, ionization chambers, diodes, etc.

D Modifying the Proton Beam

D.1
Survey

The particle beam leaving the accelerator is accepted by the beam transport system and delivered into the treatment area. In general, the physical properties (divergence, spatial dimensions, energy, energy spread, etc.) of a beam leaving the transport system are unsuitable for radiotherapy. Consequently, the beam is modified in the region between accelerator and target site.

The proton beam at the exit of an efficient beam transport system has a diameter of a few mm. Its divergence is insufficient to spread it to a size required for radiotherapy at the isocenter of the target. Exception: proton beams for eye treatment.

In general the exiting beam displays a nearly circular cross section and this shape must be modified to conform to the target outline.

It is difficult to vary the output energy of the accelerator and time consuming to change the parameters of the beam transport system to accommodate different particle energies. For this reason, the beam energy E is changed by the beam delivery system.

The energy spread $\Delta E/E$ of the exiting proton beam is of the order of 0.001. This is adequate for very small irradiation fields, e.g. in eye treatment, but the average treatment plan calls for a wider, and ideally an adjustable, energy spread.

D.2
Static Beam Shaping

D.2.1
Transverse Proton Beam Shaping

A desirable therapeutic proton beam displays at the isocenter a radiation field of up to 40 cm × 40 cm, having a dose uniformity of 2% and a dose rate of about 2 Gy/min to 4 Gy/min. The stricter the adherence to these conditions, the more complex and – unavoidably – less reliable the beam shaping system becomes.

D.2.1a
Single Scatterer

Any material in the beam's path will spread the beam by multiple scattering. As long as the material thickness encountered is very small compared with the range of the beam particles, the resulting spatial distribution will be approximately a Gaussian.

Naturally, this assumes, that the original beam is monoenergetic and that its divergence is negligible. Otherwise the original energy distribution and divergence must be convoluted with a Gaussian to find the final distribution of the beam.

To achieve the desired radiation dose uniformity across the irradiation field, only the central part of the scattered beam may be utilised. Experience shows that this is about 5% of the beam radiation intensity striking the scatterer. About 95% of the beam intensity must be discarded, producing undesirable background radiation and radioactivity of any material struck be the beam.

D.2.1b
Double Scatterer

To utilise a larger fraction of the scattered beam, its central part must be scattered again. This will produce a widened particle distribution having a relatively flat top. The second scatterer is placed downstream from the first. It either occludes the beam centrally (the central particles are scattered toward the outside), or the scatterer is ring shaped (scattering particles into the central region), or the scatterer is a combination of both. For a quantitative analysis, see Webb (1993).

It must be realised that after scattering the average particle energy will vary over the cross section of the particle beam. It is a small effect but it will increase the range straggling of the beam particles.

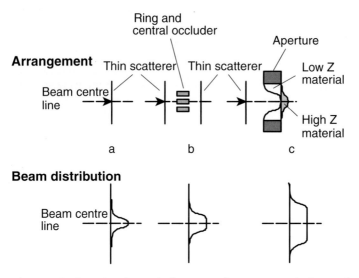

Fig. D2.1. Configurations for passive beam spreading systems. a: Single central scatterer, (b) annulus scatterer, (c) bimaterial scatterer.

A bimaterial scatterer (e.g. copper on Perspex) presents another, more elegant method for passive beam spreading (Gottschalk and Wagner 1989). The high Z material in the center flattens the beam distribution, the combined thickness ensures that the energy loss inside the scatterer is uniform over the entire beam cross section. A well designed double scatterer utilises of the order of 10% of the total particle beam fluence.

Lining up the complete scattering system is time consuming. It is sensitive to minor changes in the direction and the energy of the incident proton beam.

A radical solution to achieve a uniform irradiation field and a high beam utilisation factor ($\geq$ 90%) would be to employ a set of adjustable quadrupoles and octupoles. However, this would require a drift space of about 100 m, very rarely available.

D.2.1c
Apertures

Apertures (collimators) shape the beam's cross section in such a way that it conforms to the target's outline. Aperture design is non-trivial because the steep lateral dose fall-off of the proton beam should be affected as little as possible. Obviously, the aperture's thickness must exceed the particle range.

The aperture's material exposed to the beam becomes radioactive, predominantly emitting gamma-rays. Typically, a medium Z material displays an activity having a half-life of about 5 min.

Fixed Aperture. This aperture conforms to the projected and fixed contours of a specific target. In general it is cast from a low melting point and reusable alloy (e.g. Corrobend, melting point 70 °C). Its mould is made by an automatic milling machine receiving instructions from the radiotherapy planning program.

Variable Aperture. Designed to overcome the labour-intensive fixed aperture it uses sliding absorbers to achieve variable field sizes. Example: An appropriately arranged pair of width-adjustable and sliding slits can outline any rectangular aperture.

Multileaf Aperture. Sets of absorber leafs – in general made out of steel – are moved individually by an actuator. This allows to design many aperture shapes by remote control. In addition, the entity can be rotated around the beam axis. A problem to be solved for each arrangement is to block the unavoidable radiation leakage between the individual aperture leafs. The multileaf aperture is an economic solution, in addition it avoids the problems connected with the removal of activated apertures.

D.2.2
Longitudinal Proton Beam Shaping

D.2.2a
Shifting the Bragg Peak

Energy Degrader (or Range Shifter). To shift the dose maximum to a pre-determined depth inside the body being irradiated, an absorber (energy degrader) must be placed within the beam's path. Any material in the beam path will reduce the beam energy proportionally to its thickness. Although this avoids the lengthy task of changing the output energy of the accelerator and all the settings of the beam transport system, there is a price to be paid: The FWHM of the Bragg peak remains at the value observed for the original particle beam. Although the absolute width of the particle spectrum remains practically constant, the relative spectral energy width $\Delta E/E$ increases. This is a serious drawback, especially for proton radiotherapy of the eye.

The energy degrader should be made of a very uniform and low Z material in order to keep multiple scattering low. It is convenient to have an energy degrader of remotely controlled, variable thickness.

Example: Schreuder et al. 1999 described two identical carbon wedges moving in opposite directions across the proton beam path. Wedge angle 11.9 degrees, step width 0.1 mm water equivalent.

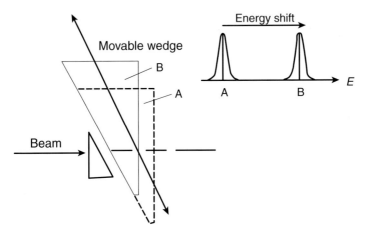

Fig. D2.2. Remotely controlled, double-wedge energy degrader.

Inevitably, the energy degrader as well as the apertures are sources of neutrons. It should be placed as far upstream of the isocenter as possible in order to reduce the number of neutrons reaching the patient.

D.2.2b
Spread Out Bragg Peak (SOBP)

The central particle beam leaving the scattering system displays an almost monoenergetic energy spectrum. Entering tissue, this beam will produce a depth dose distribution characterised by the Bragg peak. For use in radiotherapy this dose distribution has two shortcomings: the dose distribution displays a pronounced maximum and its FWHM is fixed (about 10 mm to 20 mm), rendering it unsuitable for targets longer than about 15 mm in the beam direction.

To irradiate an extended target, a dose distribution with a uniformity of better than 10% over the entire target volume is required. This can be achieved by overlapping Bragg distributions of different energies and various proton intensities. The resulting dose distribution is called a Spread Out Bragg Peak (SOBP).

It should be noted that this longitudinal beam spreading substantially decreases the ratio peak radiation dose/entrance radiation dose.

Along the beam direction x the resulting radiation dose $D(x_i)$ at depth x_i is the sum of the doses contributed by the individual Bragg distributions at position x_i:

$$D(x_i) = \sum_{i=1}^{n} W_i D_i(x_i) \qquad \text{(D2.1)}$$

where

n : number of contributing Bragg distributions
W_i : relative intensity of the i'th particle beam (beam weight)
D_i : dose at x_i for the i'th Bragg distribution.

Taking into account the dose-averaged linear energy transfer (LET), Chu et al. 1993 calculated W_i for particles of various LET.

Measurements can determine the shape of the individual Bragg distributions utilised to construct a SOBP. However, a more general approach is feasible:

Assuming that a power function describes the energy-range relation, Bortfeld and Schlegel 1996 approximate the shape of the proximal part of the Bragg distribution, see Section C4.1. They calculate a beam weight function $W(R)$ which depends on the beam range, the spacing of the individual contributions and the plateau length. After convoluting $D(x)$ with $W(R)$ the authors present an analytical expression for the SOBP distribution. This rather lengthy formula can be approximated by

$$D_{SOBP}(x) \approx D_o/(1 + 0.44r^{0.6}) \qquad \text{(D2.2)}$$

where

$$r = (x_a - x)/(x_b - x_a) \qquad \text{(D2.3)}$$

and

$D_{SOBP}(x)$: relative radiation dose at depth x
D_0 : relative dose at plateau of SOBP
x_a : proximal depth of SOBP
x_b : distal depth of SOBP.

For protons this approximation for the SOBP distribution holds remarkably well. Its maximum deviation from the exact value is 5% of D_0, its mean deviation is about 2%.

Bortfeld and Schlegel 1996 observe that the formula remains valid for any heavy charged particle beam and any substance penetrated.

To estimate the relative radiation dose received by the region covered by the SOBP, the following ratio is useful:

$$D_{norm} = \frac{\text{dose absorbed proximal to the SOBP}}{\text{dose absorbed within the SOBP}} \qquad \text{(D2.4)}$$

According to Bortfeld and Schlegel 1996:

$$D_{norm} \approx a/(1 + 0.277a^{0.55}) \qquad \text{(D2.4)}$$

where

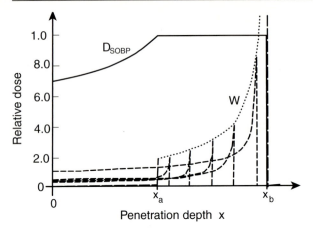

Fig. D2.3. SOBP constructed from individual Bragg distributions. Solid line: SOBP distribution D_{SOBP}. Dotted line: weight function W. $x_b - x_a$: plateau length. After Bortfeld and Schlegel 1996.

$$a = x_a/(x_b - x_a)$$

Example: For a plateau length of 50% of R, $D_{norm} = 0.78$ and for 25% of R, $D_{norm} = 2.0$. In the first case the region covered by the SOBP receives 28% more dose than the region proximal to it, about 56% of the total dose. In the second case the SOBP region absorbs half the dose received by the proximal region, about 33% of the total dose.

D.2.2c
Generating a Spread Out Bragg Peak

To generate a SOBP the particle beam must traverse various energy degrading layers, one after the other. The thickness of each layer determines the depth position of the appropriate Bragg peak. The exposure time assigned to each energy degrader represents the weight W of the individual Bragg distribution. Thicknesses and time spans determine the plateau length of the SOBP and its dose uniformity. The maximum plateau length is the full particle range for the unobstructed particle beam.

There are various, practical techniques to spread out the Bragg peak, e.g. see Chu et al. 1993:

Propeller. The cross sections of a set of propeller-like blades made of Perspex and having a width of about three times the beam diameter, are shaped in such a way as to produce a SOBP of a fixed plateau length. This rather bulky arrangement rotates at about 1000 rpm through the particle beam.

Bar Ridge. The cross section of a parallel set of metallic bar ridges is shaped appropriately. The entire set oscillates through the particle beam or the beam itself wobbles across it. In general this device is used for charged particle beams other than proton beams.

Spiral Ridge. The cross section follows a step function. the thickness of each step determines the local position of its individual Bragg peak, the step length its relative weight. The beam penetrates the spiral ridge off axis.

D.2.2d
Problems connected with the SOBP

The main disadvantage of utilising a SOBP is the increased entrance radiation dose, which may reach up to 100% of the plateau dose. However, there are additional problems:

a. The particle beam penetrates relatively thick layers of material. Consequently, the changes in the dose distribution due to inelastic scattering must be taken into account.

b. The RBE (Relative Biological Effectiveness) is a function of particle energy, i.e. penetration depth, see Coutrakon et al. 1997. Consequently the physical radiation dose distribution along the plateau must be shaped accordingly to achieve a uniform biologically effective dose distribution. This influence is especially important for heavy particle beams other than proton beams, see Coutrakon et al. 1997.

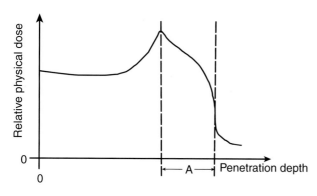

Fig. D2.4. A typically physical dose distribution for a He^{++}-beam designed to achieve a uniform biologically effective dose over region A.

c. A potentially serious problem was pointed out by Levin et al. 1988. Their calculations demonstrate that the separation between adjacent contributing Bragg peaks must be ≤ 6 mm to achieve the required plateau dose uniformity of 10%. In addition, the relative position of each contributing Bragg peak must be accurate to about 0.2 mm. Otherwise, unacceptable hot and cold radiation dose spots will develop. Taking into account the (unavoidable) motion of the target region during irradiation, this accuracy cannot be achieved with presently available techniques. In addition, this problem seems to prevent successful radiotherapy using a particle beam scanning system.

D.2.2e
Distal Isodose Shaping Device (DISD)

The DISD is a material shaped in such a way that the deposited dose will follow a preselected distribution. The DISD is made of low Z material and placed directly after the final aperture. It should be positioned as close as possible to the patient's surface to minimise the influence of multiple scattering. Sisterson et al. 1989 investigated the influence of an air gap on the isodose distribution and concluded that as long as the gap is less than 12 cm, the anticipated shift of the isodose contour remains within the margins of accuracy of the treatment plan.

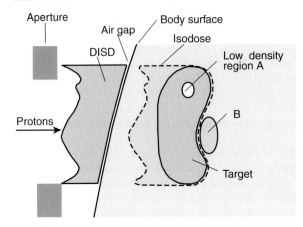

Fig. D2.5. Cross section of a DISD designed to take into account the influence of a structure A inside the target and to minimise the dose received by a distal radio-sensitive region B.

The three-dimensional DISD design is usually generated by the radiotherapy planning program.

In general a DISD significantly simplifies the irradiation procedure by often allowing single field treatment.

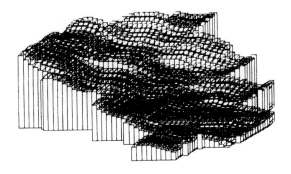

Fig. D2.6. Centre piece of a computer-generated DISD designed for eye treatment by i-PROTEUS (a proton planning system). The beam is fully absorbed outside the region covered by the DISD.

D.2.3
Beam Shaping and the Penumbra

After introducing the above described beam shaping devices, the originally steep penumbra will degrade. The extent of this widening of the penumbra depends on actual size and mutual separation of the beam shaping components. According to Monte Carlo calculations by Urie et al. 1986 the increase of the penumbra of a proton beam is dominated by: size of the air gap between beam aperture and patient, mean thickness of the DISD and the distance between the patient's surface and the target region.

D.3
Dynamic Radiation Field Shaping

It is difficult to move a patient through a narrow proton beam in such a way that an extended and uniform radiation field results. Using two magnetic dipoles with field lines orthogonal to the charged particles' direction, the beam can be dynamically spread out in such a way, that – in principle – it creates any desired radiation field shape while the patient position remains unchanged. This method was first successfully tried by Larsson et al. 1959. For a detailed description see Chu et al. 1993.

To move the particle beam dynamically and consequently to shape the radiation field without employing a static beam shaping system presents a number of advantages and disadvantages.

At present, dynamic longitudinal beam shaping is unfeasible using a conventional proton accelerator.

D.3.1
Principle of Operation

A narrow particle beam enters the field of a set of two orthogonal magnetic dipoles having magnetic field lines perpendicular to the beam direction. The time variation of the electric current applied to the dipoles determines the resulting beam pattern in any plane orthogonal to the beam. A predetermined 3D beam pattern, layer by layer, can be achieved by changing the beam energy after each complete 2D sweep. However, although most of the radiation is deposited in the narrow region of the Bragg peak, a considerable amount is deposited proximal to it.

D.3.2
Beam Scanner

The shape of the created radiation field depends on the amplitude and time pattern of the magnetic fields.

D.3.2a
Wobbler

The strength of the two magnetic fields vary continuously with time in a sinusoidal pattern having the same maximum value but shifted 90° in phase. The result is a circular radiation field. Its diameter is a function of the maximum magnetic field strength.

If the ratio of the two frequencies is an integer greater than 1, the beam describes a Lissajous pattern eventually achieving an approximately rectangular radiation dose distribution.

To create a uniform dose distribution over the entire radiation field, the wobbler has to repeat its pattern often.

D.3.2b
Linear Scanner

Each of the orthogonal magnetic field strengths follows a fixed time regime (e.g. linear, saw-tooth, step-function, etc.). The particle beam spot describes an appropriate pattern. By changing the time structure different radiation dose distributions can be achieved.

Since in general the pattern is set by a slow and a fast scan, it is possible to replace the function of the slowly scanning magnetic dipole by moving the patient support, see PSI (1995).

Utilising a narrow Bragg distribution, the scanned beam irradiates the entire target volume through a set of parallel layers. The position of each new layer is determined by changing the settings of the beam energy degrader. The scanning pattern must be synchronised with the time regime of the accelerator output. This is easily done, if the duration for the complete scan of one layer is the same as one beam spill. If the accelerator output fluctuates during treatment, many repeat scans of the same layer are indicated to cancel out short intensity variations.

The linear scanner can irradiate a cylindrical volume having an (almost) arbitrary cross section. Any steps in the lateral dose distribution caused by the scanning pattern are automatically smoothed out by the ever present elastic scattering.

The main problem associated with a linear scanning system is to match the beam edges of one line scan with the next in such a way, that the absorbed dose radiation distribution produced by adjacent scans is uniform.

Pixel Scanning. The beam is laterally limited by a system of slits, creating a (more or less) rectangular beam spot. This beam spot is moved in discrete steps within a grid pattern and remains at each position until its designated spot dose has been deposited. In general, the grid size matches the spot size. Since the volume to be treated can be scanned layer by layer, pixel scanning is a truly 3D treatment method. Within limits, any radiation dose distribution – including holes – can be achieved. With a fast and sensitive particle intensity monitor, accelerator output fluctuations may be compensated.

The edge matching from spot to spot is critical for pixel scanning. A fuzzy spot does not solve the problem because the fuzziness would extend to the lateral fall-off of the radiation field, resulting in a clinically unacceptable penumbra.

A typical pixel scanning system will irradiate up to 100 pixels in about 3 min. Consequently, for a 10 mm × 10 mm pixel size and a (10 × 10 × 10) pixel radiation field, the irradiation time exceeds 30 min.

Spot Scanning. This is a simplified version of the pixel scanner. The beam spot rests for the same period of time in all the positions within the irradiation pattern. While the spot is being moved, the beam is swept rapidly aside by a fast kicker magnet. A typical on-off switching time is 0.1 ms.

The spatial resolution of spot (and pixel) scanning is determined by the minimum achievable spot size (at best 5 mm diameter), the stability of the magnetic field strengths and the width of the Bragg peak.

D.3.3
Advantages and Disadvantages

Advantages. a. The radiation background in the treatment area is substantially reduced because the beam does not encounter any scattering material in its path. The background becomes especially low by dynamically shaping the beam so that there is no need for an aperture.

Although the energy degrader is a strong source of background radiation, it can be shielded and placed far upstream of the treatment area.

b. The beam energy spread is unchanged and distal and lateral radiation dose fall-off remain steep.

c. Beam utilisation increases substantially.

d. The spreading of the beam can be achieved over a short path length, making it possible to position the beam shaping system into a gantry having a reasonable size.

e. Beam alignment is not as critical.

f. It is possible to achieve a radiation field having a predetermined non-uniform dose distribution.

Disadvantages. a. To keep treatment duration short, the proton fluence must be very high. Consequently each position inside the radiation field is exposed for a very short period of time only. This makes accurate monitoring of the received radiation dose difficult.

b. According to Chu (1999) the instantaneous proton radiation dose rate in spots can be several orders of magnitude larger than in scattering radiation treatment systems.

c. For reliable results, on-line checks of the radiation dose delivered per voxel, beam position, beam shape and beam energy are required.

d. There is a strong coupling between scanning procedure and the time regime of the accelerator output. Consequently, the design of scanning systems is strongly influenced by the specific characteristics of the radiation source.

e. Dynamic beam shaping is complex. If the beam fails to advance, serious overdosing could be the result.

D.3.4
Summary

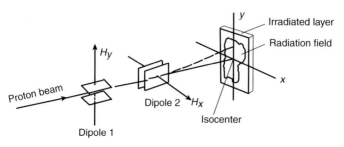

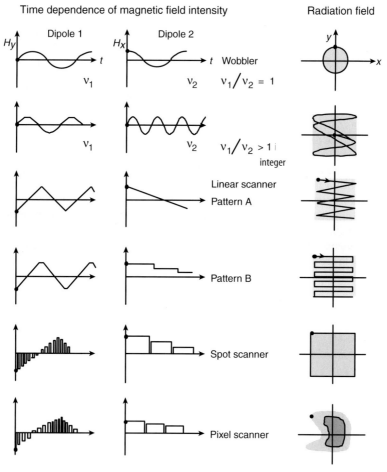

Fig. D3. Summary of dynamic radiation field shaping systems. Top: Schematics of a beam scanning system. Both magnetic dipole field lines are orthogonal to each other and to the charged particle beam line. Below: The six main methods for dynamic radiation field shaping.

E Conformal Proton Radiotherapy Planning

E.1
Introduction

Conformal radiotherapy planning tries to match a tumoricidal dose to the target volume, including a safety margin. At the same time this dose distribution must deliver a radiation dose as low as possible to normal or radio-sensitive tissues. Planning is thus one of the centre pieces of proton radiotherapy. To justify the very high expectations and the large costs of proton therapy, it should be significantly more successful than the conventional therapeutic modalities. It is difficult to attain these expectations, especially since conventional radiotherapy is progressing rapidly.

Proton radiotherapy planning, especially planning for full 3D treatment, is barely ten years old. One of the advantages of this late-comer is, that by now compact but powerful computers became available. In general there is no need for mainframes and batch processing. Work-stations and even PCs are sufficient to compute and optimise a 3D irradiation plan within minutes.

Consequently, the costs of the computer hardware is very low compared with the costs of the software.

The development of planning systems has been an individual task; most planning systems are designed for a unique proton facility. Therefore they are not easily convertible. In addition, fully 3 D planning systems still lack all desired details, for not all factors influencing the dose distribution are taken fully into account.

This section will present only an overview, for further details consult the cited literature. The following three subsections – and especially Sect. E.3 – present important aspects of conformal proton radiotherapy planning.

E.1.1
The Role of Inhomogeneities

In conventional X-ray therapy planning, tissues traversed by the radiation are in general assumed to be of uniform density. The influence of naturally occurring density differences on the dose distribution of X-rays inside the body rarely results in dose shifts of more than a few percent. In contrast, proton dose distributions are very sensitive to small density differences of material in the proton's path.

In addition, for precision planning it is important, where the density inhomogeneity is situated within the proton's path.

Example: The range of a 200 MeV proton in soft tissue (density about 1.0 g/cm^3) is 26.2 cm. If the same protons pass through a 2 cm layer of bone (density about

1.85 g/cm^3) imbedded in the soft tissue and positioned right at the entrance point, the central range will be reduced by 1.4 cm to 24.8 cm.

If that same bone is situated at a depth of 10 cm, the proton range will be reduced to 24.6 cm. The resulting difference of 2 mm, about 1% of the proton's range, is claimed to be significant in proton radiotherapy.

Materials and air gaps (e.g. caused by a DISD) upstream of the patient should also be treated as inhomogeneities. In general this influence is taken into account by using an effective source size and an additional lateral beam spread.

Thin inhomogeneities (thickness ≪ proton range), *not* extending across the full width of the proton beam, are the cause of dose variations in their shadows and at their lateral margins. Calculating the changes in the dose distribution is complex, some methods are presented by Goitein (1978).

Thick inhomogenities (thickness ≤ proton range), *not* extending across the full beam width, cause very significant local shifts in the proton range and distort the Bragg peak. To compute the changes of the proton distribution behind thick inhomogeneities, time consuming Monte Carlo computations are required.

E.1.2
Target Movements

Even if the body is fixed in position by an immobilisation system, the target will move about a mean position. There are three types of movement (analysed in detail by Okumura et al. 1995); only one can be compensated for. Movements as extensive and non-reproducible as those of the alimentary tract are not included in the following considerations.

Diagnostic and treatment positions differ. CT scans in general are taken in the supine position while treatment may be carried out in positions anywhere between vertical and horizontal. Consequently, the target region will shift due to gravitational forces. These shifts can be large and unpredictable for thoraco-abdominal targets, preventing proton treatment altogether. Intracranial movements can be as large as 4 mm for a 90° rotation of the head (Breuer and Wynchank 1995).

Movement due to respiration. Even shallow respiration causes time dependent target movements in the cranio-caudal direction exceeding 2 cm for thoraco-abdominal targets.

Example: MRI studies by Moerland et al. 1994 show respiration induced movement of the kidneys of 2 mm to 30 mm.

Movements of this magnitude are larger than the safety margins assigned during planning, so they have to be taken into account. It is feasible to gate and synchronise the proton beam intensity with the respiratory cycle. The remaining movement of a few mm may be accommodated by an enlarged safety margin, see e.g. Tsujii et al. 1995. Active breathing control will substantially reduce the effective target movement, e.g. to less than 1 mm for liver (Wong et al. 1999).

Long-term movements. Target regions may move between treatment sessions. This will cause dose uncertainties near the target's edge and possible irradiation of radio-sensitive regions. Investigations by Hanley et al. 1997 and Stroom et al. 1999 demonstrate e.g. a movement of the prostate, in the course of a complete treatment regime, of 2 mm to 7 mm. This is a significant shift for proton radiotherapy. In principle those movements can be checked by observing the positions of metallic implants determined radiologically, making it possible to change the irradiation position accordingly. However, this is rarely done.

Table E Organ movements, induced mainly by respiration.	Organ	Range of movement (in mm)
	Bladder	up to 15
	Diaphragm	10 to 40
	Kidney	10 to 40
	Liver	10 to 40
	Pancreas	10 to 30
	Prostate	2 to 7

The table demonstrates, that target movements will take place even if an immobilisation system is employed. The target shift should be taken into account to utilise the accuracy of proton radiotherapy fully.

E.1.3
The Influence of Multiple Scattering

Multiple scattering of charged particles is covered exhaustively by Molière's theory (Molière 1948), partly presented in Sect. C.2. It is worthwhile to investigate its influence on practical aspects of proton radiotherapy.

The elastic multiple scattering of protons is dominated by proton-electron interaction. It causes small angular deflections from the initial flight direction of the protons; besides a very small energy loss per scattering event. Consequently, the beam's penumbra is significantly enlarged inside the patient and the steepness of the distal dose fall-off decreases. In addition scattering smoothes the isodose lines inside the irradiated region.

The widening of a parallel proton beam entering a patient was calculated by Hong et al. 1996. Their results differ insignificantly from those of Chu et al. 1993.

Assuming that the multiple scattering distribution is a Gaussian, the rms (root mean square) radius for a pencil beam increases almost linearly with penetration depth.

Figure E1.1 presents only the spreading of a proton beam due to elastic multiple scattering inside the patient. To calculate the total rms radius of the beam additional influences must be taken into account:

a. Radial emittance due to physical source size
b. Scattering at the apertures (collimators)
c. Scattering inside the energy degrader
d. The air gap due to the DISD, etc.

If the diameter of the entering parallel beam is reduced below a certain limit (about 5 mm to 10 mm for a 200 MeV beam), too many protons are scattered out of the beam. Consequently the relative height of the Bragg peak decreases, possibly to such a degree that proton therapy looses its advantages, see e.g. figure E1.2.

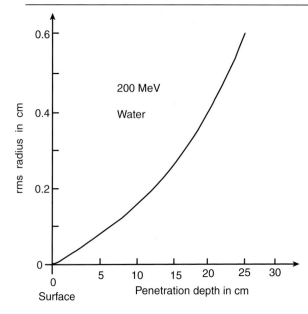

Fig. E1.1. Increase of the rms radius of a proton beam with penetration depth. Lateral spreading of the initially parallel 200 MeV beam is caused by multiple scattering. Reducing the initial energy to 150 MeV will increase the rms radius by about 50%. Modified after Hong et al. 1996.

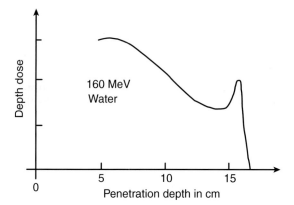

Fig. E1.2. Measured depth dose distribution for a 0.48 cm diameter proton beam in water. Modified after Hong et al. 1996.

Petti (1996) investigated in detail the influence of multiple scattering on the proton dose distribution inside an absorber including complex inhomogeneous structures. As expected, the isodose distribution contours are smooth and the steep fall-off at the end of the particle range is degraded.

An unexpected consequence of multiple scattering on SOBP distributions is the possible appearance of hot and cold spots in the shadow of complex inhomogeneities. This can change the local radiation dose in the plateau region by about ± 5%. The effect is enhanced if the proton beam passes through air cavities.

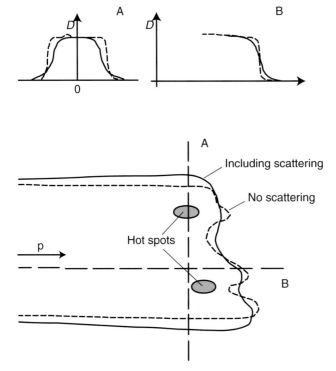

Fig. E1.3. Proton radiation dose distributions inside water containing inhomogeneities with (——) and without (-----) the influence of multiple proton scattering. A: Dose cross section. B: Depth dose.

E.2
Planning Methods

E.2.1
Data Input

Particle radiotherapy planning systems handle large amounts of data. Most input data are extracted from CT scans in addition to the particle beam dose distribution values measured in water tanks. All the data are collected from 3D arrangements.

Example: A set of 50 CT slices, each having a resolution of 512 × 512 pixel contains a matrix with 1.31×10^7 elements. Besides positional information, each matrix element carries a CT number accurate enough to reveal its electron density to three significant digits.

Modalities supplying additional data – e.g. magnetic resonance imaging (MRI), positron emission tomography (PET) and single photon emission computed tomography (SPECT) – are also employed. Input to the planning program must be able to accommodate and convert all the data from the various imaging modalities into a common frame of reference (image fusion). There may be also a need to shift, rotate and change the scale of the entire data set. In addition distorted and warped data need rectifying. Naturally, all facilities delivering data will have different resolutions, demanding conversion of their input data. Last but not least, all positional data have to be converted into the reference frame of the treatment set-up.

The amount of information to be handled by the input system is drastically reduced for shoot-through arrangements. The same applies for eye treatment planning, except if a very high resolution CT scanner is available.

All the input data are finally combined to create a 3D outline of the target, of the radio-sensitive structures to be avoided and of the density matrix describing the contents of the volume between beam entrance and target.

E.2.1a
Ultrasound

Ultrasound data are mainly employed to determine external contours like the outline of an eye, chest wall thicknesses, etc.

E.2.1b
X-rays

This anatomical imaging system mainly supplied 2D input data before CT data became available (about 1972). Target outline and target area were constructed by hand from the radiograph. Positional input data were entered into the planning device manually, as were the very few data regarding densities in the expected beam path. This input method was sufficient as long as treatment plans were constructed for one image plane only.

E.2.1c
Computer Tomography (CT)

The use of this anatomical imaging device increases the amount of input data by orders of magnitude. In return it delivers a 3D CT number matrix of the entire volume of interest. The individual CT layers are longitudinally related to each other via a scout view, i.e. a planar radiograph which can be produced by the CT scanner with the rotation switched off. In general diagnostic transaxial CT scanners are utilised. However, simplified scanners which deliver input data only sufficiently accurate for treatment planning are also employed.

The selected thickness of each CT slice and thus the amount of input data is a trade-off between spatial resolution and patient throughput.

The local density for each pixel within each CT slice – the most important quantity for proton radiation planning – is determined from the pixel's CT number. Unfortunately the relation between CT number and density is not unique but influenced by a number of factors, notably the energy of the X-rays employed by the CT scanner and the age of the X-ray tube. Data from dual energy CT scanners improve the accuracy but increase the input data flow.

Most proton planning systems do not take into account the CT numbers from each individual pixel, but utilise CT numbers averaged over the entire penetration length of a pencil beam. This considerably reduces data input and computing time, but it can lead to distortions in the distal region of the dose distribution.

Although the input CT number matrix constitutes an overwhelming proportion of input data, the clinician supplies the most important input data, e.g. outlines of the target and of the radiosensitive structures, safety margins, etc.

E.2.1d
Magnetic Resonance Imaging (MRI)

Data input from this functional imaging device complements the CT data. Features invisible on the CT image are often clearly displayed, especially tumour outlines. The basic resolution of both modalities is about the same, however, due to the longer scanning times MRI images are much more sensitive to patient movement. The differences in resolution and reproducibility must be taken into account if MRI input data are to be utilised.

Non-coplanar MRI images display a higher resolution than the corresponding CT images, because MRI image points are extracted directly from the input data matrix.

Alexander et al. 1995 found systematic deviations (mean value: 4 mm) comparing corresponding MRI and CT coordinates.

E.2.1e
Fusion of Anatomical and Functional Data

For planning purposes it is helpful to compare CT and MRI images, especially in regions of low density contrast. To overlay CT and MRI images is non-trivial due to their different formats (image size, voxel size) and the spatial orientation of the layers to be compared. In addition the different physical principles used by each modality means that features clearly used as position reference point in one modality (e.g. a bony feature in CT, or a fat/muscle interface in MRI) may be unrecognisable in the other, see figure E2.1.

If the scanning position of the patient differs for both modalities, additional problems arise: anatomical landmarks or external markers or both must be matched for regions of interest or for both sets of data. In general, planning parameters like position and pixel density are extracted from the CT data set, while matching of isodose lines and appropriate target contours takes place on the MRI image.

To bypass the considerable difficulties in matching, CT and MRI images are often displayed side by side and visually compared. Webb (1993) presents in detail the various methods for matching anatomical and functional data sets.

E.2.2
Algorithms

An important component of any proton radiotherapy planning system is the planning algorithm. Most of the time it is designed for a given treatment machine and its set-up. However, general approaches are becoming available.

Comparing the various algorithms, one realises that a compromise is needed. Ray tracing algorithms yield radiation treatment plans within a few seconds but their accu-

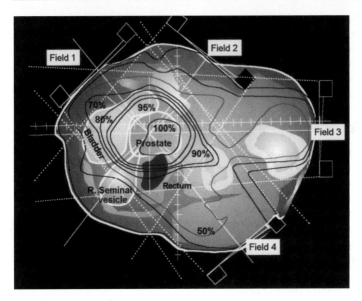

Fig. E2.1. CT-MRI fusion image achieved by a commercial software package (Picker AcQSIM). MRI: 256 × 256, 0.7 mm pixel size. CT: 512 × 512, 0.9 mm pixel size, 4 mm slice thickness. Positioning was supported by tattoo markers. Bony landmarks were employed to correlate the images. Four-field X-ray planning. Note the close proximity of the radiosensitive rectum and the bladder to the target (prostate). After Lau et al. 1996.

racy is limited. On the other hand, algorithms based on Monte Carlo techniques yield high accuracy plans but may take about twenty hours to complete a single plan. A reasonable compromise is to achieve a rapid overview within seconds by employing ray tracing, select an optimal approach and design the final treatment plan within minutes by employing an algorithm based on a differential pencil beam algorithm.

Besides computing the energy losses and the scattering of the protons entering and penetrating the patient, any algorithm should take into account the contributions from the components of the proton beam transport and beam shaping system:

1. The influence of the beam energy degrader.
2. The energy loss and scattering caused by a range modulator employed to create a SOBP.
3. The change of the beam due to collimators and/or blocks used for passive shaping of the beam's cross section.
4. Range modification and angular spread of the proton beam caused by a distal isodose shaping device (compensating bolus).

E.2.2a
Monte Carlo Method

This statistical method was initially applied to X-ray treatment planning, then extended to radiotherapy planning for fast electrons. Goitein and Sisterson 1978 employed the Monte Carlo method to investigate the influence of thick inhomogeneities on charged particle beams. For a recent application of the Monte Carlo technique to proton radiotherapy planning see Petti (1992, 1996) or Carlsson et al. 1997.

The Monto Carlo method applied to particle radiotherapy planning traces a moving particle's history due to ionization energy losses and elastic scattering. It tracks the individual particle from one point of interaction to the next.

In practice, the volume of interest is subdivided into rectangular voxels forming a 3D matrix. The calculation ends as soon as the particle's remaining track length is less than the voxel size (grid constant). Generally, this corresponds to a proton energy of about 2 MeV. A pencil beam dose distribution within the 3D matrix is achieved by adding the deposited doses of many tracks starting at the same position. Summing up the locally deposited energies along a very large number (more than a million) of initially parallel particle tracks will yield the dose distribution produced by a particle beam of finite diameter.

The scattering process is modelled according to Molière theory. Sometimes – in order to save computation time – the quantity B in Molière's formula (see Eq. C2.1) is replaced by Highland's approximation (Highland 1979). In addition, the effective atomic numbers and atomic weights in the immediate surroundings of the interaction points are taken to be those of water. Another time saving approximation employs the ionization potential of water at each interaction point irrespective of the substance involved.

Petti (1996) concluded, that the influence of the approximations generally used on the resulting dose distribution is small. The inaccuracy is smaller than the voxel size of standard CT slices.

If all factors influencing the history of the penetrating particles are properly taken into account, the Monte Carlo method yields very accurate dose distributions. Those dose distributions are utilised as bench-marks to evaluate the results of other proton radiotherapy planning methods. However, at present Monte Carlo computations are rarely employed for routine planning purposes because the computation time for one proton beam is many hours.

Example: Petti (1996) quotes a computation time (workstation AXP 3000) of 22 h for a 4 cm diameter proton beam. Parameters: Pixel size 1.56×1.56 mm, 8 CT slices with a spacing of 3 mm, 4×10^6 proton histories. The standard deviation of the dose deposited in each voxel in the central beam was $\leq 1\%$.

E.2.2b
Ray Tracing

This is a one-dimensional method. The input is a proton depth dose distribution in water. This distribution may be taken from a measurement or it could be computed by the Monte Carlo method. The input is placed into a look-up table. The proton beam is divided into a number of parallel and very thin (in general the width of one CT pixel) proton rays. While progressing through the inhomogeneous medium pixel by pixel, each individual ray is to suffer only energy losses, for scattering is neglected. That means, proton rays travel in a straight line and do not influence the dose deposited by a neighbouring ray. The water-equivalent depth of a ray is calculated using the integrated average electron density along the ray's direction. The dose at this point is then extracted from the look-up table. The final dose distribution is the sum of the doses deposited by each individual ray.

The electron density could be taken into account pixel by pixel; however, this would increasing the computing time considerably.

The influence of a beam limiting device (e.g. an aperture) can be taken into account as follows: The edge is assumed to coincide with the 50% isodose line. The dose gradient to both sides of the appropriate ray is assumed to be a Gaussian distribution, its standard deviation is a free parameter, e.g. 2 mm.

Ray tracing yields dose distributions of reasonable accuracy as long as only simple inhomogeneities are encountered by the tracing rays. Its main disadvantages are:

a. It cannot indicate hot and cold spots in the dose distribution.
b. The inevitable widening of the beam and of the beam's penumbra while penetrating through the medium are not represented.
c. Ray tracing does not predict the change in the distal dose fall-off caused by multiple inhomogeneities encountered.

E.2.2c
Pencil Beam

The concept of the pencil beam was originally developed for X-ray planning, then applied to charged particle radiation (electrons) by Hogstrom et al. 1981 and finally refined for proton radiotherapy planning by Petti (1992). Hong et al. 1996 rounded off the pencil beam algorithm by including the modifying influences of finite source size, effective source – target distance and the effects of all beam shaping devices positioned between source and patient surface.

The extension of the proton pencil beam algorithm to heavier charged particles is straightforward.

It is justified to employ the pencil beam algorithm to calculate the dose deposited by a wide proton beam, because: (a) The resulting dose distribution is almost as accurate as that calculated by the Monte Carlo algorithm; (b) the required computation time is reduced by about three orders of magnitude.

The pencil beam algorithm is significantly more accurate than the ray-tracing algorithm.

A **pencil beam** enters the medium as an infinitesimal narrow particle beam. Its energy may be spread out into a narrow spectrum. While penetrating the pencil beam spreads laterally. For planning purposes a wide beam is approximated by a set of parallel pencil beams.

A **differential pencil beam** is the differential dose distribution deposited by a scattered pencil beam. The entire dose deposited by a pencil beam can be calculated using a Monte Carlo algorithm (e.g. Petti (1992), Carlsson et al. 1997, Deasy (1998)) or can be analytically modelled (Hong et al. 1996, Carlsson et al. 1997).

The dose deposited by a wide beam is the integral over all its differential pencil beams.

The optimal separation between pencil beams is 1.2 times the rms radius of the pencil beam. This ensures a 1% dose uniformity over the entire wide beam, Brahme (1982).

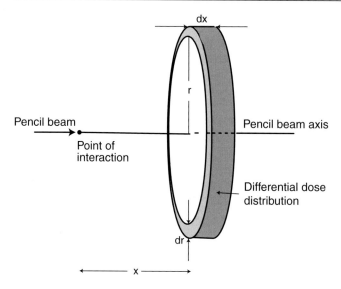

Fig. E2.2. Differential pencil beam dose distribution deposited in annual rings at distances x from a point of interaction. Homogeneous medium. Typical bin widths: $dr = 0.5$ mm, $dx = 2.5$ mm.

The computational effort is significantly reduced by the small scattering angles involved. Inhomogeneities in the beam path are taken into account by employing an effective particle range, which results from averaging the densities encountered over the entire pathlength of the pencil beam.

In general (see e.g. Hong et al. 1996) the dose D at the point of interest P (x,y,z) is a combination of two terms: (a) a central-axis term which is the depth-dose distribution at P measured along the central-axis in water, sometimes taking into account the changing effective distance from the source; (b) an off-axis term which is calculated from a Gaussian distribution. This Gaussian has a width determined by contributions due to finite source size, beam modifying devices and effective penetration depth.

$$D(x, y, z) = \int_0^{y_{max}} \int_0^{z_{max}} \Phi_o(y, z) C(x) O(x, y, z) dx dy dz \qquad (E2.1)$$

where

D : dose at point of interest P having the Cartesian coordinates x,y,z
$\Phi_0(y,z)$: proton intensity profile across the proton beam which enters the beam delivery system
$C(x)$: measured central-axis depth dose distribution
$O(x,y,z)$: off-axis dose distribution
y_{max}, z_{max} : maximum values for y, z.

A typical computation time (DEC 5000/240 work-station) for a 2500 data point dose distribution in a plane orthogonal to the beam axis is about 6 min (Hong et al. 1996).

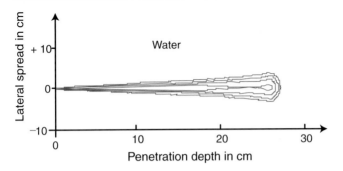

Fig. E2.3. 200 Mev pencil beam dose distribution in water calculated by a Monte Carlo algorithm. Iso-doses lines for 100%, 75%, 50% and 25%. From Carlsson et al. 1997, modified.

E.2.2d
Broad Beam

Although pencil beam algorithms are significantly faster than Monte Carlo algorithms, they are still not fast enough to use for the an initial design of the irradiation plan. For this purpose some special and very fast algorithms exist to calculate the dose distributions of broad proton beams. In many instances those algorithms are sufficiently accurate to be utilised for the final irradiation plan.

V-TREAT broad beam, Hong et al. 1996. The authors simplified their pencil beam algorithm by considering only the multiple scattering contributions from the most narrow of all beam-limiting devices in the beam line. Alternatively, the authors lump together the influences of all beam-limiting devices.

This broad beam algorithm reduces the computation time for a 2D dose distribution to about 2% of that of a pencil beam algorithm. In general, the dose distributions calculated by either algorithm agree to within 2%. Note, however, that the V-Treat broad beam algorithm becomes very inaccurate for beam diameters $\leq$ 20 mm .

PROTEUS algorithm, Breuer (1994). Inputs to this algorithm are the measured 3D dose distributions in water of a number of standard proton beams. The actual size of the broad beam employed is interpolated from those data. The algorithm combines ray-tracing and pencil beam approach to compute a 3D absorbed radiation dose distribution for a given broad beam of a given arbitrary cross sectional shape. Inhomogeneities are taken into account voxel by voxel. The computing time for a 3D dose distribution is about 1 s (PC-586, 90 MHz, 20 × 80 × 80 CT input data points).

MARSDEN algorithm, Lee et al. 1993. Input to this algorithm is a synthesised Bragg distribution based an a measured mean range and its standard deviation for a mono-energetic proton beam in water. The algorithm separates a broad beam into a number of parallel, narrow and monoenergetic elemental beams. The contributions to the penumbra resulting from the finite source size, the distances between source, collimator and patient are neglected. The lateral spread of the employed elemental beam is calculated assuming a Gaussian distribution. Inhomogeneities are taken into account by averaging the voxel densities over the entire path length of each elemental beam. The algorithm is not applicable to beam diameters $\leq$ 30 mm.

E.2.3
Planning for Eye Treatment

Proton irradiation is a preferred method to treat e.g. uveal melanoma in the back of the eye. This is due to the favourable relation between entrance dose and target dose, and to the steep distal dose fall-off.

E.2.3a
Input

65 MeV protons have a sufficient range (36 mm) to reach any target inside the eye.

It is not feasible to achieve this energy by employing an energy degrader to a, e.g. 200 MeV proton beam. The original range straggling would remain constant, i.e. the distal dose would drop from 80% to 20% within about 6 mm. For comparison: the distal dose fall-off of the beam leaving a 65 MeV proton accelerator is less than 2 mm.

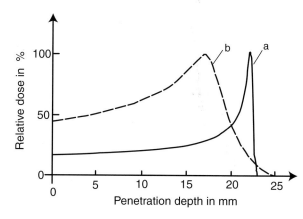

Fig. E2.4. Depth dose distributions in water observed for two different 50 MeV proton beams. (a) Protons from an accelerator having a maximum energy of 50 MeV. (b) 50 MeV protons from a 200 MeV accelerator after passing the original beam through an energy degrader. Adopted from Carlsson et al. 1997.

In general, proton beams with a maximum diameter of 20 mm and a SOBP plateau length of up to 10 mm are sufficient to fully cover the principal targets.

The physical dimensions of the individual eye and the positions of structures inside the globe are measured by optical methods or determined from images produced by ultrasound, high-definition CT or MRI. The density of the entire eye is assumed to be uniform and about (1.0 to 1.05) g/cm^3.

To facilitate treatment, the target outline is indicated by small Ta-clips sutured to the choroid. During irradiation the eye's axis is kept in position by looking at a suitably placed light emitting diode.

E.2.3b
Algorithms

Irradiation planning algorithms reconstruct the geometry of the individual eye from measured data: length of optic axis, bulbus width, anterior and posterior position of the lens, etc. The input dose distributions (Bragg curves or SOBPs) are based on measurements in water. In general, a uniform density along the beam path is assumed. Note that a density difference of only 2% will change the proton range by about 0.5 mm.

An eyelid in the beam path presents special problems, see Iborra-Brassart et al. 1999. In addition, the planning algorithm should take into account the RBE changes with depth and absorbed dose, see Paganetti (1998).

EYEPLAN, developed by Goitein and Miller 1983, was the first eye treatment planning algorithm. It is applicable only to targets in the posterior chamber. It presents the eye as a sphere, modelling the cornea as an add-on spherical segment. The eye's density is assumed to be 1.05 g/cm^3. The positions of macula and optic nerve are pre-determined and cannot be changed. The eye lid is modelled as a plate oriented orthogonal to the beam direction. The dose distribution is calculated by ray tracing, consequently the widening of the penumbra inside the eye is neglected.

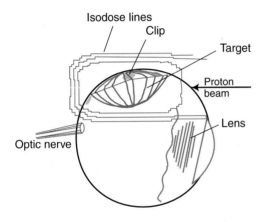

Fig. E2.5. Irradiation plan computed by EYEPLAN. SOBP, 20 mm beam diameter. A wax bolus compensates for the influence of the eye's curvature. The positions of the 3 Ta-clips are indicated. Adopted from Egger (1993).

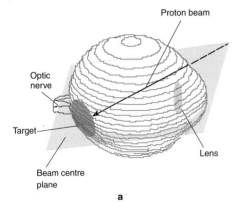

a

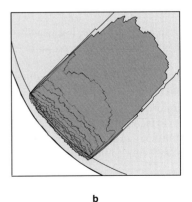

b

Fig. E2.6. i-PROTEUS. **(a)** Reconstructed eye, including target, lens, optic nerve and incident proton beam direction. **(b)** Computed isodose lines for a 54.3 MeV proton beam. The plane of the isodose lines is indicated in **(a)**. A DISD is in position.

OPTIS (Sheen 1994) is an improved version of EYEPLAN, modelling the eye as an ovoid. The eye lids are presented as adjustable spherical shells. The algorithm allows for the placement of a wedge in order to shape some parts of the distal dose distribution.

i-PROTEUS (SSI 1995) presents a modified broad beam approach, using as input the measured depth dose distribution of a 20 mm diameter proton beam. CT or MRI images of the patient's eye are utilised. If images are unavailable, the eye is reconstructed in 3D from optical measurements. The different densities of the various components (lid, lens, vitreous body, etc.) are taken into account. The algorithm can handle more than one incident proton beam and targets of any size at any position. A 3D DISD is automatically designed. See figure E2.6.

E.2.4
Comparison of Treatment Planning Algorithms

E.2.4a
Intercomparison of Different Planning Algorithms

Actual treatment plans cannot be well compared with experiments. The only available yardsticks are treatment plans employing the Monte Carlo algorithm.

This is an inconvenient standard due to the long computation times needed. It already takes many hours to compute the dose distribution generated by a single proton beam. The computation time for a complex treatment plan involving multiple beams is measured in days.

Petti et all 1996 present an enlightening comparison of the irradiation plans calculated using Monte Carlo, pencil beam and ray tracing algorithms, see figure E2.7. The pencil beam algorithm well predicts the widening of the penumbra, the ray tracing algorithm cannot. The distal dose gradient appears much too steep in the ray tracing dose distribution. The most serious discrepancy, however, is the failure of the ray tracing method to indicate the presence of the two 'hot spots' caused by the inhomogeneities present in the proton beam's path. The position and the extent of those dose extremes are well indicated by the pencil beam algorithm.

Experience shows, see Petti (1996), that if more than three proton beams are employed in the same irradiation plan, the results for pencil beam and ray tracing algorithms agree well. In those cases the superior computing speed of the ray tracing algorithm appears to be advantageous.

E.2.4b
Comparison with Simplified Measurements

The results of the various planning algorithms can be compared with experiments performed in a water phantom. Such a phantom must include structures having densities in the range 0 g/cm^3 $< \rho_e < 2$ g/cm^3. The strengths and weaknesses of the algorithms are best determined in circumstances presenting steep density gradients.

It is the development of the penumbra of a proton beam penetrating water that is most easily compared.

Ray tracing. This algorithm cannot compute the widening of the penumbra with penetration depth.

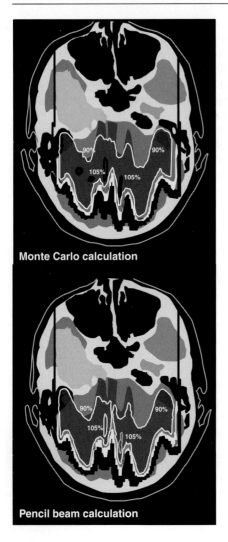

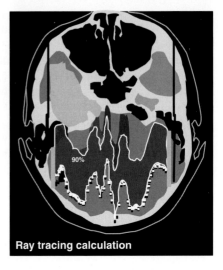

Fig. E2.7. Computed dose distributions. Proton beam: Anterior, 150 MeV, 10 cm diameter, SOBP 4 cm, no DISD. Algorithms: Monte Carlo, Pencil beam, Ray-tracing. Simplified after Petti et al. 1996.

The severe limitations of this method should disqualify it from any applications. This is not necessarily so: If all the uncertainties inherent to charged particle radiotherapy are taken into account, the results achieved by ray tracing of multiple-beam arrangements do remain inside the overall achievable accuracy. In addition, its extremely short computation times allow the planner to find the optimum beam configuration (number of beams, diameters, entrance angles, etc.) within a time interval that the other algorithms need for the design of just one or two simple irradiation plans.

Pencil beam. The pencil beam algorithm developed by Hong et al. 1996 yields optimal results, because it includes the unavoidable influence of all the beam line elements on the dose distribution.

The approach presented by Petti (1992) applies the pencil beam algorithm only after the proton beam has entered the patient.

Measurements by Hong et al. 1996 using an unrestricted proton beam indicate excellent agreement within the experimental uncertainties. Investigating laterally und longitudinally shaped proton beams the authors find, that the calculated penumbras are wider than those measured.

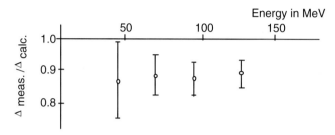

Fig. E2.8. The ratio of measured ($\Delta_{meas.}$) and calculate ($\Delta_{calc.}$) proton beam penumbra widths in water for some proton beam energies. Energy degrader and DISD are employed. The results for pencil beam and broad beam calculations concur. The error margins of the measurements are indicated. Extracted from Hong et al. 1996.

Broad beam. Only Hong et al. 1996 have presented a systematic comparison between measured and computed penumbras. The authors cannot find any significant differences between the results from pencil beam and broad beam algorithms. It is interesting to note, that the computation times for the broad beam algorithm (V-TREAT) are significantly lower.

E.2.5
Summary

Although X-rays and protons (and other charged particles) act on the tissues via secondary electrons, both modalities require entirely different methods to develop an irradiation plan. In first approximation X-ray planning considers merely the exponential attenuation of the radiation while penetrating the patient. Proton irradiation planning must take into account at least the following: (a) density changes along the beam path, (b) small target movements during and between treatments, (c) elastic (and possibly inelastic) scattering of the beam particles, (d) the influence of the edges of beam limiting devices.

Because the only advantage and justification of proton radiotherapy is its ability to deliver a desirable radiation dose distribution precisely, all the dose distribution modifying factors must be taken into account. The calculations must be carried out in all three spatial dimensions.

The earliest treatment plans applied unchanged single beam dose distributions previously measured in a water tank. Crossed beam plans overlaid the dose distributions of two or more particle beams. Although in this case the Bragg peak is not utilised, the resulting dose distributions display an entrance dose below the target dose.

Those rather simple planning methods were replaced by **ray tracing algorithms,** made possible by the introduction of a high resolution imaging method, CT. The broad particle beam is subdivided into many narrow and parallel rays. The range of each ray penetrating into the patient's body is calculated individually. Only ionisation energy losses are taken into account, scattering is neglected. The resulting dose distribution displays an unchanged beam penumbra and its lateral and distal dose fall-off is unrealistically steep. In addition, locally enhanced or decreased radiation dose regions remain hidden. Ray tracing is still widely used in planning for eye treatment.

High speed computers allow implementation of a **Monte Carlo algorithm** in order to compute the dose distribution for a given beam configuration. In this case the fate of, and the dose deposited by, individual particles is tracked while they advance into the body. Energy loss and scattering is taken into account. Summing over (at least) a million particle histories yields a dose distribution with an accuracy of about 1%. Employing very fast computer work-stations and optimised algorithms, the time needed to compute the dose distribution of one broad proton beam is many hours. Consequently, the Monte Carlo method is unsuitable – at least for the time being – for routine radiotherapy planning.

The dose distribution calculated for a **pencil beam** takes into account the contributions due to energy loss, multiple scattering and (possibly) inelastic scattering caused by nuclear interactions. This method may be extended to include the influence on the final dose distribution of individual beam line elements (scatterers, beam limiting and beam shaping devices, etc.). Theoretically, this eliminates the need to use as input data the measured cross sections or depth dose distributions of the particle beam employed.

Applied to a three-dimensional density grid – determined from a set of CT slices – and integrated, the various pencil beam algorithms yield dose distributions in adequate agreement with those calculated by the Monte Carlo method. The computation time for one particle beam decreases to a few minutes. In general, this time is still too long to design an optimal dose distribution plan for day to day routine application.

Broad beam algorithms are simplified versions of pencil beam algorithms, summing over the dose distributions computed for a number of narrow sub-beams. Introducing measured proton radiation intensity profiles, limiting the influence of beam line elements and employing look-up tables, the dose distributions calculated by broad beam algorithms deviate only a few percent from detailed pencil beam (and Monte Carlo) calculations. However, the width of the penumbra is mostly underestimated. The computation times are reduced to about a few seconds, making broad beam algorithms suitable for routine radiotherapy planning.

Particle radiotherapy can be analysed as a system. Each element of this system contributes to its overall accuracy. From this point of view, the need for very sophisticated radiotherapy planning algorithms appears doubtful: The isodose lines computed by the various algorithms all agree within the overall accuracy (see the following section).

E. 3
Overall Accuracy of Treatment Planning and Execution

E.3.1
General Considerations

High accuracy in proton radiotherapy planning is of utmost importance, as are accurate and precise execution of the treatment plan. To achieve this, each step in the long chain from planning to actual radiation treatment must be carefully analysed with respect to avoidable and unavoidable uncertainties.

Uncertainty is not related to error. Errors are avoidable in principle, uncertainties are unavoidable but may be reduced in size by studying their nature and occurrence.

An analysis is also required to avoid excessive attention to one or more steps leading to uneven strengths of the individual links in the entire chain. Unfortunately, there is no general agreement regarding the definitions of accuracy and precision. For the following considerations accuracy and precision are adapted from the definitions of Rayner (1967) – as follows:

Accuracy is a measure of the agreement between the actual (measured and/or calculated) value of the quantity of interest and its true value. Since the term 'accuracy' is here applied to radiotherapy planning, 'true value' is the value aimed for, e.g. the position of the 90% isodose contour line.

Precision or **reproducibility** is a measure of how well repeated measurements of the same quantity agree with one another.

Accuracy and precision are expressed in units appropriate to the situation, e.g. in mm or in %.

Overall accuracy combines both accuracy and precision.

In the following considerations accuracy, precision and overall accuracy refer to the spatial position of a (given) isodose line; in general 50% or 90% isodose lines are considered.

E.3.2
Factors Influencing Accuracy and Precision

E.3.2a
Accuracy

a. The **spatial resolution** in the plane of the CT slice used to determine the target's location is limited. Under the best of circumstances it is 0.4 mm to 1.0 mm (Urie 1995). Reducing the CT slice thickness improves the resolution but the noise level increases and consequently pixel density differences are less accentuated. The optimum spatial resolution orthogonal to the plane of the CT slice, is 2 mm to 3 mm for head images and 3 mm to 5 mm for body images (Urie 1995). This is a random uncertainty.

b. The **density of structures** is determined by converting the Hounsfield numbers of the appropriate CT pixels. According to Schneider at al 1996, the accuracy for the conversion is about 2% to 3%.

Taking into account CT images produced by X-ray tubes of different energy and considering the change of CT numbers with penetration depth, the above quoted accuracy could be exaggerated. An uncertain density value causes a corresponding uncertainty in the calculated proton range and in the shape of the distal dose fall-off. This is a random uncertainty.

Example: A 200 MeV proton beam penetrates a body region which includes a 2 cm length of bone. An uncertainty of 2% to 3% of the measured bone density causes an uncertainty of 0.6 mm to 1 mm in the calculated proton range.

c. The **position of a significant density change** (e.g. bone-soft tissue transition) encountered by a proton beam inside the body is not taken into account by most planning systems (except by PROTEUS). An average density over the entire path length is deemed sufficient. This is sometimes not justified.

Example: A 200 MeV proton beam encounters a 2-cm-long bone either at the entrance or toward the end of its path. The proton range computed by using an average density value differs by 1% from a range calculated by taking into account the density pixel by pixel.

This is a systematic error and could be avoided.

d. The **proton energy-range relations** tabulated by different authors (Janni 1982, ICRU 1993) vary by almost 1%. Consequently the uncertainty of the calculated range of 200 MeV protons is $\geq$ 2 mm. However, this uncertainty may be neglected in practice, if the relations between the energy settings at the accelerator and the resulting proton ranges in water are experimentally determined. A few percent deviation between the calibrated energy settings and the actual proton energy may be neglected for planning purposes.

e. The accuracy of the **dose calibration** of a proton dose meter is on average 4.3% (Vynckier 1995) or – under the best of circumstances – about 3% (Palmans et al. 1996). Taking into account the clinical environment an overall dose accuracy of – at best – 5% seems to be reasonable. A typical slope of the distal dose fall-off for a 200 MeV proton beam is about 15%/mm and about 4%/mm for the lateral fall-off, NAC (1993). That means any dose measurement achieves a positional accuracy for the distal 50% isodose contour of about 0.3 mm and about 1.2 mm for the lateral 50% isodose contour. This is a random uncertainty.

f. The **RBE** value used in proton radiotherapy planning is taken as either 1.0 or 1.1. This 5% uncertainty (1.05 ± 0.05) in the biological radiation dose causes an uncertainty of about 0.3 mm in the position of any distal isodose line. The corresponding lateral uncertainty is about 1.2 mm. This is (at present) a random uncertainty.

g. The **RBE is a function of proton energy.** Consequently, the RBE values change with penetration depth, a factor rarely taken into account. According to Paganetti et al. 1997, the RBE increases from 1.1 at the Bragg peak (or the SOBP plateau) to 1.9 toward the distal dose fall-off. Assuming a distal slope value of 15%/mm, the RBE increase will shift the 90% isodose contour by 0.15 mm (0.6 mm for the 50% isodose). This is an error and could be avoided.

h. **Transfer of the target coordinates** from the CT slice coordinate system to the treatment system frame of reference. According to Murphy (1997) this manipulation introduces an uncertainty of 0.1 mm to 1 mm per translational axis and 0.6° to 1.3° per rotational axis. This accuracy is achieved for positioning of the head, consequently it is a lower limit. It is a random uncertainty.

Murphy (1997) assumed that the diagnostic and the treatment postures coincide. If this is not the case, the uncertainty due transfer of the target coordinates will be larger.

i. **Positioning** for treatment. Webb (1993) estimates, that under optimal circumstances the positioning of a patient introduces positional uncertainties of 0.6 mm to 0.9 mm. Hanley et al. 1997 measured the same quantity as 1.7 mm to 2.0 mm. This is a random uncertainty.

k. **Target motion.** Motion caused by respiration, gravity, positional and vascular pulsation, etc. is practically unavoidable. Depending on treatment site the resulting uncertainty is about 1 mm to 4 mm for intracranial structures (Serago et al. 1992, Breuer and Wynchank 1995), 10 mm to 30 mm for liver and kidney (Okumura et al. 1995). This uncertainty can be cut down if the beam intensity at the treatment site is significantly reduced at the appropriate moments. E.g. the beam intensity could be controlled by signals triggered from the cardiac and/or the respiratory cycles, Inada et al. 1992. This is a random uncertainty.

E.3.2b
Precision

a. **Time dependence of the dosimeter.** The dosimeter response will change over the period of a radiotherapy treatment course. If the dosimeter is re-calibrated daily, a reproducibility of better than 2% over a two week period is achievable. The resulting precision for the position of the 50% isodose contour is ≤ 0.1 mm. This is a negligible contribution to the overall accuracy.

b. The **position of the patient** fixed by the positioning system, will change between treatment sessions. Hanley et al. 1997 measured in 20% of their patients a change of about 2 mm to 7 mm in the set-up positions. This indicates a value for the average reproducibility of the same order as the uncertainty of positioning, i.e. about 2 mm. If anatomical or other fixed landmarks are used to reposition the patient before each treatment session, this discrepancy becomes negligible.

c. Little is known about **internal target drift** over a time span of several weeks. A reasonable assumption is that this drift is small compared with short term target movements.

Conclusion: The uncertainty due to the precision of the entire treatment system is small compared with other uncertainties.

E.3.2c
Other Factors

Additional factors will influence accuracy and precision of proton radiotherapy: The exact shape of the same Bragg distribution differs between measurements carried out with diodes and with ionization chambers. The values of standard particle dose distributions depend to some degree an the type of the employed dosimeter, edge scattering at beam-limiting devices is not fully understood, etc.

E.3.3
Overall Accuracy

E.3.3a
General

The overall accuracy of the radiation dose delivered by a proton radiotherapy system depends on accuracy and precision achievable by its individual components. Because the various quantities are in general independent of each other, standard error analysis applies.

Accepting the values presented above for the uncertainties and employing quadratic addition, the resulting overall accuracy for the distal position of the 90% isodose line is $\pm$ 3% – under the best of circumstances. The system's overall accuracy reaches $\pm$ 5 mm if the upper limits of the analysed quantities are considered.

Most likely the average overall positional accuracy of the distal 90% isodose line for a 200 MeV proton beam is $\pm$ 4.4 mm or about 2%.

If very high resolution CT images are available, the appropriate average overall accuracy will change to about $\pm$ 3.6 mm.

Since the above considerations are almost independent of the initial proton energy, the overall accuracy for a 100 MeV proton isodose line remains approximately $\pm$ 4.4 mm, equivalent of 5.6% of the range of the proton beam.

Although the overall accuracy is conservatively evaluated here, the presented results should cause concern within the proton radiotherapy community. The estimated values jeopardise the main advantage of proton radiotherapy: positional accuracy.

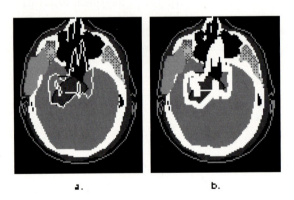

a.   **b.**

Fig. E3. The overall accuracy for the 90% and the 105% isodose lines of a 150 MeV proton beam inside the head. **a.** Standard presentation. **b.** Overall positional accuracy of $\pm$ 4.4 mm indicated by the width of the isodose lines.

E.3.3b
Overall Accuracy of Eye Treatment

The factors influencing the positional overall accuracy of proton radiotherapy of the eye are in general the same as those listed above. The actual values differ, in particular: **(a)** the dimensions of the eye are optically measured with a (claimed) accuracy of 0.1 mm; **(b)** the density of the interior of the eye is assumed to be uniformly 1.00 g/cm^3

or 1.05 g/cm^3. However, the density of the interior of the eye increases with age (see Francois 1959) and should be assigned the value 1.05 ± 0.03 g/cm^3. (c) The range-energy relation is extracted from tables, introducing an uncertainty of about 1%, i.e. 0.25 mm; (d) the uncertainty in the target positioning for treatment can be assumed as 0.2 mm.

Summary: The overall positional accuracy achievable for proton radiotherapy of the eye is about ± 1 mm, i.e. 4%. This value excludes any uncertainties introduced by the treatment planning systems employed.

References for Part I

Ahmad NR, Huq MS, Corn BW (1997) Respiration-induced motion of the kidneys in whole abdominal radiography: implications for treatment planning and late toxicity. Radiother Oncol (Ireland) 42:87-90

Alexander E, Kooy HM, van Herk M, Schwartz M, Barnes PD, Tarbell N, Mulkern RV, Holupka EJ, Loeffler JS (1995) Magnetic resonance image-directed stereotactic neurosugery: use of image fusion with computerized tomography to enhance spatial accuracy. J Neurosurg 83:271-276

Alonso JR (1995) Design Criteria for Medical Accelerators. In: Linz U (ed) Ion Beams in Tumor Therapy. Chapman and Hall, Weinheim, pp 171-180

Atomic and Nuclear Properties of Materials (1986) PhysLett 170B:38

Berger MJ (1993) Penetration of proton beams through water I. Depth-dose distribution, spectra and LET distribution. NISTIR Report 5226, Gaithersburg, USA.

Bethe HA (1930) Zur Theorie des Durchgangs schneller Korpuskularstrahlen durch Materie. Ann Phys 5:325-340

Bethe HA (1953) Molière's theory of multiple scattering. PhysRev 89:1256-1266

Bloch F (1933) Zur Bremsung rasch bewegter Teilchen beim Durchgang durch Materie. Ann Phys 16:285-320

Blosser HG (1989) Compact superconducting synchrocyclotron system for proton therapy. Nucl Instr Methods Phys Res B40/41:1326-1330

Bortfeld T (1997) An analytical approximation of the Bragg curve for therapeutic proton beams. Med Phys 24:2024-2033

Bortfeld T, Schlegel W (1996) An analytical approximation of depth-dose distributions for therapeutic proton beams. Phys Med Biol 41:1331-1339

Brahme A (1982) Physical and biological aspects in the optimum choice of radiation modality. Acta Radiol Oncol 21:469-479

Brahme A, KÑllman P, Tilikidis (1995) A development in the ion beam therapy planning and treatment organisation. In: Linz U (ed) Ion Beams in Tumor Therapy. Chapman and Hall, Weinheim, pp 290-299

Breuer H (1994) A complete proton radiotherapy planning system 50-250 MeV. XX.PTCOG, Chester

Breuer H, Wynchank S (1995) Quantitation of brain movement within the skull associated with head position: its relevance to proton therapy planning. XXIII PTCOG, Cape Town

Cambria R, Herault J, Brassart N, Silari H, Chauvel P (1997) Proton beam dosimetry: a comparison between the Faraday cup and an ionization chamber. Phys Med Biol 42:1185-1196

Carlsson AK, Andreo P, Brahme A (1997) Monte Carlo and analytical calculation of proton pencil beams for computerized treatment plan optimization. Phys Med Biol 42:1033-1053

Chu WT, Ludewigt BA, Renner TR (1993) Instrumentation for treatment of cancer using proton and light-ion beams. Rev Sci Instrum 64:2055-2122

Chu WT (1995) Radiation detectors. In: Linz U (ed) Ion beams in tumor therapy. Chapman and Hall, Weinheim, pp 234-245

Chu WT (1999) Biological effects due to high dose rates. PTCOG Beam Scanning Workshop, Cape Town, South Africa

Constable IJ, Goitein M, Koehler AM, Schmidt RA (1976) Small field irradiation of monkey eyes with protons and photons. Rad Res 65:304-314

Coutrakon G, Cortese J, Ghebremedhin A, Hubbard J, Johanning J, Koss P, Maudsley G, Slater CR, Zuccarelli C (1997) Microdosimetry spectra of the Loma Linda proton beam and relative biological effectiveness comparisons. Med Phys 24:1499-1506

Deasy JO (1998) A proton dose calculation algorithm for conformal therapy simulations based on Molier's theory of lateral deflections. Med Phys 25:476-483

Egger E (1993) Therapieplanung fÅr Augenbestrahlungen mit Protonen. PSI-Proceedings, Villingen, pp 105-109.

Fano U (1954) Inelastic collisions and the Molière Theory of Multiple Scattering. Phys Rev 93:117-120

Fowler JF (1981) Nuclear particles in cancer treatment. Hilger, Bristol

Franceis J (1959) Les cataractes congenitales. Bull Soc Fr Ophtal

Geller R, Golovanivsky KS, Michaut C, Bacal M, Buzzi J-M, Laugier A, Schwartz LH (1996) ECRIPAC for Protontherapy. Private communication

Goitein M (1978) A technique for calculating the influence of thin inhomogeneities on charged particle beams. Med Phys 5:258-264

Goitein M, Sisterson J (1978) The influence of thick inhomogeneities on charged particle beams. Rad Res 74:217-230

Goitein M, Miller T (1983) Planning proton therapy of the eye. Med Phys 10:275-283

Gottschalk B, Wagner MS (1989) Contoured scatterer for proton dose flattening. Harvard Cyclotron Laboratory Report (March)

Gottschalk B, Koehler AM, Schneider RJ, Sisterson, Wagner MS (1993) Multiple Coulomb scattering of 160 MeV protons. Nucl Instr Meth Phys Res B74:467-490

Grusell E, Isacsson U, Montelius A, Medin J (1995) Faraday cup dosimetry in a proton therapy beam without collimation. Phys Med Biol 40:1831-1840

Hanley J, Lumley MA, Mageras GS, Sun J, Zelefsky MJ, Leibel SA, Fuks Z, Kutcher GJ (1997) Measurement of patient positioning errors in three-dimensional conformal radiotherapy of the prostate. Int J Radiat Oncol Biol Phys 37:435-444

Highland VL (1975) Some practical remarks on multiple scattering. Nucl Instr Meth 129:497-499

Highland VL (1979) Erratum. Nucl Instr Methods 161:171

Hiraoka T, Kawashima K, Hoshino K, Bichsel H (1994) Energy loss of 70 MeV protons in tissue-substitute materials. Phys Med Biol 39:983-991

Hogstrom KR, Mills MD, Almond PR (1981) Electron beam dose calculations. Phys Med Biol 26:445-459

Hong L, Goitein M, Bucciolini M, Comiskey R, Gottschalk B, Rosenthal S, Serago C, Urie M (1996) A pencil beam algorithm for proton dose calculations. Phys Med Biol 41:1305-1330

Iborra-Brassart N, Herault J, Bondian PY, Courdi A, Chauvell P (1999) Treatment planning for eye tumors: problems encountered. XXX PTCOG Meeting, Cape Town, South Africa

ICRU (1993) Stopping power and ranges for proton and alpha particles. Report 49, Bethesda

ICRU (1998) Clinical proton dosimetry Part I: Beam production, beam delivery and measurement of absorbed dose. Report 59, Bethesda, USA

Inada T, Tsuji H, Hayakawa Y, Maruhashi A, Tsujii H (1992) Proton irradiation synchronized with respiratory cycle. Nippon Igaku Hoshasen Gakhai Zasski (Japan) 52:1161-1167 (Index Medicus 93027071)

Janni JF (1982) Proton range-energy tables, 1 keV–10 GeV. Atomic Data and Nuclear Data Tables 27:147-339

Karlsson U, Kirby T, Orrison W, Lionberger M (1995) Ocular globe topology in radiotherapy 33:705-712

Koehler AM, Schneider RJ, Sisterson JM (1977) Flattening of proton dose distributions for large field radiotherapy. Med Phys 4:297-301

Kortmann RD, Hess CF, Meisner C, Schmidberger H, Bamberg M (1996) Accuracy of field alignment in abdominal radiation therapy. Int J Radiat Oncol Biol Phys 35:779-783

Larsson B, Leksell R, Rexed B, Sourander P (1959) Effect of high energy protons on the spinal cord. Acta Radiol 51:52-64

Lau HY, Kagawa K, Lee WR, Hunt MA, Shaer AH, Hanks GE (1996) Short communication: CT-MRI image fusion for 3D conformal prostate radiotherapy: use in patients with altered pelvic anatomy. Br J Radiol 69:1165-1170

Lawrence JH (1957) Proton irradiation of the pituitary. Cancer 10:795-798

Lee M, Nahum AE, Webb S (1993) An empirical method to build up a model of proton dose distribution for a radiotherapy treatment-planning package. Phys Med Biol 38:989-998

Moerland MA, Bergh AC van den, Bhagwandien R, Janssen WM, Bakher CJ, Lagendijk JJ, Battermann JJ (1994) The influence of respiration induced motion of the kidneys on the accuracy of radiotherapy planning, a magnetic resonance imaging study. Radiother Oncol (Ireland) 30:150-154

Molière G (1947) Theorie der Streuung schneller geladener Teilchen I. Z Naturforsch 2a:133-145

Molière G (1948) Theorie der Streuung schneller geladener Teilchen II. Z Naturforsch 3a:78-97

Murphy MJ (1997) An automatic six-degree-of-freedom image registration algorithm for image-guided frameless stereotactic radiosurgery. Med Phys 24:857-866

NAC (1993) National Accelerator Centre Annual Report, Faure, South Africa

Okumura T, Tsuji H, Tsuji H (1995) Compensation for target motion. In: Linz U (ed) Ion beams in tumor therapy. Chapman and Hall, Weinheim, pp 308-315

Pagnetti H (1998) Calculation of the spatial variation of relative biological effectiveness in a therapeutic proton field for eye treatment. Phys Med Biol 43:2147-2157

Paganetti H, Olko P, Kobu H, Becker R, Schmitz T, Waligorski MP, Filges D, Muller-Gartner HW (1997) Calculation of relative biological effectiveness for proton beams using biological weighting functions. Int J Radiat Oncol Biol Phys 37:719-729

Palmans H, Seuntjens J, Verhaegen F, Denis JM, Vynckier S, Thierens H (1996) Water calorimetry and ionization chamber dosimetry in an 85-MeV clinical proton beam. Med Phys 23:643-650

Pedroni E, Bacher R, Blattmann H, Böhringer T, Coray A, Lomax A, Lin S, Munkel G, Scheib S, Schneider U, Tourovsky A (1995) The 200-Mev proton therapy project at the Paul Scherrer Institute: conceptual design and practical realization. Med Phys 22:37-53

Petti PL (1992) Differential-pencil-beam dose calculations for charged particles. Med Phys 19:137-149

Petti PL (1996) Evaluation of a pencil-beam dose calculation technique for charged particle radiotherapy. Int J Rad Oncol Biol Phys 35:1049-1057

PSI (1995) Paul Scherrer Institut, Annual Report, Villingen

Rayner MA (1969) A first course in biometry for agriculture students. University of Natal Press, Pietermaritzburg

Sailer SL, Bourland JD, Rosenman JG, Sherouse GW, Chaney EL, Tepper JE (1990) 3D beams need 3D names. Int J Rad Oncol Biol Phys 19:797-798

Sandison GA, Lee CC, Lu X, Papiez LS (1997) Extension of a numerical algorithm to proton dose calculations. I.Comparisons with Monte Carlo simulations. Med Phys 24:841-849

Schneider U, Pedroni E (1994) Multiple Coulomb scattering and spatial resolution in proton radiography. Med Phys 21:1657-63

Schneider U, Pedroni E, Lomax A (1996) The calibration of CT Hounsfield units for radiotherapy treatment planning. Phys Med Biol 41:111-124

Schneider U, Schaffner B, Loman T, Pedroni E, Tourovsky A (1998) A technique for calculating range spectra of charged particle beams distal to thick inhomogeneities. Med Phys 26:457-463

Schreuder AN, Kiefer N, van der Merwe J, Muller A, Langen K, Symons JE (1999) The new energy degrading system for the NAC proton therapy beam. XXX PTCOG Meeting, Cape Town, South Africa

Scott WT (1963) The theory of small-angle multiple scattering of fast charged particles. Rev Mod Phys 35:231

Segrè E (1965) Nuclei and Particles. Benjamin, New York

Serago C, Okunieff P, Gall K, Fullerton B, Urie M, Rosenthal S (1992). XVII PTCOG meeting, Loma Linda

Sheen MA (1994) Review of EYEPLAN at Clatterbridge. XX. PTCOG metting, Chester

Siebers JV (1993) Shielding measurements for 230 MeV protons. Nucl Sci Eng 115:13-23

Siebers JV(1995a) Shielding and radioprotection. In: Linz U (ed) Ion beams in tumor therapy. Chapman and Hall, Weinheim pp 191-200

Siebers JV, Vatnitzky SM, Miller DW, Moyers MF (1995b) Deduction of the air W value in a therapeutic proton beam. Phys Med Biol 40:1339-1356

Sisterson JM, (1999). PARTICLES, Newsletter of PTCOG, No. 24 (July)

Sisterson JM, Urie MM, Koehler AM, Goitein M (1989) Distal penetration of proton beams: the effects of air gaps between compensating bolus and patient. Phys Med Biol 34:1309-1315

Slater JM, Miller DW, Archambeau JV (1988) Development of a hospital-based proton beam treatment center. Int J Rad Oncol Biol Phys 14:761-775

SSI (1995) i-Proteus manual. Stellenbosch Scientific Instruments, Stellenbosch, South Africa

Stroom JC, Koper PCM, Korevaaar GA, van Os M, Janssen M, de Boer HCJ, Levendag PC, Heijmen JM (1999) Internal organ motion in prostate cancer patients treated in prone and supine position. Radiother Oncol 51:237-248

Tobias CA, Van Dyke DC, Simpson ME, Anger HO, Huff RL, Koneff AA (1954) Irradiation of the pituitary of the rat with high energy deuterons. Am J Roentgenol Radiat Ther Nucl Med 72:1-21

Tsujii H, Tsujii H, Okumura T, Onara K, Koyama S, Matsuzaki Y (1995) Proton therapy of thoraco-abdominal tumours. In: Linz U (ed) Ion beams in tumor therapy. Chapman and Hall, Weinheim pp 127-132

Urie M, Goitein M, Holley WR, Chen GTY (1986) Degradation of the Bragg peak due to inhomogeneities. Phys Med Biol 31:1-15

Urie M, Sisterson JM, Koehler AM, Goitein M, Zoesman J (1986) Proton beam penumbra: effects of separation between patients and beam modifying devices. Med Phys 13:734-740

Urie M (1995) Treatment planning for proton beams. In: Linz U (ed) Ion beams in tumor therapy. Chapman and Hall, Weinheim pp 279-289

Vatnitzky S, Moyers M, Miller D, Abell G, Slater JM, Pedroni E, Coray A, Mazal A, Newhauser W, Jaekel O, Heese J, Fukumura A, Futami Y, Verhey L, Daftari I, Grusell E, Molokanov A, Bloch C (1999) Proton dosimetry intercomparison based on the ICRU report 59 protocol. Radiother Oncol 51:273-279

Vavilov PV (1957) Ionization energy losses of high-energy heavy particles. Sov Phys JETP 5:749-751

Vynckier S, Bonnett DE, Jones DTL (1991) Code of practice for clinical proton dosimetry. Radiother Oncol 20:53-63

Vynckier S, Bonnett DE, Jones DTL (1994) Supplement to the code of practice for clinical proton dosimetry. Radiother Oncol 32:174-179

Wambersie A, Battermann JJ (1995) Socio-economic aspects of ion beam therapy. In: Linz U (ed) Ion beams in tumor therapy. Chapman and Hall, Weinheim pp 24-32

Webb S (1993) The physics of three-dimensional radiation therapy. Institute of Physics Publishing, Bristol and Philadelphia

Wilson RR (1946) Radiological use of fast protons. Radiology 47:487-491

Wong JW, Sharpe MB, Jaffray DA, Kini VR, Robertson JM, Stromberg JS, Martinez AA (1999) The use of active breathing control (ABC) to reduce margin for breathing motion. In J Radiat Oncol Biol Phys 44: 911-919

Proton Therapy and Radiosurgery

F General Aspects of Proton Therapy

F.1
General Clinical Overview

F.1.1
A Brief Medical History

Proton therapy made good progress despite the relatively few proton therapy facilities that became available during the 44 years since the first patients were treated in 1954.

The history of the medical uses of proton beams from seven facilities up to 1980 with horizontal beams has been recorded by Raju (1980).

From 1980 to 1989, only three more facilities became available to bring the total to ten. From 1989 to 1998, six more facilities were added.

New plans for commencing proton therapy are also proposed by many other institutions in the world.

Up to 1990, all beams were horizontal. Isocentric gantries became available only with the establishment of the magnificent and dedicated facility at Loma Linda in 1990.

The latest major facility with isocentric gantries is the North Eastern Proton Therapy Centre in Boston, Massachusetts, USA, completed in 1998.

A very advanced isocentric system is under construction in Villigen at the Paul Scherrer Institute. This unit will use spot scanning, and is close to completion.

The five low energy beams (up to 100 MeV) are used mainly for uveal melanoma (Chiba, Clatterbridge, Nice, Louvain la Neuve and Davis).

The higher energy beams (100–250 MeV and more) are mostly horizontal beams suitable for radiosurgery for intracranial lesions and for the treatment of para-spinal lesions.

Horizontal beams have many drawbacks for large field proton radiotherapy, because imaging and planning is highly dependent on computerised tomography (CT), where the patient is imaged in a supine position. This position must be accurately reproducible on the treatment couch for fractionated proton therapy. The patient therefore cannot be rotated on the long axis of the body for more than a few degrees without major organ shifts with horizontal beam delivery. Only isocentric proton beam gantries offer an optimal solution to this problem. There are only three such facilities presently. For brief historical overviews of proton therapy see Raju (1980) Suit and Urie (1992), Miller (1995) and Mehta (1995).

F.1.1.1
Early Proton Therapy

Palliative therapy: protons were first used as palliative therapy for patients with cancer. At the Lawrence Berkeley Laboratories (LBL) the first "radiosurgery" was for pain relief, and from 1954–1957, doses of 150–200 Gy were used for pituitary gland irradiation to reduce the secretion of some hormones to suppress the growth of hormone dependent cancers such as carcinoma of the breast. Chemical hormone suppressers have since then obviated the need for this approach, and these huge doses are now seldom if ever, employed.

Curative Therapy was used since Harvard started Bragg peak pituitary irradiation in 1963, with doses from 60–150 Gy for acromegaly, 40–110 Gy for Cushing's disease and 20–80 Gy for Nelson's syndrome.

For AVMs, historical doses ranged from 10 Gy to 40 Gy, the lower doses were reserved for the larger lesions. Here also, doses in excess of 20 Gy are of questionable value.

The skin dose with early proton therapy could be kept to below 5 Gy with prescribed doses up to 40 Gy by using 3–4 fields.

To date the majority of patients have been treated with low energy protons (65–100 MeV) for uveal melanoma, with an estimated 3600 cases up to 1998. Chondromas, chordomas and chondrosarcomas near sensitive neural structures such as the brain stem and spinal cord were the other major pathologies treated successfully, but with energies in the region of 160 MeV

Intracranial lesions like AVMs have been treated with fair results with protons, however not as good as with helium ions or even photon systems. Some newer information may explain why not, and will be discussed in Chapters I and L.

World-wide, up to 1998 an estimated 20,000 patients in 18 institutions have been treated with protons with good results. Protons do not seem suitable for the very small and discrete lesions needed for functional radiosurgery, e.g. for Parkinson's disease.

F.1.1.2
Modern Proton Therapy

A major, advanced centre in the USA commenced therapy in 1990. This was Loma Linda, the first hospital-based proton therapy facility. This magnificent facility has two horizontal beams, one for eye therapy and a second for head and neck therapy as well as 3 isocentric gantries, which can deliver 250 MeV protons from any direction like a modern linear accelerator can. This made fractionated therapy for malignant conditions at a variety of body sites possible. Treatments of patients with head and neck tumours started in March 1991, and by summer 1991, in other body sites (Slater *et al.* 1992).

A new proton therapy centre with isocentric gantries has opened in Boston Massachusetts. This is the North Eastern Proton Therapy Centre (NEPTC). Construction of this facility started in September 1995 and was completed in 1998.

Work is under way on the advanced isocentric system with spot scanning facilities at the Paul Scherrer Institute in Villigen, Switzerland.

The National Accelerator Centre in South Africa started proton therapy in 1993 with a single horizontal scattered beam of 200 MeV. A second beam line with a beam 30^0 off the vertical with spot scanning plus a scattered horizontal beam, is under construction. A special feature is the stereophotogrammetric system of immobilisation (Jones *et al.* 1995), described in Appendix P.7.

Isocentric proton therapy is still in its infancy and international co-operative comparative clinical trials can only now be undertaken *versus* isocentric photon facilities.

Table F1.1 Chronology and beam energy of proton therapy centres globally	**Institute**	**Date**	**Energy (MeV)**
	Lawrence Berkeley Laboratories (USA)	1954–1957	340
	Svedberg Laboratory Uppsala (Sweden)	1957–1973	185
	MGH/Harvard (Boston, USA)	1963	160
	Dubna	1968	200
	Moscow	1969	70–200
	Gachina	1975	1000
	Chiba (Japan) NIRS	1979	70
	Tsukuba (Japan) PRMS	1983	250
	Villigen, PSI (Switzerland)	1984	72, 200
	Clatterbridge (England)	1989	63
	Loma Linda (California)	1990	70–250
	Louvain (Belgium)	1991	85
	Nice (France)	1991	63
	Orsay (France)	1991	73, 200
	NAC (South Africa)	1993	200
	UCLA (Davis, California)	1994	65
	North Eastern Proton Therapy Centre, Massachusetts	1998	70–250

Table F1.1 shows the institutional chronology and beam energy of present facilities.

F.1.2
History of Non-proton Radiosurgery

Particle therapy initiated the basic concept of a high dose of radiation with rapid fall-off in dose, directed precisely to a small lesion volume (radiosurgery) as outlined above.

Frustration with the available time on research cyclotrons stimulated Leksell to build the confocal 201 ^{60}Co source Gamma Knife for radiosurgery in 1968. (For a vivid description of the relevant history, read Mehta 1995).

Modern linear accelerators have been adapted since the 1980's for radiosurgical work by Betti and Derichinski (1983) in Buenos Aires, Colombo *et al.* (1985) in Vicenza, Hartman *et al.* (1985) in Heidelberg and Podgorsak *et al.* (1987) in Canada.

Barcia-Salorio (1977) converted a conventional [60]Cobalt unit for radiosurgery with 30 fixed fields in 1977.

The advent of the CT scanner and magnetic resonance imaging (MRI) combined with the phenomenal growth in computing power for 3-D planning computers, stimulated an explosive development of radiosurgery (Alexander and Loeffler 1994)

F.1.3
Indications for Proton Therapy

To date, the majority of indications for proton treatment were for patients with uveal melanoma of the eye, tumours near the base of skull or spinal cord like chordomas. Part of the reason for this restricted repertoire was the relatively low energy of some beams, the lack of isocentric gantries, and the earlier relatively poor imaging facilities for intracranial lesions.

There is hardly any body site that can not benefit from proton therapy, since the major reason for using proton beams is their good physical dose distributional capabilities. A list of indications is therefore rather superfluous. Some rarer lesions treated include glomus jugulare tumours, craniopharyngiomas, retinoblastomas, ethmoid and maxillary sinus tumours. Many other sites may benefit from the inherently better dose localisation of protons as opposed to photons (Suit 1992). The body sites, outside of the cranium, that may benefit from proton therapy are discussed in Chapter F on Body Tumours. The limiting factor may be the cost of constructing proton therapy facilities.

F.1.4
Imaging and Planning Requirements

Magnetic resonance imaging (MRI) can show up lesions, often invisible on CT, but it cannot supply electron density maps essential for computing dose distributions as CT scanners can. *Image fusion of MRI and CT and stereotactic angiography where applicable, is therefore an extremely important requirement for accurate lesion localisation for planning.* Such systems have been described (Kooy *et al.* 1994).

Some spatial distortion in the x-y axis (up to 4 mm) with MRI due to magnetic field variation (sometimes due to metal artefacts in the patient) makes MRI less accurate than CT scanning and unsuitable for planning. For an excellent overview see Alexander and Loeffler (1994).

Henkelman (1992) summarised the advantages of MRI and CT in Table F1.2

Cerebral angiography, especially a stereotactically obtained angiogram, is very important in the localisation and imaging of vascular anomalies in the brain such as arteriovenous malformations or aneurysms (Bova and Friedman 1991; Alexander and Loeffler 1994).

PET scanning can give information on the metabolic state of a lesion, but its spatial resolution is poor.

Planning computers

Table F1.3 summarises the requirements for planning computers

Table F1.2 Advantages and disadvantages of MRI and CT scanning for radiotherapy planning

MR Imaging for precision radiotherapy	
Advantages	**Disadvantages**
Good soft tissue imaging	No density information
Tumour specific contrast	Potential spatial distortion
3-D representation	
Excellent resolution	

CT scanning for precision radiotherapy	
Advantages	**Disadvantages**
Good bone imaging	3-D information suboptimal
Good density information	
No spatial disorder	

Table F1.3 Basic requirements for proton therapy planning computers

- Accommodation of adequate CT and MRI data
- Capability to fuse or register MRI, CT and angiography
- Non-coplanar beams 3-D display
- Beams eye view displays
- Digitally reconstructed radiographs
- 3-D dose calculation and display
- Dose volume histograms
- Reliable algorithm for predicting proton dose distributions (scattered beams and spot scanning)
- Printouts for collimator and compensator manufacture
- Special software for spot scanning systems
- User friendly, direct dose readout

Read also the section on planning in the relevant chapter in Part 1. The comments on planning by Alexander and Loeffler (1994) are very informative.

Published comparative plans illustrating the superiority of proton plans may no longer be valid, as most of the published comparative plans were made with 2-D coplanar photon plans. New comparisons are required with 3-D protons *versus* the best 3-D conformal photon plans (Bonnett 1993) (see also H.3.11).

It would be useful to have, instead of percent isodose lines, the direct dose (Gy) values for specific dose values. The formula is given in Appendix P.3. This formula should be considered for inclusion in planning algorithms.

It would be more useful to know, for example, where the 10 Gy line is, rather than to know where the 20% (for example) isodose line is.

The formula

$$\frac{\text{required dose}}{\text{prescribed dose}} \times \text{prescription dose}$$

will give position of the isodose line with the required dose. This could easily be built into the planning computer algorithm.

F.1.5
Beam Delivery Requirements

Existing proton therapy beam lines are usually horizontal beam lines of 70–250 MeV. The lower energies are used for eye therapy using mainly scattering systems. Modern units utilise one or more gantries for isocentric beam delivery.

Gantry and spot scanning: The merits of isocentric beam delivery are indisputable, as mentioned above.

The principles and advantages of spot scanning have been discussed in detail by Pedroni et al. (1995).

Proton therapy systems can in principle achieve good conformal dose distributions by a combination of couch movement and depth modulation of the beam by spot scanning techniques, which may make the need for isocentric proton gantries less obvious. Some doubt has been expressed as to the mathematical feasibility of spot scanning (Levin et al. 1988). The large computing powers of modern computers seem to have overcome this potential obstacle.

The reliability of treatment units for cancer patients is a very important consideration, and down times less than that of a linear accelerator should be aimed at.

Number of beams: It is wise to use a minimum of 3–4 beams in most cases with protons to obtain good conformation and to reduce the plateau dose per beam. For example, if 25 Gy is delivered to a lesion via only 2 beams, then the plateau dose may be as much as 30–40%, or 8–12.5 Gy, which may be a dangerously high dose to too large a volume of normal brain (Voges et al. 1996); no cranial nerve should be exposed to a single dose larger than 8 Gy, especially the optic nerve, which is the most sensitive of the cranial nerves. For more than two beams the plateau dose is reduced porportionally.

Beam Shaping: See also the section on physics.

Motorised multileaf collimators (MLCs) have been developed which allow conformation of the beam shape to the shape of the lesion outline from any arbitrary angle. They eliminate the need for casting shielding blocks, but they do not eliminate compensators. They are time saving "state of the art" devices for linear accelerators. MLCs for proton therapy have been made (Miller 1995) but these may be eclipsed by the development of spot scanning systems (Pedroni et al. 1995). Spot scanning allows field shaping and depth modulation, resulting in almost perfect conformal dose distribution to target. Spot scanning techniques are only possible with heavy charged particles, and offers the ultimate in 3-D dose distribution capability.

A special generation of 3-D planning computers is needed to model the dose distributions for discrete spots of radiation, and these are under development at PSI and elsewhere.

F.1.6
Patient Positioning and Immobilisation

Positioning devices include the regular radiotherapy beds, computerised chairs, body casts, frames and special stereotactic frames for radiosurgery.

Relocatable frames and masks: Easily relocatable frames enable repeated, accurate and convenient replacement of the frame, so that multiple fractions can be delivered if desired, for example Jones et al. (1995), (SPG mask), Gill and Thomas (1989), Lyman *et al.* (1989), and Fabrikant *et al.* (1992). The SPG system (Jones *et al.* 1995) is described in Appendix P.7. Fractionation spares the normal tissues and reduces the risk for acute radiation reactions, usually due to oedema of the irradiated tissues. These principles are more fully explained in Chapter H on Radiobiology.

F.1.7
Positioning for Extracranial Lesions

An example of a sophisticated system for extracranial immobilisation, is the PSI system (Pedroni *et al.* 1995). Patient handling comprises the treatment gantry, the table and also a special support for head treatments (the so-called "Top Rot" system). Facilities for X-ray imaging for simulation and positional verification are catered for. (Fig. F1.1)

The patient is immobilised in the supine position in his individually moulded couch. The patient couch is in turn transported in a special "patient transporter".

In the treatment room, the patient's couch is coupled mechanically to the gantry table. This table is so designed that the patient will always be treated in exactly the same supine position as during data collection – for example, CT slices for treatment planning, which is also done with the patient in his mould on the transporter.

The table has been designed to provide three translations: 25 cm for x and y and 80 cm for z, with a relative positioning precision better than 0.1 mm.

Scanning the patient in the same position that he will be treated is very important to avoid gravity induced organ shifts.

Fig. F1.2 shows a proposed beam line at NAC in South Africa: One 30° off vertical combined with the horizontal beam line, both to be fitted with spot scanning systems. (Schreuder *et al.* 1998)

F.1.8
The Composition of Tissues and Proton Therapy Planning

Water makes up 65% of the body mass in adults. Proton beams are very sensitive to changes in tissue density, and the major elements disturbing the basically watery composition of the body, are calcium in bone and air in the bony sinuses and lungs.

Oxygen makes up 65% of the body mass, carbon 18% hydrogen 10% and nitrogen 3%. The rest, 4%, consists of small quantities of electrolytes and trace elements.

Hydrogen comprises 63% of all the atoms in the body (making MRI so very effective and useful to image hydrogen in its various physical states), oxygen 26% carbon 9% and nitrogen 1%.

Calcium is the most abundant mineral element in the body, and the most obstructive to the passage of low energy X-rays, making CT scanning and X-ray photography possible and so very useful. Bone-air interfaces as found in the sinuses (mastoid, frontal, ethmoid and maxillary) tax the algorithms for proton planning computers severely, and it is unwise to rely on the distal end of the Bragg peak to stop millimetres away from the spinal cord or brain stem after having traversed bone or bone-air combinations such as for example, the mastoid air cells.

Computerised tomography can map the electron density of tissues, and this information is used for predicting dose distributions.

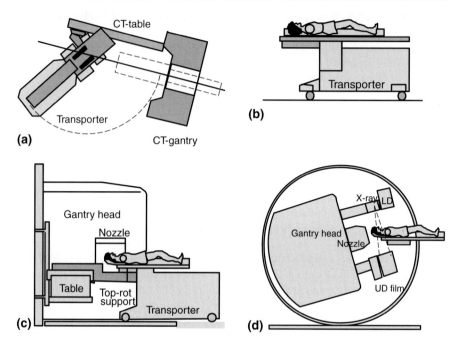

Fig. F1.1 Overview of the patient handling system under development for PSI proton therapy facility. (a) Patient positioning in CT room *(view from top)*. The patient will be prepared for treatment outside of the treatment room. Before each fraction the positioning of the patient, lying in this couch, will be controlled by taking scout view images with a modified CT unit. The CT table has been modified to permit a mechanically reproducible coupling of the couch from the patient transporter to the CT table. (b) Transport to treatment room. After being successfully positioned, the patient will be moved into the treatment room using a special carriage system. (c) Coupling of the couch to the proton gantry *(side view)*. In the treatment room the couch will be coupled to the gantry in the same way as for the CT table. After removing the patient transporter from the gantry platform the dynamic scanning of the beam will be started under complete computer control. (d) Control of patient positioning on the gantry *(front view)*. If necessary X-ray images of the patient in the treatment position will be taken directly on the gantry (X-ray tube and film position are given in the picture). The possibility of verifying the position of the patient on the gantry with the proton beam using transmission proton radiographs is provided by two boxes (the upper detector UD and lower detector LD) which can be rotated from the side into the beam and which contain the detector systems for proton radiography. (Redrawn from Eros Pedroni et al. 1995, Med Phys 22:37–53)

Magnetic Resonance Imaging (MRI) can map the distribution of hydrogen atoms very well, and this quality is very useful for demonstrating oedema and extravasated fluid, but MRI is of no use to determine proton dose distribution directly, although it can be useful to image the oedema induced by radiosurgery and thus to verify the proton dose distribution and location.

F.1.9
Optimised Proton Beams *versus* Photon Based Radiosurgery Beams

The collimator sizes for the Gamma Knife varies from 4 mm (very suitable for radiosurgical treatment of functional disorders) to 18 mm.

Two collimator sizes in-between are 8 and 14 mm. Multiple isocentres (2–6) can be used for larger lesions, but then the dose inhomogeneity may give rise to complications (Nedzi *et al.* 1991).

The linear accelerator collimators vary from 5 mm diameter to 50 mm diameter, with sharp fall-off – typically about 15% per mm (Wasserman *et al.* 1998). (Fig. F1.2).

For very small lesions, protons are probably unsuitable as the minimum useful beam diameter for plateau therapy is about 10–15 mm, for Bragg peak therapy about 15–20 mm. For small diameter proton beams the penumbra is almost as large as for the larger diameter fields. Thus the ratio of the area (volume) inscribed by small diameter proton beams relative to the penumbral width is unfavourable (Table F1.4)

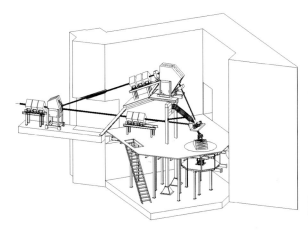

Fig. F1.2 A proposed beam line at NAC in South Africa

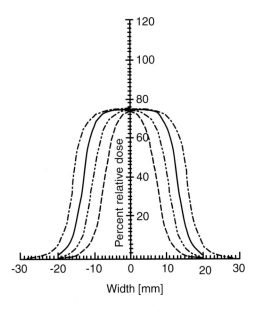

Fig. F1.3 Representative static beam dose profiles in water from Barnes-Jewish Hospital of St Louis. Varian Clinic 6/100 beams modified by divergent secondary circular collimators. Curves correspond to apertures with 15 mm (*dotted line*), 20 mm (*dash dot dot dash line*), 25 mm (*solid line*), and 30 mm (*dash dot dash line*) diameters. The dose gradient is typically about 15% per mm at the field edge. (Redrawn from TH Wasserman *et al.* 1998, In: Principles and Practice of Radiation Oncology, pp 387–404)

Table F1.4 Ratio of penumbral width to the diameter of the prescription isodose for protons

Prescription isodose	3 cm diameter	5 cm diameter	10 cm diameter
100%	0.14	0.44	0.55
90%	0.33	0.53	0.73
80%	0.44	0.66	0.78

also see fig. P3.1

A proton beam of 2.5×5 mm^2 had been used for cross-firing (plateau therapy) for very small lesions. Doses of 200 Gy produced a necrotic lesion within weeks. Girolami *et al.* (1996) compared, by means of Monte Carlo simulations, the radial dose distribution of photons and protons and showed that (for suitable photon fluxes) radiosurgery with 1–100-MV photon beams will be possible with a precision comparable to plateau radiosurgery with 200–580 MeV proton beams. As far as Bragg peak therapy is concerned, the authors remark that the Bragg peak "disappears" due to multiple scattering in narrow proton beams. The accuracy of cross-firing with proton beams may have an attainable precision very similar to that of a Gamma Knife.

The dose fall-off for proton beams can vary depending on residual range, hardware in the beam, proximity of the final collimator to the patient and the "phase-space" of the accelerator. A narrow phase-space window ensures that mainly homoenergetic protons will enter the accelerator.

The dose fall-off is steep in the plateau area of the beam, and from Lee *et al.* (1993) a modelled 200 MeV proton beam will have a penumbra of 4.1 mm (90% to 10% isodose) and near the end of the SOBP at 200 mm depth, 13 mm (90% to 10% isodose). The distal fall-off is 10 mm from the 90% to the 10% isodose, these values represent dose fall-offs of 19.5%, 6.1% and 8% per mm respectively, which are not as good as is obtainable with the photon systems with typical fall-offs of 10–15% per mm.

According to Podgorsak *et al.* (1989) the Gamma Knife dose will fall from 90% to 10% in 5 mm to 22 mm maximum, representing dose fall-off from 16% per mm to 3.6% per mm. Dynamic rotation with the linear accelerator achieves fall-offs of from 5 mm to 17 mm, or 16% per mm to 4.7% per mm.

The width of the 90% isodose (that will cover the target) relative to the penumbral width for proton beams are indicated in Table F1.4 and shows that for narrow proton beams this ratio is particularly poor and may explain why very narrow proton beams are not very useful for very small lesions – too much normal tissue is being irradiated relative to the target, unless homogeneity is sacrificed and the prescription isodose adjusted downwards from the 90% isodose to a suitable lower value. (See Chapter I on Dose-Volume Relationships)

For larger fields the ratio 90% width to penumbra becomes very favourable for protons and may explain the increased utility for protons for the larger radiosurgical lesions (> 25 cm^3) (Phillips *et al.* 1990) and for larger lesions elsewhere in the body. Figure F1.4 shows proton beam isodose curves for 200 MeV protons with a residual range of 11.5 cm, and should be studied in conjunction with Table F1.4. Figure G3.2 shows the isodose distributions for similar lesion diameter for protons (plateau beam) and for the isodose distribution of a linear accelerator adapted for radiosurgery.

The largest linear accelerator collimator (50 mm diameter) can treat a maximum tissue volume of 65.4 cm^3, 21 times the volume (3.1 cm^3) of the largest Gamma Knife collimator of 18 mm (Alexander, Loeffler and Kooy 1994). For helium ions the Bevatron accelerator modified for stereotactic radiosurgery (165 MeV/U) had a 90% to 10% distal fall-off of 2–3 mm (26–40% per mm) and a lateral fall-off 1 cm proximal to the distal edge of a beam with 7 cm residual range and 2 cm SOBP of 2.5 mm or 32% per mm (Fig. F1.5a). Figures F1.5b, F.1.5c and F1.5d show the beam profiles for the Gamma Knife (14 mm beam), a 30 mm proton Bragg Peak beam, and a 20 mm linear accelerator beam for comparison. The helium ion beam profile shows a much sharper dose fall-off per millimetre and this may explain why helium ions appear to allow higher doses for AVMs without complications – because much less surrounding brain will be irradiated with helium ions compared to protons. (See Chapter I on Dose-Volume Relationships). This facility was unfortunately shut down in 1992.

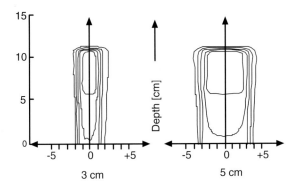

Fig. F1.4 (a) Isodose distribution for a 200 MeV proton beam degraded to have a residual range of 11.5 cm for a 3 cm and 5 cm beam. Note that the ratio of the 90% zone is unfavourable for the smaller beam (see Table A1.4).

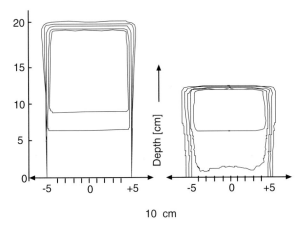

Fig. F1.4 (b) Comparison of a calculated 10-cm diameter beam (Lee et al. 1993) with a 200 MeV proton beam degraded to have a residual range in water of 11.5 cm. The 90%, 70%, 50%, 30% and 10% isodoses are shown.

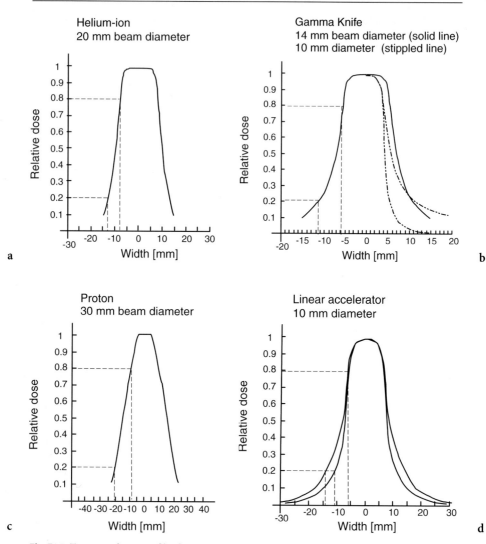

Fig. F1.5 Transverse beam profiles for:

(a) A 20 mm diameter Bragg Peak 165-MeV/U helium-ion beam at the Bevatron accelerator at the University of California, Berkeley, Lawrence Berkeley Laboratory, modified for stereotactic radiosurgery of an intracranial AVM. The penumbra (80%–20%) is 4.6 mm.

(b) A 14 and 10 mm diameter photon beam for the Gamma Knife. The penumbra (80%–20%) is 5.3 mm, 1.4 and 7.3 mm respectively.

(c) A 30 mm diameter Bragg peak 200 MeV proton beam with 11.5 cm residual range, the penumbra (80%–20%) is 11.6 mm. The penumbra for a proton beam (except for very small beams) is independent of the field size.

(d) A 10 mm diameter beam for a linear accelerator at Heidelberg (Podgorsak *et al.* 1989). The penumbra (80%–20%) is 5.5 mm and 8.9 mm for the 2 axes respectively.

Note that the x-axes are not all drawn to the same scale. The penumbral width of proton beams is largely independent of the beam size, in contrast to photon beams.

F.1.10

Summary

Although proton therapy has a relatively long history (44 years since 1954) fewer than 20 clinically useful centres have been constructed globally up to 1998. These include about five units only suitable for eye therapy, eight facilities with sufficient energy mainly for intracranial and paraspinal work, and only three units for isocentric beam delivery for all types and locations of tumours. The availability of several isocentric facilities heralds a new era for extracranial proton therapy.

Modern planning requires sophisticated multi-imaging techniques to ensure adequate lesion localisation, dose delivery, and immobilisation. Since the rationale for the use of protons is based on dose distributions superior to those currently available for photons, image fusion of MRI, CT and stereotactic angiography are absolutely essential to ensure accurate proton therapy planning.

Existing published comparative plans for photon *versus* protons can no longer be considered valid, since the older comparative studies did not compare proton therapy plans to modern 3-D photon plans and new comparisons are needed.

Spot scanning may have to be compared *versus* photons and scattered proton beams; there is a dire need for globally conducted and integrated co-operative prospective randomised clinical trials to answer many questions.

Although there are arguments that proton dose distributions are so superior that clinical trials may be considered unethical, I do not agree: randomised trials should then show significant differences soon and can be stopped early. For some situations like chordomas, the results for historical controls are so inferior that trials are probably no longer justified. On the other hand, pure dose escalation may not be relevant, e.g. carcinoma of the prostate. (See Chapter K.4.2)

Proton therapy may have an advantage over photons in most clinical situations where a large dose to a lesion is required and a low to moderate dose to sensitive adjacent normal tissues.

CT scanners can measure electron density distributions essential for planning. Hydrogen is the most abundant element in the body, and is important in the imaging of tissues by MRI. Bone (calcium) is dense and bone-air interfaces perturb the path length of protons considerably and such perturbations are difficult to model in planning computers.

Modern removable immobilisation systems make fractionated proton radiosurgery ("stereotactic radiotherapy") and proton radiotherapy possible and comfortable. An example of such a sophisticated system is the stereophotogrammetric system at the National Accelerator Centre in South Africa.

A minimum number of 3 beams per intracranial lesion are advisable for large single doses to ensure that the plateau doses to large volumes of brain are kept low for intracranial radiosurgery with protons.

Spot scanning or multileaf collimators may obviate the need for expensive and time-consuming custom-made collimators for proton beams.

The Gamma Knife can treat very small lesions (smallest collimator 4 mm), the smallest collimator of a linear accelerator is 5 mm, and the smallest useful Bragg peak beam for protons is 15–20 mm. The 90% isodose width is very small for such beams compared to the penumbra in the Bragg peak zone, and this makes protons less suitable for high doses to small lesions near critical structures.

The cost of constructing proton therapy centres remains very high. Protons may become very popular if the cost of suitable accelerators could be drastically reduced.

The reliability of beam availability and the user friendliness of any radiotherapy installation are of paramount clinical importance to avoid serious patient and clinician frustration.

F.1.11
References

Alexander E, Loeffler JS, Kooy H (1994) Steretactic Radiosurgery. In: Pell M, Thomas DGT (eds) Hand-
    book of Stereotaxy using the CRW Apparatus. Williams and Wilkins pp 179–191
Barcia-Salorio JL, Broseta J, Hernadez G et al. (1979) Radiosurgical treatment in huge acoustic neuro-
    mas. In: Szilka (ed) Stereotactic cerebral irradiation. INSERM Symposium No 12, Amsterdam, Else-
    vier, North Holland, Biomedical Press pp 245–249
Betti O, Derichinsky VE (1983) Irradiation stereotacique multifaisceau. Neurochirurgie 29:295–298
Bonnett DE (1993) Current developments in proton therapy: a review. Phys Med Biol 38:1371–1392
Bova FJ, Friedman WA (1991) Stereotactic angiography: An inadequate database for radiosurgery? Int
    J Radiat Oncol Biol Phys 20:891–895
Colombo F, Benedetti A, Pozzo F (1985) External stereotactic irradiation by linear accelerator. Neuro-
    surgery 16:154–160
Fabrikant JI, Levey RP, Steinberg GK et al. (1992) Charged particle radiosurgery for intracranial vascu-
    lar malformations. Neurosurg Clin of North Am 3:99–139
Gill SS, Thomas DGT (1989) A relocatable frame. J Neurol Neurosurg Psychiatry 52:1460–1461
Girolami B, Larsson B, Preger M et al. (1996) Photon beams for radiosurgery produced by laser Comp-
    ton back-scattering from relativistic electrons. Phys Med Biol 41:1581–1596
Hartman G, Schlegel W, Sturm V et al. (1985) Cerebral radiation surgery using moving field irradiation
    at a linear accelerator facility. Int J Radiat Oncol Biol Phys 20:1185–1192
Henkelman M (1992) New imaging technologies: prospects for target definition. Int J Radiat Oncol Biol
    Phys 22:251–257
Jones DTL, Schreuder AN, Symons JE Rüther, Van der Vlugt G, Bennett KF, Yates ADB (1995) Use of
    stereophotogrammetry in proton radiation therapy. Proceedings FIG Commission 6. International
    FIG Symposium, Cape Town
Kooy H, van Herk M, Barnes PD, Alexander E III et al. (1994) Image fusion for stereotactic radiothera-
    py and radiosurgery treatment planning. Int J Radiat Oncol Biol Phys 28:1229–1234
Lee M, Nahum AE, Webb S (1993) An empirical method to build up a model of proton dose distribu-
    tion for a radiotherapy treatment-planning package. Phys Med Biol 38:989–998
Levin CV, Gonin R, Wynchank S (1988) Computed limitations of spot scanning for therapeutic proton
    beams. Int J Biomed Comput 23:33–41
Lyman, JT, Phillips MH, Frankel KA et al. (1989) Stereotactic frame for neuroradiology and charged
    particle Bragg peak radiosurgery of intracranial disorders. Int J Radiat Oncol Biol Phys
    16:1615–1621
Mehta M (1995) The physical, biologic and clinical basis of radiosurgery. In: Current Problems in Can-
    cer Vol XIX, Mosby Yearbook Inc St Louis pp 267–328
Miller DW (1995) A review of proton beam radiotherapy. Med Phys 22:1943–1954
Pedroni E, Bacher R, Blattmann H et al. (1995) The 200 MeV proton therapy project at the Paul Scher-
    rer Institute: Conceptual design and practical realisation. Med Phys 22:37–53
Phillips MH, Frankel KA, Lyman JT et al. (1990) Comparison of different radiation types and irradia-
    tion geometries in stereotactic radiosurgery. Int J Radiat Oncol Biol Phys 18:211–220
Podgorsak EB, Oliver A, Pla M et al. (1987) Physical aspects of dynamic stereotactic radiosurgery. Appl
    Neurophysiol 50:263–268
Podgorsak EB, Pike GB, Olivier A et al. (1989) Radiosurgery with high energy photon beams: a com-
    parison among techniques. Int J Radiat Oncol Biol Phys 16:857–865
Raju MR (1980) Heavy Particle Radiotherapy. Academic Press
Schreuder AN, Jones DTL, Conradie JL et al. (1998) The non-orthogonal fixed beam arrangement for
    the second proton therapy facility at the National Accelerator Centre. 15th Conference on the appli-
    cation of accelerators in commerce and industry. American Institute of Physics.
Slater JM, Archambeau JO, Miller DW et al. (1991) Int J Radiat Oncol Biol Phys 22:383–389
Suit H (1992) Editors note. NCI proton workshop. Int J Radiat Oncol Biol Phys 22:233–235
Suit H, Urie M (1992) Review: Proton Beams in Radiation Therapy. J Natl Cancer Inst 84:155–164

Voges J, Treuer H, Sturm V, Buchner C, Lehrke R, Kocher M, Staar S, Kuchta J, Müller RP (1996) Risk analysis of linear accelerator radiosurgery. Int J Radiat Oncol Biol Phys 36:1055–1063

Wasserman TH, Rich KM, Drzymala RE *et al.* (1998) Stereotactic Irradiation. In: Perez CA, Brady LW (eds) Principle and Practice of Radiation Oncology. Lippincott-Raven Publishers, pp 387–404

G The Rationale for Proton Therapy

G.1
Introduction

Protons have superior dose distributional qualities compared to X- or gamma rays, which is the major advantage.

The superior dose distribution of protons is due to a unique quality of heavy charged particles, depositing the maximum radiation dose at a specific depth, in a narrow zone called the Bragg peak. The dose may be four times as high as the entrance dose at the Bragg peak. The depth at which the Bragg peak occurs is energy dependent. (See section on physics)

Beyond the Bragg peak, no radiation energy is deposited, so that the tissues beyond the target are totally spared, in contrast to a photon beam that deposits a substantial percentage of its energy in the tissues in front of as well as beyond the target. (See Physics, Part I, Chapter B.1.1)

The plateau region of the Bragg peak can be profitably utilised for therapy for lesions smaller than 15–20 mm in diameter, where the penumbra for Bragg peak therapy is too large relative to the area or volume covered by the 90% isodose zone (Table F1.4, Chapter F.1.8). Proton therapy can therefore be divided into "Bragg peak" therapy and "plateau" therapy.

G.2
Bragg Peak Therapy

The properties of protons have been described and their use in the treatment of disease have been reviewed regularly (Koehler and Preston 1972; Raju 1980; Verhey and Munzenrider 1982; Bonnett 1990, 1993; Webb 1993).

Figure G2.1 shows the depth dose curves schematically for 16 MeV X-rays and 230 MeV protons.

Optimal beam characteristics are essential to optimise the benefits of proton therapy. This includes the optimal energy for the task in hand, e.g. about 70 MeV for eye lesions, 160 MeV for intracranial lesions, and 250 MeV for tumours like the prostate gland or the uterine cervix. Excess energy for the task in hand leads to an unnecessarily large penumbra. Other factors for optimising a beam are mentioned in Chapter F.1.9.

Figure G2.2 shows that the Bragg peak is poorly developed for small diameter beams, making proton beams of < 1.5 cm not very useful for Bragg peak therapy, also because the penumbra is relatively wide for small beams. (See Chapter I)

The special qualities of protons are discussed below.

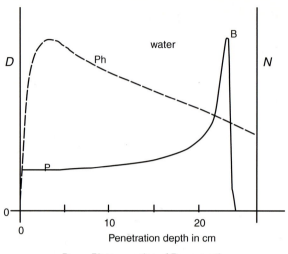

Fig. G.2.1 Characteristic depth-dose curves for 16 MeV photon beam and protons (230 MeV).

P = Plateau region of Bragg peak
B = Bragg curve peak (230 MeV)
Ph = 16 MeV photon beam absorption curve

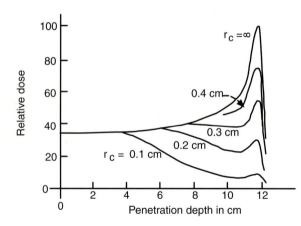

Fig. G.2.2 Relative dose as a function of depth on the central axis of a uniform circular proton beam of initial range 12 cm in water; rc is the radius of the collimator. The curve $r_c = \infty$ is an experimental depth-dose curve, and the other curves are calculated. (From Preston and Koehler, 1968) In practice, for a 200 MeV scattered proton beam, the minimum usable diameters are about 10 mm for a plateau beam and 20–25 mm for a spread out Bragg peak. For small 4–5 mm intracranial lesions for radiosurgery, the Gamma Knife and linear accelerator are more suitable.

Table G.2.1 The advantages of a proton peak therapy compared to photon beams, PTV = planning target volume, CTV = clinical target volume

Conformity index:	Planning target volume to clinical target volume ratio (PTV/CTV) for protons
Inhomogeneity Co-efficient:	Dose difference across the target $(D_{max} - D_{min})/D_{min} \times 100$ for protons
Localisation factor:(LF):	Improved dose ratio to target relative to whole brain dose for radiosurgery (integral dose target)/(integral dose to the brain)

Table G2.1 summarises the qualities of proton beams that will be discussed in this section.

Table G2.2 The average conformity index (CI). LA 1: linear accelerator 1 isocentre, LA 2: linear accelerator complex planning, GK 1: Gamma Knife 1 isocentre, GK 4: Gamma Knife 4 isocentre, N/A: data not available or not applicable, Table adapted from Verhey *et al.* (1998)

Lesion volume (cm^3)	Conformity index (CI)				
	Proton	LA 1	LA 2 complex	GK 1	GK 4
1.0	1.47	1.76	1.35	1.42	1.26
6.0	1.43	2.07	1.43	1.29	N/A
6.5	1.34	N/A	1.62	1.61	N/A
14.5	1.26	2.35	1.26	1.54	N/A
26	1.10	1.56	1.27	1.33	N/A

G.2.1
The Conformity Index

Verhey *et al.* (1998) defined the conformity index (CI) as the *volume* inscribed by the prescription isodose divided by the target volume:

$$CI = \frac{[\text{volume inscribed by the presciption isodose}]}{[\text{target volume}]}$$

They compared radiosurgery treatment modalities (linear accelerator, Gamma Knife and protons) based on the physical dose distributions for lesions of irregular shape for volumes of 1 cm^3 to 26 cm^3. Table G2.2 is based on their data.

Table G2.2 shows that for small volumes (1–6 cm^3), proton beams are no better than the photon beams. From 6.5 cm^3 and upwards, protons have a better conformity index than photons.

Hamilton *et al.* (1995) compared static conformal fields with multiple noncoplanar arcs to a single isocentre based on linear accelerator technology. The volume receiving the prescription isodose was found to be more than 3.5 times larger than the target volume for all the plans investigated. This may indicate that for irregularly shaped targets, a conformity correction factor of about 3 should be considered for photon systems, but much less for protons (about 1.5). The volume obtained from the computer for the planning target volume may be more prudent to use for determining dose-volume relationships. (See Chapter I on Dose-Volume Relationships)

G.2.2
The Inhomogeneity Coefficient and Its Effects

The inhomogeneity co-efficient (IC) reflects the *dose differences* across the target area and is defined as follows:

$$IC = \frac{\text{Maximum dose minus the minimum dose}}{\text{the minimum dose}} \times 100$$

(Phillips *et al.* 1994)

If a dose of 10 Gy is specified at 80% then the maximum dose would be 100/80 × 10 Gy = 12.5 Gy and the IC would be 12.5–10 Gy/10 Gy × 100 = 25%

The inhomogeneity co-efficient for commonly used prescription isodoses for the various modalities are reflected in Table G2.3.

Table G2.3 Inhomogeneity coefficients for commonly used prescription isodoses

	Prescription isodose (%)					
	100	90	80	65	50	37
Protons	0	5.3	25			
Linear accelerator			25	54		
Gamma Knife				54	100	170

Inhomogeneity in dose can lead to far greater biological damage than intended, reflected in the "double trouble" of both a higher total dose and a higher dose per fraction in the treatment volume (Withers 1994). This very important problem is discussed in Chapter C.1.9 on Radiobiology.

In this regard, Nedzi *et al.* (1991) found that tumour dose inhomogeneity correlated very strongly with complications for primary and secondary brain tumours.

G.2.3
The Localisation Factor

Phillips *et al.* (1990) introduced the concept of the localisation factor (LF). This factor is defined as the *ratio of target integral dose to total integral dose* to the brain:

Table G2.4 Localisation factor for various lesion volumes (*AVM*). Data from Phillips *et al.* (1990)

Volume (cm³)	Location	Beam	LF	Ratio Proton LF/ Photon LF
0.8	Central	Proton	0.013	
		Photon	0.009	1.4
1.6	Peripheral	Proton	0.057	
		Photon	0.032	1.8
5.0	Central	Proton	0.10	
		Photon	0.06	1.7
5.7	Peripheral	Proton	0.14	
		Photon	0.06	2.3
28	Central	Proton	0.21	
		Photon	0.13	1.6
56	Peripheral	Proton	0.38	
		Photon	0.20	1.9

LF = integral dose to the target volume/Integral dose to the entire brain
The integral dose is expressed in units of cm³. Gy.
Table G2.4 is an abbreviated adaptation from the data of Phillips *et al.* (1990)

The conclusion is that for all volumes examined, the 150 MeV protons deliver a relatively larger dose per cm³ to the target than to the brain, compared to photons. *This advantage increases with increasing target size, and the LF is especially favourable for protons for lesion sizes over 5 cm³* – about 22 mm diameter. The results are graphically illustrated in Fig. G2.3 by means of dose-volume histograms (DVHs). See also DVHs for photon radiosurgery system, Chapter N, Fig. N1.1.

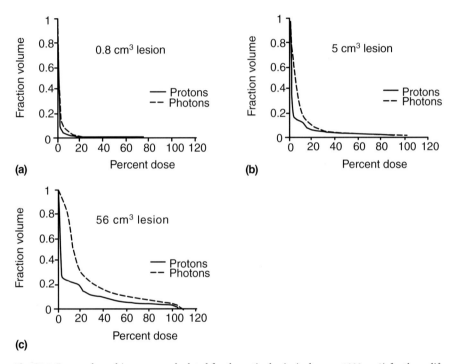

Fig. G2.3 Dose-volume histograms calculated for the entire brain (volume = 1300 cm3) for three different sizes of target volumes. The target volumes are 0.8, 5.0 and 56 cm³. The histograms are shown for protons and photons. (Redrawn from MH Phillips *et al.* 1990, Int J Radiat Oncol Biol Phys 18:211–220)

Phillips *et al.* (1990) compared the 3-D dose distributions of different radiation types, and found charged particles (including protons) to be better than photons from the Gamma Knife or linear accelerator.

The LF may not however, be the determining factor in the formation of complications, as an important discriminator may be the volume of brain receiving 10 Gy (Voges *et al.* 1996) or 12 Gy (Flickinger *et al.* 1997), which may be heavily dependent on the penumbra of a beam, and the prescription isodose. (See Chapter I on Dose-Volume Relationships)

Nedzi *et al.* (1991) also found that the total dose as well as the number of isocentres correlated strongly with the development of complications, because an increased number of isocentres can increase the dose inhomogeneity almost three fold.

The development of miniature multileaf collimators may remove the need for multiple isocentres with the linear accelerator, simultaneously improving the homogeneity of dose and reducing the side effects. (See Chapter I on Alternatives to Proton Therapy)

The above qualities of proton beams (IC, LF, and CI) lead to an improved **therapeutic ratio (TR)**. (See Chapter H.1.3)

The Gamma Factor: A second conclusion that can be drawn from the improved localisation, homogeneity and conformal qualities of proton beams is that a higher dose may be given to a tumour, because the complication rate may be kept constant, where the complication rate for a given tumour is low, but the cure rate is not satisfactory. The gamma factor predicts that if a usually tolerated dose could be increased by, say 10%, then for a gamma factor of 2 the local control rate could be expected to be 20% higher. The gamma factor is discussed in Chapter H.1.8 on Radiobiology for Fractionated Proton Therapy.

G.3
Plateau Therapy

For very small lesions, Bragg peak therapy is not optimal, because with very narrow beams the Bragg peak is not fully developed (Preston and Koehler 1968). (Fig. G2.2)

The minimum diameter for Bragg peak therapy is about 15 mm. For very small fields with protons, the plateau part of the depth dose curve needs to be utilised.

A small (< 1 cm diameter) lesion near sensitive structures, like, for example, the optic nerve with a lesion in the cavernous sinus, may be better treated with coplanar plateau beams, because this part of the beam has the steepest lateral fall-off in dose (about 19% per mm).

The drawbacks with plateau therapy are that the localisation factor is much reduced, since the beam energy must be high enough to ensure that the Bragg peak will fall outside of the head, at some point in space. Even then the exit dose will be higher than the entrance dose, and if three intersecting fields are used, if the dose to the lesion normalised at 100%, each "track" will receive 33.3% of the dose or more on the exit side. Care must be taken that the Bragg peak falls <u>outside</u> the head. (Fig. G3.1)

The advantages of plateau therapy relative to photon radiosurgery, are the economy in time using only 3 to 4 fields, the penumbra is good and very small lesions can be irradiated homogeneously.

Photon therapy offers an alternative to proton therapy for very small lesions.

The Gamma Knife has circular collimators of 4, 8, 14 and 18 mm available. For the linear accelerator, the available collimators range from 5 mm to 50 mm. The high dose regions have an aspherical shape and may fail to spare the optic chiasm sufficiently in the example quoted above, if the target volume extends well outside the sella turcica. A heavy particle approach may be accomplished with two lateral beams, avoiding the chiasm (Alexander and Loeffler 1994).

For protons, collimators from 5 mm (plateau) to 100 mm or larger for extracranial therapy, are available.

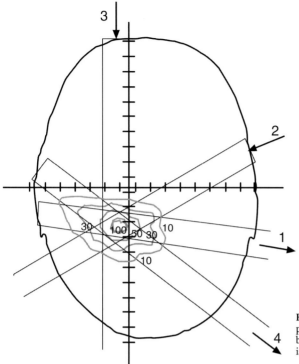

Fig. G3.1 Treatment plan for proton plateau irradiation of a brain lesion. The beam diameter is 20 mm.

Plateau therapy has one more advantage over Bragg peak therapy. The relative biological effectiveness (RBE) in the plateau is stable, whereas there is an increase in the RBE with depth in the distal Bragg peak area, which makes the dosimetry in this critical area more uncertain. (See Chapter H.1.4)

Figure G3.2 compares the dose distribution for a 9 arc linear accelerator field with that of a 3-field plateau proton beam, for beam diameter of 25 mm (linear accelerator) and 20 mm beam diameter coplanar proton plateau distribution (protons).

G.4
Definition of Radiosurgery and Stereotactic Radiotherapy

"Radiosurgery" is a term used to indicate a single large radiation with very steep fall-off in dose away from the lesion, to a very small volume, originally intended to cause necrosis in intracranial lesions. "Stereotactic radiotherapy" (SRT) is a term used to indicate super-accurate 3-dimensional fractionated radiotherapy (Brada and Graham 1994). SRT offers improved localisation and delivery of radiation to brain lesions and is best described as stereotactically guided conformal radiotherapy. The stereophotogrammetric method of patient immobilisation for proton therapy at the National Accelerator Centre is an easy way of reproducibly positioning the patient repeatedly with great comfort (Jones and Schreuder 1995).

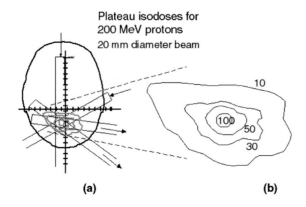

(a)   **(b)**

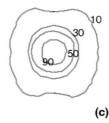

(c)

Fig. G3.2 **(a)** Plateau isodoses for 200 MeV protons for 20-mm diameter beam. **(b)** Isodoses from **(a)** enlarged. **(c)** Representative linear accelerator isodoses for a 26-mm diameter beam. 90%, 50%, 30% and 10% isodoses are shown. The beam diameters from **(b)** and **(c)** are on the same scale. The volume in **(c)** is spheroid, that of the proton beam more discoid, which is an advantage in areas like the pituitary fossa. (Also see L4.1)

G.5
Large Field Proton Therapy

A distinct advantage of Bragg peak proton therapy is the fact that even only a simple 2-field arrangement can give a very good dose distribution for large field irradiation. Figure G5.1 shows the very good coronal, sagittal and transverse dose distributions for two 200 MeV beams, uncompensated.

Figure G5.1 is an example of large field proton therapy and it shows that the field arrangements can be more economical than photon beams. For example, for an equivalent photon plan, 4–8 beams with a linear accelerator may be needed. Special volumes of the International Journal of Radiation Oncology biology and Physics have been devoted to comparative planning, and special reports on this subject have been submitted to the National Cancer Institute in Bethesda, from where it may be obtained. The TERA Project brochure contains much relevant information on comparative planning (Amaldi and Silari 1995).

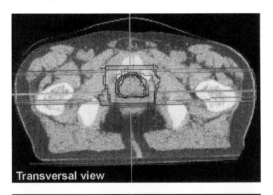

Transversal view

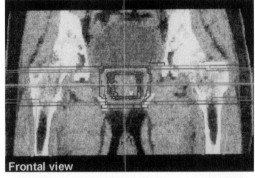

Frontal view

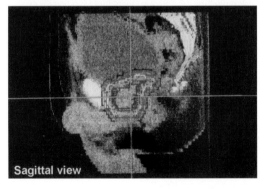

Sagittal view

Fig. G5.1 A single uncompensated, yet well collimated plan for protons for a carcinoma of the prostate, 200 MeV protons. Only lateral beams were utilised. For conformal photon therapy, 4–8 beams are required.

G.6
Summary

Bragg peak proton therapy allows the delivery of well-defined doses of radiation energy, confined largely to the lesions treated.

This allows either higher doses keeping the complication rate constant, or keeping the cure rate constant and reducing the complication rate. Quantification of these parameters recently became available as the conformity index, localisation factor, gamma factor, and inhomogeneity co-efficient.

Protons are suitable for radiosurgery (especially for lesions larger than 5 cm^3) stereotactic radiotherapy, and for large volume therapy. Protons should perform better than photons because of better homogeneity of dose across the target, and a better conformation compared to the photon or gamma ray therapy units. The integral dose to the adjacent normal organs can be much reduced by proton therapy, compared to photon or gamma ray techniques, since fewer beams are required, and because of the unique qualities of the Bragg peak dose distribution.

For very small lesions close to sensitive structures like the optic nerve, plateau therapy may be considered, because the Bragg peak is not well developed for very narrow proton beams, and in such situations the penumbra for a suitable Bragg peak beam may bee too large to avoid the optic nerve.

G.7.
References

Alexander E, Loeffler JS, Kooy H (1994) Stereotactic Radiosurgery. In: Pell M, Thomas DGT (eds) Handbook of stereotaxy using the CRW apparatus. Williams and Wilkins pp 179–191

Amaldi U, Silari (eds) (1995) The TERA Project, Vol I and II. INFN-LNF Publishers

Bonnett DE (1990) The role of protons in radiotherapy. In: Vourvopoulos G, Paradellis T (eds) Applications of nuclear techniques. World Scientific, Singapore, pp 109–30

Bonnett DE (1993) Current developments in proton therapy: a review. Phys Med Biol 38:1371–1392

Brada M, Graham JD (1994) Stereotactic external beam radiotherapy in the treatment of glioma and other lesions. In: Tobias JS, Thomas PRM (eds) Current radiation oncology, Vol 1. Arnold, London, pp 85–101

Fabrikant JI, Levy RP, Steinberg GK et al. (1992) Charged particle radiosurgery for intracranial vascular malformations. Neurosurg Clin North Am 3:99–139

Flickinger JC, Kondziolka D, Pollock BE et al. (1997) Complications from arteriovenous malformation radiosurgery: Multivariate analysis and risk modelling. Int J Radiat Oncol Biol Phys 38:485–490

Hamilton RJ, Kuchnir FT, Sweeney P, Rubin SJ et al. (l995) Comparison of static conformal field with multiple non-coplanar arc techniques for stereotactic radiotherapy. Int J Oncol Biol Phys 33:1221–1228

Jones DTL, Schreuder AN, Symons JE Rüther et al. (1995) Use of stereophotogrammetry in proton radiation therapy. Proceedings FIG Commission 6. International FIG Symposium, Cape Town

Koehler A, Preston WM (1972) Protons in radiation therapy. Med Phys 4:297–301

Luxton G, Petrovich Z, Jozsef G et al. (1993) Stereotactic radiosurgery: principles and comparison of treatment. Neurosurgery 32:241–259

Nedzi L, Kooy H, Alexander E et al. (1991) Variables associated with the development of complications from radiosurgery of intracranial tumours. Int J Radiat Oncol Biol Phys 21:591–599

Phillips MH, Frankel KA, Lyman JT et al. (1990) Comparison of different radiation types and irradiation geometries in stereotactic radiosurgery. Int J Radiat Oncol Biol Phys 18:211–220

Phillips MH, Steltzer KJ, Griffin TW et al. (1994) Stereotactic radiosurgery: a review and comparison of methods. J Clin Oncol 12:1085–1099

Preston WM, Koehler AM (1968) The effects of scattering on small proton beams. Internal report

Raju MR (1980) Heavy particle radiotherapy. Academic Press, New York

Suit HD, Westgate SJ (1986) Impact of improved local control on survival. Int J Radiat Oncol Biol Phys 12:453–458

Suit H (1992) Editors Note, NCI Proton Workshop: potential clinical gains by use of superior radiation dose distribution. Int J Radiat Oncol Biol Phys 22:233–234

Verhey LJ, Munzenrider JE (1982) Proton beam therapy. Ann Rev Biophys Bioeng 11:331–357

Verhey LJ, Smith V, Serago F (1998) Comparison of radiosurgery treatment modalities based on physical dose distributions. Int J Radiat Oncol Biol Phys 40:497–505

Voges J, Treuer H, Sturm V et al. (1996) Risk analysis of linear accelerator radiosurgery. Int J Radiat Oncol Biol Phys 36:1055–1063

Webb S (1993) The physics of three-dimensional radiation therapy. Institute of Physics Publishing, Bristol, pp 172–212

Withers HR (1994) Biology of radiation oncology. In: Tobias JS, Thomas PRM (eds) Current Radiation Oncology. Vol 1 pp 5–23

H Radiobiology

H.1
Radiobiology for Fractionated Proton Therapy

H.1.1
Introduction

Fractionated therapy with protons is becoming more common and as a general principle, the smaller the dose per fraction, the lower the risk for complications.

The rather more drastic effects of single large doses will be discussed in the Chapter H.2 on Radiobiology of Radiosurgery.

A basic understanding of the likely radiobiological effects may help to guide clinical decision making, therefore an understanding of the "biologically effective dose" (BED) is very useful for any person involved in the field of radiotherapy. The BED will be discussed in a separate chapter (H.3) for easy reference, as the BED will be used to illustrate many aspects of practical proton therapy. Generally, the biological effects of a dose of radiation are dependent on the type of radiation, oxygen status of the lesion, lesion nature, volume, total dose, fraction size, dose inhomogeneity and treatment schedule.

Fractionation (delivery of a particular total dose chosen in multiple increments or fractions) is very important in the management of malignant lesions; less so with lesions which are themselves "late reacting" for example, arteriovenous malformations or meningiomas.

Because of the nature of dose-response curves, it is very difficult to avoid complications totally with curative radiotherapy procedures and any substantial dose of radiation carries with it the risk of complications – this has important medico-legal implications.

H.1.2
Linear Energy Transfer

Linear energy transfer (LET) is a term referring to the energy transferred from the irradiation beam to the medium, expressed as kilo electron volt of energy lost (keV) per micrometer of track length of a charged particle. Protons, like photons and electrons, are classed as sparsely ionising radiation, in contrast to particles like neutrons, carbon nuclei and alpha particles, which are densely ionising. Densely ionising tracks cause much greater biological damage per unit track length than sparsely ionising tracks, and are much more likely to break both strands of the DNA double helix than sparsely ionising beams, which are more likely to break only single strands of DNA.

Single strand breaks are repaired much more easily and precisely than double strand breaks by the usual repair enzymes.

Table H1.1 shows typical LET values for different radiation types.

Table H1.1 Typical LET values of different types of radiation. Modified from: Hall EJ (1994), [a] Miller (1995)

Radiation type	LET (keV/micron)
[60]Cobalt	0.2
250 keV X-rays	2.0
10 MeV protons	4.7
150 MeV protons	0.5
Very slow protons[a]	80.0
2.5 MeV alpha particles	166.0

For most biological systems the RBE (see below) increases with increasing LET to reach a maximum value at about 100 keV/(m. There is a component of high LET in proton beams, which makes continued research particularly important because it is relevant to the radiobiology and fractionation regimens for proton therapy. In the penumbral area, which is the area impinging on the normal tissues, a higher than expected RBE may detract from the utility of proton beams.

H.1.3
The Therapeutic Ratio

According to Paterson (1963) this ratio is a balance between the lethal dose of radiation to a tumour (TLD) and the normal tissue tolerance (NTT), and can be represented as:

TR = TLD/NTT

The NTT is not a fixed value, but it is a clinically useful term for the dose, which yields an acceptable probability of a complication for an acceptable probability of cure. It is an elastic value which varies with the nature of the complication, prognosis, wishes of the patient and other considerations specific to each clinical situation (Withers 1994).

The TR can be modified in principle by better conformation of prescription isodose to target, sensitising tumour cells by radiosensitisers (e.g. misonidazole) or selectively protecting the normal tissues, e.g. amifostine (Grdina *et al.* 1995; Capizzi RL 1996).

The value of this ratio, to be clinically useful, should always be greater than 1.

The good normal tissue sparing characteristics of proton beams offer an opportunity to improve the "therapeutic ratio" with proton therapy relative to photon therapy, but the dose fall-off characteristics of the beam and the isodose distributions on the treatment plan are other very relevant parameters to scrutinise when planning. Some photon or gamma ray radiosurgical systems have a very favourable dose fall-off, even when compared to proton therapy.

The therapeutic ratio can be interpreted in radiobiological terms as well. The differential effect of the dose to the target relative to the dose to the normal tissues is far larger than the numerical doses suggest. This is due to the effects of fractionation. (See Chapter H.3 on BED)

For example, if the dose is normalised to 100% over the tumour area for a conventionally irradiated four field "box" technique for carcinoma of the cervix, and the dose to the tumour is prescribed at 2 Gy per fraction, the biologically effective late damage to the target area will be, for 50 Gy total dose, equivalent to $BED_2 = 100$ Gy. If the dose to the normal tissues outside of this area is 1 Gy per fraction, then the total late damage to the normal tissues will not be halved (25 Gy/50 Gy) = 100% lower but will be $BED_2 = (37.5$ Gy$/BED_2 = 100$ Gy$) = 166.6\%$ lower. If the tumour is not conformally covered by the 100% isodose line, a lot of normal tissues around the tumour will be exposed to 66.6% more irradiation than necessary which will simply contribute to the severity of late complications. The excellent conformity and localisation achievable with protons for large lesions should therefore in principle, ensure low complications.

H.1.4
The Relative Biological Effectiveness

The relative biological effectiveness (RBE) is a ratio comparing the effects of a beam of uncertain biological effect to the effects of a reference beam of known biological effect.

Definition: The RBE of some test irradiation (r) compared with ^{60}Co is defined by the ratio $D^{60}Co/D_r$ where $D^{60}Co$ and D_r are, respectively, the doses of ^{60}Co gamma rays and r is the test radiation required to render equal biological effect.

The RBE does not have a fixed value. Its value depends on the LET, radiation dose, number of fractions, dose rate and on the biological system or the biological end point under investigation (Hall 1994). Some texts use 250 kV X-rays as the reference radiation. It is essential to make sure which reference irradiation was used to determine a specific RBE value, because ^{60}Cobalt is significantly less effective biologically than 250 keV X-rays.

The RBE for charged particles is proportional to Q^2/V, where Q is the charge of the particle (1 for protons) and V is the velocity of the particle. The RBE for protons is therefore proportional to $1/V$ (Hall 1994), and is thus inversely proportional to the velocity of the protons, and protons near rest should therefore have a large RBE. Miller *et al.* (1995) confirmed this experimentally.

Measured RBE values for protons are shown in Table H1.2.

The RBE of protons in the plateau region is widely accepted as 1–1.1 and in the Bragg peak area 1.1–1.2 confirmed by Paganetti *et al.* (1997) who measured an RBE = 1.0 in the plateau region, and RBE = 1.1 in the centre of the Bragg Peak for a 250 MeV beam (early intestinal tolerance in mice).

The RBE for protons relative to ^{60}Co has been found to be 1.09–1.32 (Urano *et al.* 1984), with RBE values increasing with decreasing proton energy. RBE values of 1.0 at 31 MeV, 1.4 at 12 MeV, and 1.5 at 8 MeV in the distal fall-off zone of a high-energy proton beam have been measured.

Paganetti *et al.* (1997) measured the RBE at 1.9 for a 70 MeV beam (Chinese hamster V79 cells). In the lateral direction, they found virtually no variation in the RBE. These authors concluded that for therapy planning with protons it might be wise to take into account the possibility of a depth dependence of the RBE for protons, especially at lower energies. Lower energies, e.g. 70 MeV, are typically used for the treatment of uveal melanoma in eyes where the preservation of vision is a major consideration.

Clinically the effect of an RBE increase in the dose fall-off zone may be tantamount to the distal "penumbra" expanding by 2 mm or more, which may be clinically important in neuroradiosurgery with protons and eye therapy (See also Chapter I on Dose-Volume Relationships and Section E)

Table H1.2 The RBE of Protons. *CH* = Chinese hamster

Author	Proton energy	Biological system	Depth	RBE
Urano (1984)	31 MeV 12 MeV 8 MeV	Various murine normal and tumour tissues	Distal peak	1.0 1.4 1.5
Paganetti (1997)	250 MeV	Intestinal intolerance	Peak	1.1–1.2
Tang (1997)	65 MeV	(CH – ovary)	2 mm 10 mm 18 mm 23 mm	1.05 1.1 1.12 1.19
Robertson (1994)	100–250 MeV	V79 CH	Peak	1.1–1.3
Paganetti (1997)	70 MeV	V79 CH	Peak	1.9

Tang *et al.* (1997) examined the change of the RBE in the spread-out Bragg peak (SOBP) of beam of 65 MeV protons.

They exposed Chinese hamster ovary (CHO) cells at 2 mm depth, corresponding to the entrance, and 10, 18 and 23 mm depths, corresponding to different positions in the SOBP.

Cell survival curves were generated with the in vitro colony formation method and fitted to the linear-quadratic model, with ^{137}Cs gamma rays as the reference irradiation.

The relative biological effectiveness (RBE) values for a surviving fraction (SF) level of 0.1 are 1.05, 1.10, 1.12 and 1.19 for depths of 2, 10, 18 and 23 mm respectively. There was a significant dependence of RBE on depths in modulated proton beams at the 0.1 surviving fraction level ($P < 0.05$). Moreover, the rise of RBEs significantly depended on increasing SF level or decreased irradiation dose ($P = 0.0001$). They concluded that, in order to maintain uniformity of radiobiological effectiveness for the target volume, careful attention should be paid to the influence of depth of beam and irradiation dose.

H.1.5
Dose Response Curves

An example of a typical dose response curve for cells in culture is shown in Fig. H1.1 illustrating that increasing radiation doses kill increasing numbers of cells, also that cells in different phases of the cell cycle have different sensitivities to the same radiation doses (Sinclair WK 1968).

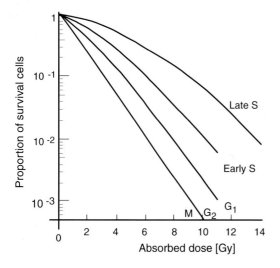

Fig. H1.1 Survival curves of Chinese hamster cells irradiated in different phases of the mitotic cycle, showing that cells have different sensitivities to irradiation in different phases of the cell cycle. (Redrawn from Sinclair WK, 1968. In: Tubiana M, Dutreix J, Wambersie A (eds). Introduction to Radiobiology)

Withers (1982) has shown that the dose response curve for late reacting tissues curves faster than the dose response curve for early reacting tissues, with the result that the curves tend to cross each other. (Fig. H1.2)

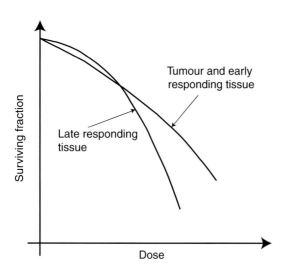

Fig. H1.2 The dose-response relationship for late-responding tissues is more curved than for early-responding tissues. In the linear quadratic formulation this translates into a larger α/β ratio for early than for late effects. The ratio α/β is the dose at which the linear (α) and the quadratic (β) components of cell killing are equal: that is $\alpha D = \beta D$. (Redrawn from the concepts of HD Withers, 1994. In: Eric J Hall (ed) Radiobiology for the Radiologist, LB Lippincott pp 211–229)

The effect of this is that in the low dose, small fraction zone before the crossover takes place, small fractions (individual small doses) cause less damage to the late reacting tissues than to early reacting tissues. A fractional dose beyond the crossover region will cause more damage to the late than the early reacting tissues.

Tissues irradiated *in vivo* (as opposed to cells in culture) respond in different ways, depending on the tissue type and the fractionation pattern. Withers (1982) has identified this phenomenon, based on clinical data, and could separate tissues into "early reacting tissues" and "late reacting tissues", from which the above curve was derived.

Large doses per fraction are invariably unkind to late reacting tissues, including tissues like the brain, lung, kidney, eye and spinal cord, whereas small doses per fraction spare the normal tissues and also help to sensitise tumours, due to the fact that re-oxygenation, and with it re-sensitisation and redistribution of cells into the sensitive phase of the cell cycle, should take place.

Typical clinical derived dose effect curves are depicted in Fig. H1.3

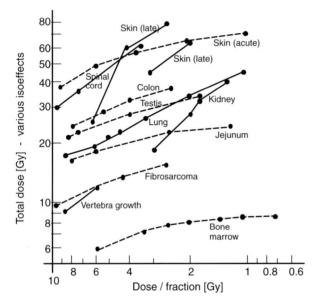

Fig. H1.3 Isoeffect curves in which the total dose necessary for a certain effect in various tissues plotted as a function of dose per fraction. Late effects are plotted with *solid lines*, acute effects with *dotted lines*. The data were selected to exclude an influence on the total dose of regeneration during the multifraction experiments. The main point of the data is that the isodoses for late effects increase more rapidly with decrease in dose per fraction than is the case for acute effects. (Redrawn from HR Withers, 1985, Cancer 55:2086–2095)

Dose effect curves from cell cultures are sigmoid with a sharp increase in cell death on the linear portions of the curve (Fig. H1.4).

A tumour is assumed to be more sensitive than normal tissues, for example seminoma of the testis, and is represented by the curve on the left. From the figure it follows that a dose delivered at A will result in zero complications but a very low probability of cure. At dose B the complication rate will be low, as will be the cure rate. The cure rate can be high by giving a very large dose, as at C, but then the complication rate will be totally unacceptable.

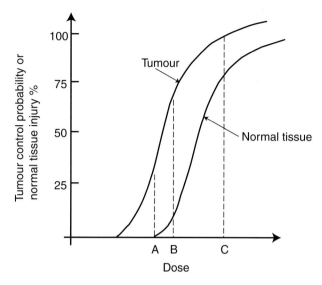

Fig. H1.4 Illustrative sigmoid dose-response curves for tumour control probability and normal tissue sequelae. The dose at *A* will invoke no complications, but will cure only about 27% of the particular tumour. The dose at *curve C* will cure nearly 100% of the particular tumour, but will cause complications in about 77% of patients. The dose at *B* will represent a reasonable clinical compromise

An important practical, ethical and medico-legal implication of Fig. H1.4 is that some incidence of complications is inevitable in the best practice of radiotherapy (Withers 1994). Some tumours may be more resistant to radiation than normal tissues. In such a case, very careful exclusion of as much normal tissue as possible may make it possible to still deliver a tumouricidal dose.

H.1.6
The Importance of Fractionation

Fractionation is a key strategy in conventional radiotherapy where it has proved its ability to spare normal tissues whilst simultaneously doing optimal damage especially to *malignant* tumours. This is due to several radiobiological effects associated with fractionation, like re-oxygenation of anoxic components in tumour tissue, re-entry of tumour cells into a more radiosensitive phase of the cell cycle, and fundamental differences in the DNA repair patterns of tumour cells and "late reacting" normal tissue cells. Rapid repopulation between fractions can negatively influence tumour control (especially in malignant tumours), and the repopulation potential of tumours needs to be taken into account, for example in the treatment of primary and secondary malignant tumours. In rapidly growing tumours it may be advantageous to deliver relatively large doses of radiation per day, but in small doses per fraction to as high a total dose as is commensurate with an acceptable complication rate. Delivering more than one fraction per day without interruption to a tolerably high total dose is termed hyper-fractionation.

H.1.7
The Oxygen Enhancement Ratio – The OER

Anoxic cells are difficult to kill by radiation.

OER = radiation dose needed to kill anoxic cells/dose needed to kill oxygenated cells

Even small malignant tumours contain a percentage of anoxic cells, which can be considered less radio-responsive by a factor of 2 or more. Radiation damage done to well-oxygenated tumours or tissues is larger than the damage inflicted by the same dose of radiation to the same type of tumour containing anoxic cells. This is true for all sparsely ionising radiation like ^{60}Co X-rays, electron- and proton beams.

Tumours over about 1 cm^3 may contain up to 10% of anoxic cells, which may need twice, or even three times the dose required to kill oxygenated cells.

Fractionated radiotherapy, however, offers the opportunity for malignant tumours to reorganise and re-oxygenate and thus to become vulnerable again to lower doses of irradiation.

The OER is higher at high single doses (e.g. 10 Gy or more). At these doses, the OER may be 3.5. At lower (fractionated) doses the OER may have a lower value, typically about 2. Single large doses may therefore be disadvantageous if the target tissue is known to be anoxic (Palcic and Skarsgard 1984).

The OER may be important when normal tissue tolerance, e.g. brain, is considered, since the brain tissue surrounding a tumour may be compressed and anoxic, and will thus be relatively protected (Larson *et al.* 1993). In this regard, the protection offered will be better for photon or gamma rays (linear accelerator or Gamma Knife) than for protons, since the protection may be reduced by a high LET component in the distal dose fall-off region of a proton beam, where the RBE may be as high as 1.5.

Positron emission tomography (PET) is able to give information on the oxygen status of tumours and normal surrounding brain. Where PET is available, it may help to determine a fractionation strategy.

H.1.8
The Gamma Factor, Malignant Lesions and Fractionated Proton Therapy

Malignant lesions are likely to require well-fractionated therapy, this may not be necessary for benign lesions like arteriovenous malformations (Hall and Brenner 1993).

According to Suit (1986, 1992) any increase in the dose delivered using the superior localising qualities of protons is likely to lead to improved local control of the tumour, and improved survival.

The gamma factor is a dimensionless number, which describes how large a change in tumour control probability can be expected for a given relative increase in absorbed dose.

A dose increase of 1% on the linear part of the dose-response curve will result in an increase in tumour control probability of γ per cent (Brahme 1984).

The gradient of the dose-response curve varies with various tumour types, and the gamma factor for, for example, the nasopharynx for T1 and T2 tumours is 2.85, for T3 larynx 3, and for Hodgkin's disease 0.4.

It follows that, if the dose to a tumour could be increased by 20 per cent, then the local control probability will be improved by 40% for a tumour with a gamma factor of 2.

Suit and Westgate (1998) have shown that improved local control of a tumour may translate to a better survival.

Some mean gamma factor values are found in Table H1.3.

Table H1.3 Mean Gamma factors for a variety of tumours

Tumour site	Stage	Gamma	D_{50} (Gy)
Larynx	T1	3.2	51.7
	T3	4.2	67
Bladder	T1–2	1.1	60.2
	T4	2.1	63.2
Prostate	Stage B	4.2	52.7
	Stage C	5.0	63.3
NSCLC	All stages	1.0	49.2
Breast	T2–3	3.4	77.2
Lymphoma		1.0	25.7
Hodgkin		0.4	14

D_{50} is the dose that will control 50% of the tumour

In the above examples, if a 10% dose escalation can be achieved, then T1 and T2 nasopharyngeal tumours should have an increase in local control for a 10% increase in dose of $(10 \times 2.8) = 28\%$.

Hodgkin's disease will, with a 10% increase in dose and with a gamma factor of 0.4, only achieve an improved local control rate of $10 \times 0.4 = 4\%$.

H.1.9
Inhomogeneity of Dose and its Effects

Significant heterogeneity of dose distribution will lead to an increased risk of injury, particularly in late responding normal tissues. This increased risk reflects the "double trouble" of both a higher total dose and a higher dose per fraction in the treatment volume. For example, if a tumour dose is prescribed at the 80% isodose contour, then the total dose and dose per fraction in tissues receiving D_{max} would be 25% (not 20%) higher. A tumour dose per fraction of 2 Gy would deliver 2.5 Gy at D_{max}. The BED, for an α/β ratio of 2 Gy would be equal to 100 Gy for a homogeneous dose of 2 Gy of 25 fractions, but for 25 fractions of 2.5 Gy a part of the lesion would receive a BED dose of 158.6 Gy for an α/β ratio of 2 Gy. In large volumes of irradiated tissue, the severity of the late effect may then be wrongly ascribed to some vague volume effect, whereas it is in fact an effect of inhomogeneity of dose (Withers 1994).

Nedzi et al. (1991) found that for radiosurgery with a linear accelerator, the complication rate correlated very strongly with the large dose inhomogeneity encountered when multiple isocentres were used for treating brain tumours too large for a single isocentre. This issue is important and needs study, as "hot spots" may be beneficial, e.g. to initiate obliteration in AVMs.

H.1.10
Radiosensitisers/Radioprotectors

Radioprotective agents are under investigation in an effort to improve the therapeutic ratio; unfortunately some of these substances, like amifostine, do not penetrate the blood brain barrier.

However, for fractionated therapy for protons or photons in other body sites, amifostine (Grdina *et al.* 1995; Capizzi RL 1996) may be of real value. It is a prodrug, and depends on alkaline phosphatase present in normal cells to activate the prodrug to the active sulphydryl containing radioprotector, which can enter the cell. Malignant cells are defective in alkaline phosphatase, and hence the prodrug is not activated and the active part cannot enter these cells, which are therefore not protected. Amifostine can be given subcutaneously just prior to irradiation before each fraction, and this promising drug may help to enhance the efficacy of fractionated (proton) therapy still further.

Radiosensitisers could turn protons into "the poor man's pions" if they could sensitise tumour cells selectively. The reader is referred to radiobiology texts covering this subject.

H.1.11
Summary

Proton beams have the potential of superior dose localisation, with a consequent increase in the ability to spare normal tissues, and a simultaneous opportunity to escalate the dose. This may lead to improved local control and survival opportunities, especially for malignant lesions. The gamma factor is a dimensionless number indicating the potential escalation in local control rate that may be obtained from a given percentage increase in dose to a malignant lesion.

Protons, like photons, are sparsely ionising and have only a slightly larger relative biological effectiveness (RBE) of 1.1 compared to photons, which are also sparsely ionising. However, there may be a component of more densely ionising slow protons immediately beyond the Bragg peak.

Dose response curves indicate not only the general radiosensitivity of cells and tissues, but also their sensitivity to dose per fraction.

Dose-effect relationships teach us that no dose is totally safe, each attempt at cure carries with it a certain degree of risk. An important practical, ethical and medicolegal implication of this fact is that some incidence of complications is inevitable in the best practice of radiotherapy.

Protons can deliver a homogeneous dose over the target area if the dose is prescribed at the 100% isodose, thus eliminating the trouble of a higher fraction and disproportional large biologically effective dose at D_{max} compared to D_{min} in the target area. Achieving homogeneity across the target however, will expose a larger volume of normal tissues to the penumbra, which in addition may have an RBE larger than 1.1. In the brain this may be of critical importance.

Fractionation has undoubted benefits for the sparing of late reacting tissues and is more effective in eradicating malignant tumours because of re-oxygenation and other phenomena occurring during the protracted treatment process.

Since normal brain tissue is very sensitive to radiation damage and single large doses are especially so, it may help to reduce complications by fractionating the dose wherever possible.

H.1.12
References

Brahme A (1984) Dosimetric precision requirements in radiation therapy. Acta Radiol Oncol 23:379–391

Capizzi RL (1996) The preclinical basis for broad-spectrum selective cytoprotection of normal tissues from cytotoxic therapies by amifostine (Ethyol). Eur J Cancer 32A Suppl 4:S5–16

Grdina DJ, Shigematsu N, Dale P et al. (1995) Thiol and disulphide metabolites of the radiation protector and potential chemopreventive agent WR-2721 are linked to both its anti-cytoxic and anti-mutagenic mechanisms of action. Carcinogenesis 16:767–774

Hall EJ, Brenner DJ (1993) The radiobiology of radiosurgery: Rationale for different treatment regimes for AVMs and malignancies. Int J Radiat Oncol Biol Phys 25:381–385

Hall EJ (1994) Radiobiology for the radiologist, 4th edn., Lippincott, Philadelphia

Larson DA, Flickinger JC, Loeffler JS (1993) The radiobiology of radiosurgery. Int J Radiat Oncol Biol Phys 25:557–561

Lea DE, Catcheside DG (1942) The mechanism of the induction by radiation of chromosome aberrations in tradescantia. J Genet 44:216–245

Miller DW (1995) A review of proton beam radiotherapy. Med Phys 22:1943–1954

Nedzi L, Kooy H, Alexander E et al. (1991) Variables associated with the development of complications from radiosurgery of intracranial tumours. Int J Radiat Onc Biol Phys 21:591–599

Paganetti H, Olko P, Kobus H et al. (1997) Calculation of the relative biological effectiveness for proton beams using biological weighting functions. Int J Radiat Oncol Biol Phys 37:719–729

Palcic B, Skarsgard LD (1984) Reduced oxygen enhancement ratio at low doses of ionising radiation. Radiat Res 100:328–339

Paterson R (1963) The treatment of malignant disease by radiotherapy, 2nd edn. Arnold, London

Robertson JB, Eaddy JM, Archambeau et al. (1994) Relative biological effectiveness and dosimetry of a mixed energy field of protons up to 200 MeV. Adv Space Res 14:271–275

Sinclair WK (1968) Cellular effects of ionising radiation. Cell survival curves. In: Tubiana M, Dutreix J, Wambersie A (eds) Introduction to radiobiology. pp 86–124

Suit HD, Westgate SJ (1986) Impact of improved local control on survival. Int J Radiat Oncol Biol Phys 12:453–458

Suit H (1992) Editors note. Proton Workshop: potential clinical gains by use of superior dose distribution. Int J Radiat Oncol Biol Phys 22:233–234

Tang JT, Inoue T, Yamazaki H et al. (1997) Comparison of radiobiological effective depths in 65-MeV modulated proton beams. Br J Cancer 76:220–225

Urano, M Verhey LJ, Goitein M et al. (1984) Relative biological effectiveness of modulated proton beams in various murine tissues. Int J Radiat Oncol Biol Phys 10:509–514

Withers HR, Thames HD, Peters LJ (1982) Differences in the fractionation response of acutely and late responding tissues. In: Karcher, Kogelnik, Reinartz (eds) Progress in radio-oncology, vol 2. Raven Press, New York, pp 287–296

Withers HR (1985) biologic basis for altered fractionation schemes. Cancer 55:2086–2095

Withers HR (1994) Biology of radiation oncology. In: Tobias JS, Thomas PRM (eds) Current radiation oncology vol 1. pp 5–23

H.2
The Radiobiology of Single Large Fractions

H.2.2
Introduction

Protons are also used for radiosurgical purposes.

The radiobiology of radiosurgery is the radiobiology of single large doses of radiation. The biological damage caused by single large doses is intense and severe, therefore there is understandably a trend away from single large fractions towards multifraction therapy and towards lower effective single doses in order to reduce both acute and late complications.

The rationale for fractionated therapy for malignant lesions is strong on current radiobiological grounds, but not for benign lesions, which themselves consist of late reacting tissue types.

In the past, single doses of 45 Gy were not uncommonly used for radiosurgery, but there is now a trend towards much lower single doses, for example 12–15 Gy for meningiomas.

The increase in the relative biological effectiveness (RBE) of protons with increasing depth in the penumbral zone has been discussed (Chapter H.1.4) and relevant aspects will be discussed further in this chapter.

The oxygen effect is larger for single large fractions than for conventional fractions (up to 3.6).

Tables of fractionated doses to replace single radiosurgical doses for both malignant lesions and non-malignant lesions like AVMs will be discussed.

Since the threshold dose for brain necrosis may be as low as 14 Gy, and since 15 Gy may be the minimum dose needed for the obliteration of AVMs, there is obviously a very narrow therapeutic window, and some complications in many clinical situations may be inevitable.

H.2.2
The Effect of the RBE Variation in the Penumbra of Proton Beams

The RBE has been discussed in the previous chapter on the radiobiology for fractionated proton therapy. In this chapter, the implications of the RBE variation with depth in the Bragg peak zone are emphasised.

Figure H2.1 shows the likely late effect dose for a constant RBE at 1.1 compared to a regularly increasing RBE from 1.1 at the 100% isodose to 1.5 at the 10% isodose for a biologically effective dose (BED) with an α/β ratio = 2. The BED is discussed in Chapter H.3.

Figure H2.2 shows that abnormal metaphases in cells are peaking beyond the Bragg peak (redrawn from Larsson and Kihlman, 1960)

These graphs are illustrative only and should not be used clinically unless specific RBE data can be obtained from the institutional radiobiologist.

The RBE strictly compares the dose of an unknown radiation type to the dose of a known radiation type to do the same biological damage and it should *not be used to compare the effects of different fractionation schemes.* Another term the *radiosurgical*

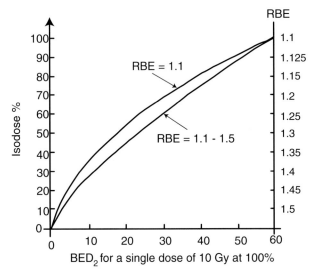

Fig. H2.1 Illustrative influence of the RBE variation in the distal penumbral zone on the biologically effective dose (BED) for late reacting tissues, ($\alpha/\beta = 2$) assuming that the RBE is 1.5 for protons near rest. For a single dose of 10 Gy; 15 Gy; 20 Gy; 25 Gy or 30 Gy, multiply the BED_2 value by 1.0; 1.97; 3.39; 5.20 and 7.40 respectively. The top curve assumes a non-changing RBE for protons with RBE = 1.1. For example, for a single dose of 30 Gy, the BED_2 will be ~163 Gy for the RBE = 1.1, as compared to a BED_2 of ~ 230 Gy at the 60% isodose at RBE = 1.25. Note that no measured data exist for specific % isodose lines. This graph assumes a linear increase of RBE from the 90% to 10% isodoses. See also Table H1.2, Fig. H2.2

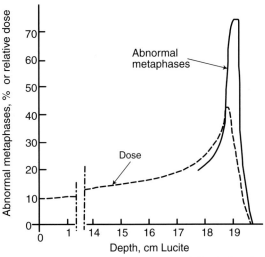

Fig. H2.2 Per cent abnormal metaphases (*solid line*) plotted as a function of depth in Lucite compared with depth-dose distribution (*dotted line*) (Redrawn from Larsson and Kihlman, 1960)

factor (RSF) should rather be introduced to avoid confusion. This is discussed further in Chapter H.3.15.

H.2.3
The Cobalt Gray Equivalent Dose

The dose prescribed for protons and helium ions are expressed in Cobalt Gray Equivalent (CGyE). This abbreviation will be used for the cobalt Gray equivalent throughout this book.

CGyE = Proton dose × proton RBE

Conversely, if a photon dose of 20 Gy is prescribed, the proton dose would be 20/1.1 = 18.2 Gy.

Also see L1.2.13.

H.2.4
The Oxygen Enhancement Ratio and radiobiological effects of Large Single Doses

The oxygen enhancement Ratio (OER) is higher, in the order of 3.5, for single large fractions of 10 Gy or more. Malignant tumours contain anoxic cells in the majority of tumours larger than 1 cm^3. (See Chapter H.1.7). At lower (fractionated) doses the OER may have a lower value, typically about 2. Single large doses may therefore be disadvantageous if the target tissue is known to be anoxic. (Palcic and Skarsgard 1984). A single large dose also does not allow redistribution of cells into a more radiosensitive phase of the cell cycle. (See Chapter H.1.6)

Figure H2.3 illustrates the huge biological effects of single large doses *versus* fractionated equivalent doses for both early and late effects.

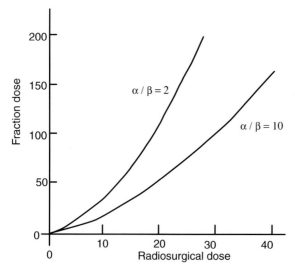

Fig. H2.3 Radiosurgery dose *(horizontal axis)* versus total fractionated radiotherapy dose at 2 Gy per fraction necessary to produce the same radiobiological effect *(vertical axis)*, both for late ($\alpha/\beta = 2$) and for early-responding ($\alpha/\beta = 10$) tissue (Larson et al. 1993)

H.2.5
Inhomogeneity of Dose and Its Effects; the Volume Effect

According to Withers (1994) significant heterogeneity of dose may mean an increased risk of injury, particularly in late responding normal tissues. The inhomogeneity effect may be blamed for complications in large tumour volumes. This effect is discussed in Chapter H.1.9, and in Chapter H.3.7, on the BED.

H.2.6
Fractionated Dose Equivalents to Single Large Doses

Brenner *et al.* (1991) and Hall and Brenner (1993) have suggested fractionated dose equivalents for recurrent brain tumours. This table is given in Appendix P.5.

This table is not suitable for AVMs and we have prepared a table based on the linear-quadratic model first used by Lea and Catcheside (1942) for use with AVMs. The BED_2 can be used directly to calculate the equivalent fractionated doses in stead of using the tables (table P6).

H.2.7
Categories of Lesions in the Brain

Larson *et al.*(1993) and Loeffler *et al.*(1995) divided lesions in the brain into four categories, which are conceptually very useful.

Table H2.1 classification of radiosurgical target types. Modified from Loeffler *et al.* (1995)

Class	Probable α/β ratio of tissue type	α/β of normal tissue in treated volume
AVM	0.6–2	2
Meningioma	2	2
Astrocytoma	10	2
Metastatic	10	2

H.2.7.1
Category 1: AVMs and Similar Lesions

The model target is late responding tissue intertwined with or imbedded within late responding normal tissues.

The vessels of an AVM are late reacting and these vessels do not supply blood to the brain. In AVMs with a compact nidus, these vessels may be separated by only a few glial cells and will be surrounded by normal brain or somewhat anoxic brain tissue. Fractionation is unlikely to confer any benefit. See Chapter H.3 on the BED in this regard.

Because of the vascular nature of AVMs, radiation damage to their vessels is as likely to cause extravasation of protein rich fluid like the vessels of the brain itself. The oedema induced by radiosurgery is ascribed to the localised breakdown of the blood-brain barrier (Mehta *et al.* 1995). This may be the reason for the observation that the volume of tissue, *including the AVM*, receiving a dose of 10 Gy should not exceed 10 cm^3 (Voges *et al.* 1996). An equivalent fractionated dose may nonetheless help to avoid acute oedema and its effects.

AVM-nidi probably contain no functional brain tissues.

H.2.7.2
Category 2: Meningiomas and Similar Lesions

A meningioma is often surrounded by fibrous tissue, not by brain, hence it is less likely to cause symptoms than AVMs (Larson *et al.* 1993). This is borne out by the later work of Voges *et al.* (1996). There is little need for a wide rim of tissue around the target; isodose lines can be drawn tightly around a meningioma or acoustic neuroma and only a single fraction may suffice, although it may be beneficial to treat in two or more fractions simply to avoid acute effects.

The reported results for radiosurgery with these tumours are favourable – 100% actuarial progression free survival at 2 years (Larson *et al.* 1993).

H.2.7.3
Category 3: Low Grade Astrocytoma and Similar Lesions

The model here is that of early responding target tissue embedded within late responding tissues, in which case both normal glial cells and malignant glial cells reside within the target volume. This situation is clearly an indication for fractionated therapy as it is the familiar, usual situation that the radiation oncologist encounters in his or her daily practice. Brenner *et al.* (1991) appreciated that fractionation is beneficial for brain tumours and published a table for equivalent fractionated doses. (See Appendix P.5 and Chapters H.3.8 and H.3.9)

Glioblastoma may infiltrate widely, therefore for primary brain tumours it seems more prudent to fractionate conventionally otherwise the anoxic cells in the tumour that are not killed, will cause regrowth.

H.2.7.4
Category 4: Metastatic Lesions

Fractionation would seem the better course of action. However, a case can be made for a single dose for palliative situations like metastatic lesions. The dose will depend on the volume irradiated and on the amount of normal tissues exposed, as well as on the life expectancy of the patient.

Since metastatic lesions are often small and near spherical, and have little infiltration into the normal brain, no margin may be needed around the lesion. The clinical target volume (CTV) and the planning target volume (PTV) can be identical and a single large dose may be used. Radiosurgery is valuable to control metastatic lesions of all histologies and is especially valuable where the patient's life span may be short. A short life span can be expected if the patient has an uncontrolled primary tumour or multiple metastases extracranially. (See Chapter L.6)

The fractionated equivalent doses of Brenner (table P5.1) could be used.

H.2.8
Summary

Proton beams are sparsely ionising in the plateau region, but this may not be true for protons nearing the end of their range. Therefore the RBE may gradually increase in the distal dose fall-off zone. Since the iso-RBE line may extend further than the isodose lines, this will effectively enlarge the distal fall-off zone, and possibly the entire fall-off zone (penumbra) on treatment plans, depending on the field arrangement. This exposes more brain tissue than intended to unacceptably high doses.

Clinicians should familiarise themselves with the RBE values in the penumbra of their institution's proton beam, and take this into account in determining the volume of normal tissues irradiated.

Single large doses are extremely potent and damaging. It will be prudent to use the simple BED formula (Chapter H.3.3) to calculate the equivalent doses in terms of conventional fractionation in order to assess the biological effects realistically.

Fractionated radiosurgery appears to be beneficial especially for the treatment of malignant tumours.

The BED formalism forms the basis for inter-relating single large doses and the (possibly) equivalent fractionated regimens. Caution is needed in applying any biological model or formula and fine clinical judgement is required at all times.

H.2.9
References

Brenner DJ, Martel, MK, Hall EJ (1991) Fractionated regimes for stereotactic radiotherapy of recurrent tumours in the brain. Int J Radiat Oncol Biol Phys 21:819–824

Fowler JF (1989) The linear-quadratic formula and progress in fractionated therapy. BJR 62:679–694

Hall EJ, Brenner DJ (1993) The radiobiology of radiosurgery: Rationale for different treatment regimes for AVMs and malignancies. Int J Radiat Oncol Biol Phys 25:381–385

Larson DA, Flickinger JC, Loeffler JS (1993) The radiobiology of radiosurgery. Int J Radiat Oncol Biol Phys 25:557–561

Larsson B, Kihlman BA (1960) Chromosome aberrations following irradiation with high energy protons and their secondary irradiation: a study of dose distribution and biological efficiency using root tips of Vicia faba and Allum cepa. Int J Radiat Oncol Biol 2:18–19

Lea DE, Catcheside DG (1942) The mechanism of the induction by radiation of chromosome aberrations in tradescantia. J Genet 44:216–245

Loeffler JS, Larson DA, Shrieve DC, Flickinger JC (1995) Radiosurgery for the treatment of intracranial lesions. In: De Vita, Hellman S, Rosenberg A (eds) Important advances in oncology. JB Lippincott Company, Philadelphia pp 141–156

Mehta M (1995) The physical biologic and clinical basis of radiosurgery. In: Current problems in cancer Vol 19 No 5, Mosby Yearbook St Louis pp 267–328

Palcic B, Skarsgard LD (1984) Reduced oxygen enhancement ratio at low doses of ionising radiation. Radiat Res 100:328–339

Voges J, Treuer H, Sturm V, Buchner C, Lehrke R, Kocher M, Staar S, Kuchta J, Müller RP (1996) Risk analysis of linear accelerator radiosurgery. Int J Radiat Oncol Biol Phys 36:1055–1063

Withers HR (1994) Biology of radiation oncology. In: Tobias JS, Thomas PRM (eds) Current radiation oncology Vol 1 pp 5–23

H.3
The Biologically Effective Dose and Fractionation

H.3.1
Introduction

Single large doses of irradiation have drastic effects, especially on late reacting tissues.

The biologically effective dose (BED) is a very useful yardstick for the clinician to gauge the effects of the different fractionation regimens used for a variety of conditions. This should help the reader to compare the regimens more intelligibly, or enable him or her to assess the influence of changing a regimen.

Chapter H.1 on the Radiobiology of Fractionated Proton Therapy should preferably be read before this chapter.

H.3.2
Notational Convention for the BED

Throughout this book, the relevant α/β ratio is indicated as a subscript. For example, BED_2 means the biologically effective dose for an α/β ratio = 2, and BED_{10} will mean the biologically effective dose for an α/β ratio = 10.

The BED replaced the TDF (time dose fractionation) CRE (cumulative radiation effect) and NSD (nominal standard dose) formalisms (Fowler 1989). The α/β ratio is briefly discussed in Chapters H.3.3 and H.3.4.

For a formal discussion on the LQ-model, from which the BED is derived, the reader is referred to several fine textbooks on radiobiology, and the excellent review articles of Fowler (1989) and Wheldon (1998).

H.3.3
The Linear Quadratic Model of Cell and Tissue Response to Radiation and the BED

Lea and Catcheside (1942) first introduced the LQ model describing the effect of radiation on *tradescantia*. The model is now used widely in day to day radiotherapy practice (Thames and Hendry 1987; Fowler 1989; Whithers 1992; Bentzen 1993) to predict the biological impact of different total doses and changing doses per fraction.

The BED formula is derived from the LQ-model

$$BED = Nd \left(1 + \frac{d}{\alpha/\beta}\right)$$

BED is the biologically effective dose which indicates the amount of damage that a particular fractionation schedule is likely to inflict on a tissue with a particular α/β ratio.

N is the number of fractions

d is the dose per fraction

The α/β ratio is a ratio defining the sensitivity of tissues to the dose per fraction.

The α/β ratio can be inferred from multi-fraction experiments in nonclonogenic systems. The α/β ratio is the dose at which cell killing by the linear (α component) and the quadratic (β components) are equal (Hall 1994).

The BED formula is very easy to use and calculations can often be done by mental arithmetic although for safety's sake they should always be controlled by a second person (Fowler 1989).

H.3.4
Some Commonly used Values for the α/β Ratio

Table H3.1 Some commonly used values for the a/b ratio

α/β Values (Gy)	Site
Acute reacting tissues	
7.0–10.0	Malignant tumours
8.6–12.5	Skin desquamation
6.0–10.7	Small intestine, jejunum clones
8.0–13.0	Colon
Late reacting tissues	
2.3–4.9	Cervical spinal cord
2.3–4.9	Lumbar spinal cord (Fowler 1989)
1.2–1.3	Eye for cataracts
1.6–2.0	Retina
0.6	AVMs (Brenner and Hall 1993)

The α/β ratio for AVM obliteration may be 0.55 Gy assuming an RBE for protons of 1.1. Hall and Brenner (1993) found an α/β ratio of 0.46 for helium ions (RBE = 1.3)

For early effects, a time factor may be included in the calculation of the BED, but the time factor has a very small impact on the BED for late effects.

Biological effective doses for different α/β ratios are not comparable. The BEDs for tissues with different α/β ratios are not to be compared; for example the BED_{10} = 100 Gy and BED_2 = 100 Gy are not at all identical. The actual fractionated schedule for 100 Gy for a BED_{10}, assuming 2 Gy fractions will be obtained from about 42 fractions. The schedule for 100 Gy for a BED_2 assuming a 2 Gy fractions will be obtained from 25 fractions.

The BED is expressed in Gy.

Because of the uncertainties about the values of the α/β ratios, the BED formula should be used with caution and circumspection, and it should not override clinical judgement.

H.3.5
Inhomogeneity of Dose and the Relative Damage

The effects of inhomogeneity of dose for fractionated radiotherapy have been discussed in Chapter H.1.9.

In radiosurgery this effect is amplified, as the inhomogeneity co-efficient can vary from 25 at the 80% prescription isodose (frequently done with linear accelerator radiosurgery) to as much as 170, if the dose is prescribed at the 37% isodose level, at times prescribed with the Gamma Knife.

If the α/β ratio for brain damage is assumed to be $= 2$ Gy, then the inhomogeneity index can be expressed also in terms of the relative damage to late tissues by calculating the biologically effective dose (BED_2) for the D_{max} and dividing it by the BED_2 for D_{min}. This will give an indication of the late damage that can be expected in the lesion centre *versus* the late damage at D_{min}, the prescribed peripheral dose.

Inhomogeneity coefficients (IC) for example for a 10 Gy dose, with the resultant *relative damage* (RD) defined as BED_{2max}/BED_{2min} are shown in Table H3.2.

Table H3.2 The relative damage (*RD*): The effect of inhomogeneity of dose due to varying the prescription isodose, in terms of the biologically effective dose for late reacting tissues expressed as the relative damage, BED_{2max}/BED_{2min}

Prescription isodose percent	D_{max} (Gy)	D_{min} (Gy)	Inhomogeneity co-efficient (IC)	BED_{2max}/BED_{2min} = RD
35	28.6	10	186	7.3
50	20.0	10	100	3.7
65	15.4	10	54	2.2
80	12.5	10	25	1.4
90	11.1	10	11	1.2
100	10.0	10	0	1.0

These values are illustrative only, and they are not substantially different for single doses larger or smaller than 10 Gy.

It can be seen that at the 65% prescription isodose, already more than twice the late damage can be expected in the central area compared to the periphery of the lesion.

H.3.6
Brain Tolerance

Table H3.3 summarises the data discussed below, and the BED is used to compare the data. A fair agreement between widely divergent fractionation schemes and brain tolerance can be discerned. No compensation for the volumes of brain irradiated has been attempted.

Table H3.3 Brain tolerance for single and fractionated doses

Author	Author	Tolerance dose (Gy)	Fraction size (Gy)	BED$_2$
Loeffler	1990	15.5 (mean)	15.5 (mean)	135.6
Engenhart	1994	12–14	12–14	84–112
Marks	1991	60–70	2	120–140
Fulton	1994	80	1 × 3/day	120
Sheline	1986	12–14	12–14	84–112
		35	3.5	96.3
		60	1.71	111.4
		70	1.23	110.8

Loeffler *et al.* (1990) found no case of symptomatic brain necrosis in 18 patients where the treatment volume was small (up to 23 cm^3, diameter 3.5 cm); the median radiosurgical dose was low, 15.5 Gy, median BED$_2$ = 136.5 Gy

Brain tolerance may be as low as 12–14 Gy for single radiosurgical fractions, BED$_2$ = 84–112 Gy. (Engenhart *et al.* 1994).

For conventional fractionation, the risk of brain necrosis increases rapidly with doses above 60–70 Gy, BED$_2$ = 120 Gy to 140 Gy. (Marks *et al.* 1991)

Fulton *et al.* (1992) could achieve doses of up to 80 Gy at 1 Gy fractions three times a day without serious complications (BED$_2$ = 120 Gy), however it is possible that for fraction sizes < 1.2 Gy late tissue sparing may not occur, due to a failure of such a low dose to switch on the repair enzymes (Wheldon *et al.* 1998).

Loeffler *et al.* (1990) experienced significant radionecrotic complications with volumes up to 113 cm^3 (diameter 6 cm) irradiated by single doses of about 22 Gy equivalent, BED$_2$ = 264 Gy.

Brain tolerance has been estimated by Sheline (1986) to be approximately 10–14 Gy in 1 fraction, 35 Gy in 10 fractions, 60 Gy in 35 or 70 Gy in 60 fractions. The BED$_2$ for these regimens are 112 Gy, 96.25 Gy, 111.4 Gy and 110.8 Gy respectively, which affirms the ability of the linear quadratic model to predict late cerebral damage. If these doses are exceeded, the end result will be cerebral necrosis, which usually is a serious and undesirable complication.

It seems that for a variety of fractionation schemes a BED$_2$ of 110 Gy to 120 Gy should be safe, for fractionated or single dose. Whole brain tolerance may be as low as BED$_2$ = 84 Gy.

H.3.7
Optic Nerve and Retinal Tolerance

Table H3.4 summarises the data.

Optic Nerve: For a good review of the radiopathology for conventional radiotherapy, the reader is referred to Alberti *et al.* (1991).

Fraction sizes over 1.9 Gy carries a 47% risk for doses larger than 60 Gy compared to a risk of 11% for fraction sizes < 1.9 Gy each (Parsons 1994) to induce neuropathy.

Table H3.4 Comparative relative biologically effective doses for retinal and optic nerve tolerance.
(r), retinal tolerance
(o), optic nerve tolerance

Author	Date	Dose (Gy)	Fraction number	$BED_{1.6}$ (Gy)
Duke-Elder (r)	1972	35	± 18	78 (tolerance)
Parsons (r)	1983	50	27–20	108–128 (tolerance)
		60	27–20	143–173 (almost all patients developed retinopathy)
Kinyoma (r)	1984	40	10	140 (retinopathy in 3/4 patients with Grave's disease)
Leber (o)	1995	7.5–15	1	43–156
Lunsford (o)	1995	8–9	1	48–57 (tolerance for single dose)
Aristizabal (o)	1977	50	25–20	112–128 (12.5–22% optic nerve damage)
Suit (o)	1992	70	5	682 (50% damage)
Parsons (o)	1983	69	± 38	147 (tolerance to optic nerve for uveal melanomas therapy)
Harris & Levene (o)	1976	42–70	21–35	95–158

Leber *et al.* (1995) found that the optic apparatus was not damaged with single large doses between 7.5 Gy to 15 Gy, or a $BED_{1.6}$ of 43 Gy to 155.6 Gy provided that the nerve was normal and not compromised prior the radiosurgery. The consensus however from many experienced clinicians puts the single fraction tolerance for the optic nerve at 8 Gy.

Optic neuropathy increases sharply after doses over 60 Gy conventionally fractionated therapy ($BED_{1.6} = 135$ Gy). It seems that the doses used for the treatment of uveal melanoma (70 GyE in 5 fractions, 14 GyE per fraction) are bound to cause blindness if the optic nerve is in the field.

Retina: There is a wide range in the clinical severity of retinopathy from little impairment to complete loss of vision. *Pain occurs only if neovascular glaucoma is present at the same time.*

There is a large discrepancy between the single dose tolerance of the retina and the optic nerve compared to conventionally fractionated therapy, despite the predictions of the linear quadratic model, which may therefore underestimate the damage to the optic (and probably other cranial nerves) for single large doses by almost 130%. This means that the BED formalism is not appropriate for large single doses for the optic nerve. For single doses it seems to be wise not to exceed 8 Gy, and for conventionally fractionated doses (2 Gy per fraction or less) 45 Gy–50 Gy. Fractions larger than 2 Gy are especially dangerous.

Since the retinal tolerance is lower than that of the nerve, a dose such as used for treating uveal melanoma (14 GyE × 5) is likely to destroy the retina in the irradiated field. (See Table H3.4)

H.3.8
A Comparison of the Various Dose Levels used to Treat Uveal Melanoma

Table H3.5 The biologically effective dose for late reacting tissues ($BED_{1.6}$) and tumour (BED_{10}) for uveal melanoma CGyE Cobalt Gy equivalent = proton dose × proton RBE

Dose (CGyE)	Fraction number	Fraction Size (CGyE)	$BED_{1.6}$ (Gy)	BED_{10} (Gy)	$BED_{10}/BED_{1.6}$ ratio
50	5	10	362	100	0.27
60	4	15	623	150	0.24
70	5	14	683	168	0.25
80	7	11.4	688	171	0.25

The addition of chemotherapy may potentiate the effects of radiation on the retina. Radiation retinopathy usually manifests within 3 years after radiotherapy (Alberti *et al.* 1991).

Radiation retinopathy is characterised by microaneurysms of the capillaries with "cotton wool spot" intraretinal haemorrhage and leakage from the retinal vessels with hard exudates. Progressive occlusion of small retinal vessels with secondary ischaemia and oedema can be observed subsequently. Chronic changes include vitreous haemorrhage, retinal detachment and optic nerve atrophy with blindness. The fovea is the most sensitive part of the retina.

Parsons *et al.* (1983) discovered two types of radiation optic neuropathy (RON). (1) Injury to the distal end of the nerve which produces an ischaemic neuropathy with disc pallor, oedema and haemorrhages on or around the disc, and (2) more proximal injury producing retrobulbar optic neuropathy without detectable disc oedema and or haemorrhage. Visual loss occurs suddenly and may be complete or partial with progression over a period of several months. Kline *et al.* (1985) reported four cases of RON within 3 years with doses of 46–63.4 Gy in 25–47 fractions.

Nahum *et al.* (1994) is doing a study comparing 70 GyE in 5 fractions (14 Gy × 5) with 50 GyE in 5 (10 Gy × 5) fractions with the aim of reducing normal tissue complications for the same level of control (table H3.8). Even a "small" dose of 50 Gy in 5 fractions is still biologically brutal and it is only because of the very tiny volumes of tissue involved that these doses can yield acceptable clinical results.

H.3.9
Age Related Macular Degeneration

Luther Brady (1996) concludes in an editorial that "Age related macular degeneration represents an exciting new area of potential application of radiation therapy technology in the treatment of a significant and important problem in the United States".

There are potential advantages in using protons instead of photons, as reported by Yonemoto *et al.* (1996). The advantages include sparing of the brain, sinuses or opposite eye. A single lateral proton beam is used, as for photon plans, or a single anterior beam (Moyers *et al.* 1999). We converted doses already published for ARMD to BED values.

Table H3.6 compares the biological impact on the retina and nerve with radiation regimens used up to 1998.

Table H3.6 $BED_{1.6}$ doses for age related macular degeneration (ARMD).
Sas. = Sasai, Bers = Berson, Frei = Freire, Berg = Berginck, Yon = Yonemoto (proton therapy). Bold letters: Probable optic nerve tolerance. Berginck et al. produced some evidence for a dose-response of ARMD lesions. The single dose tolerance for the optic nerve seems to be 8 Gy, $BED_{1.6} = 48$

Patient	No.	Dose (Gy)	Fraction number	Response %	$BED_{1.6}$
Sas	18	10	5	28	23
Bers	52	15	8	79	32.5
Frei	41	15	8	71	32
Sas	18	20	10	39	45
Berg	**10**	**8**	**1**	**50**	**48**
Yon	**19**	**8**	**1**	**58**	**48**
Berg	**10**	**12**	**2**	**70**	**57**
Berg	10	18	3	60	85.5
Berg	10	24	4	80	114.0

H.3.10
The RBE of Protons

This has been discussed in Chapter H.2.2. The relative biological effectiveness (RBE) of a proton beam, increasing with depth, may cause a larger volume than intended to be irradiated and thus to an increase in complications. The impact of the RBE on dose-volume relationships in proton therapy merits careful further study.

H.3.11
The Dose-Volume Histogram

Most treatment plans deviate by 5% or more from the mean dose across the plan. Wheldon *et al.* (1998) point out that the radiobiological effects of inhomogeneities should be built into the algorithms of computer systems so that a biological, and not a physical dose distribution will be presented to the radiotherapist. This perhaps should be a concern of the compilers of future algorithms for planning systems for proton radiotherapy and radiosurgery. In addition, RBE variations and the biological effects should probably be examined in the same context. (See also F1.4)

H.3.12
Summary

The biologically effective dose (BED) is a useful reference value to compare the late *or* early effects of two different fractionation schemes. The resultant "dose" has no real clinical validity as such; it is simply a very useful yardstick taking the effects of fractionation and the α/β ratios of various tissues or organs into account.

Many examples that may be of practical use have been included for ready reference and a framework for the comparison of other fractionation regimens that may be contemplated. The BED illustrates that single large doses can be expected to be relatively ineffective for the treatment of malignant tumours, and have very harsh biological effects.

The BED is useful to emphasise the effects of inhomogeneity of dose across a target. It also shows that an increase in the RBE with depth in the distal penumbra of a proton beam may lead to much more serious late effects in this zone than may be anticipated.

Lastly, the radiobiological implications of variations in dose and RBE in the dose-volume histogram (DVH) should get the attention of the writers of algorithms for planning computers, in order to reflect not only physical dose but biological dose distributions across the area of interest.

H.3.13
References

Alberti W, Aug KK, Calvo W *et al.* (1991) In: Scherer E, Streffer C, Trott KR (eds) Radiopathology of organs and tissues. Springer, Berlin Heidelberg New York

Aristizabal S, Caldwell WL, Avita J (1977) The relationship of time-dose-fractionation factors of complications in the treatment of pituitary tumours by irradiation. Int J Radiat Oncol Biol Phys 2:667–673

Bentzen SM (1993) Quantitative clinical radiobiology. Acta Oncol 32:259–275

Berson AM, Finger PT, Sher DL *et al.* (1996) Radiotherapy for age related macular degeneration: preliminary results of a potentially new treatment. Int J Radiat Oncol Biol Phys 36:861–865

Bergink GJ, Deutman AF, Broek JE van den *et al.* (1995) Radiation therapy for age related subfoveal choroidal neovascular membranes. Doc Ophthalmol 90:67–74

Brady LW (1996) Radiotherapy in macular degeneration. (editorial) Int J Radiat Oncol Biol Phys 36:936

Brenner DJ, Martel MK, Hall EJ (1991) Fractionated regimes for stereotactic radiotherapy of recurrent tumours in the brain. Int J Radiat Oncol Biol Phys 21:819–824

Duke-Elder S (1972) System of ophthalmology, vol 14, part 2. Injuries: nonmechanical injuries Mosby, St Louis, pp 985–999

Engenhart R, Wowra B, Debus J *et al.* (1994) The role of high dose single-fraction irradiation in small and large intracranial arteriovenous malformations. Int J Radiat Oncol Biol Phys 30:521–529

Fowler JF (1989) The linear-quadratic formula and progress in fractionated therapy. BJR 62:679–694

Freire J, Longton WA, Miyamoto CTS *et al.* (1996) External radiotherapy in macular degeneration: technique and preliminary subjective response. Int J Radiat Oncol Biol Phys 36:857–860

Hall EJ (1994) Radiobiology for the radiologist, 4th edn. Lippincott, Philadelphia

Hall EJ, Brenner DJ (1993) The radiobiology of radiosurgery: Rationale for different treatment regimes for AVMs and malignancies. Int J Radiat Oncol Biol Phys 25:381–385

Harris JR, Levene MB (1976) visual complications following irradiation for pituitary adenomas and craniopharyngiomas. Radiology 120:167–171

Kinyoma JL, Kalina RE, Brower SA *et al.* (1984) Radiation retinopathy after orbital irradiation for Grave's disease. Ophthalmology. 102:1473–1476

Kline LB, Kim JY, Ceballus (1985) Radiation optic neuropathy. Ophthalmology 92:1118–1126

Lea DE, Catcheside DG (1942) The mechanism of the induction by radiation of chromosome aberrations in tradescantia. J Genet 44:216–245

Leber KA, Bergloff J, Langman G *et al.* (1995) Radiation sensitivity of visual and oculomotor pathways. Stereotact Funct Neurosurg 64 [Suppl 1]:233–281

Loeffler JS, Alexander E (1990) The role of stereotactic radiosurgery in the management of intracranial tumours. Oncology 4:21–31

Lunsford LD, Witt TC, Kondziolka D *et al.* (1995) Stereotactic radiosurgery of anterior skull base tumours. Clin Neurosurg 42:99–118

Marks LB, Spencer PD (1991) The influence of volume on the tolerance of brain to radiosurgery. J Neurosurg 75:177–180

Moyers MF, Galindo RA, Yonemoto LT, Loredo L (1999) Treatment of macular degeneration with proton beams. Med Phys 26:777–782

Nahum AE, Deanaley DP, Steel GG (1994) Prospects for proton beam radiotherapy. Eur J Cancer 30A:1577–1583

Paganetti H, Olko P, Kobus H *et al.* (1997) Calculation of the relative biological effectiveness for proton beams using biological weighting functions. Int J Radiat Oncol Biol Phys 37:719–729

Parsons JT, Fitzgerald CR, Hood CI *et al.* (1983) The effects of radiation on the eye and optic nerve. Int J Radiat Oncol Biol Phys 9:609–612

Parsons JT, Bova FJ, Fitzgerald CR *et al.* (1994) Radiation optic neuropathy after megavoltage external-beam irradiation: analysis of time-dose factors. Int J Radiat Oncol Biol Phys 30:755–763

Paterson R (1963) The treatment of malignant disease by radiotherapy, second edition. Arnold, London

Sasai K, Murata RM, Mandai M, *et al.* (1997) Radiation therapy for ocular neovascularisation (phase I/II study): Preliminary report. Int J Radiat Oncol Biol Phys 39:173–178

Sheline SE, Wara WM, Smith V (1986) Therapeutic irradiation and brain injury. Int J Radiat Oncol Biol Phys 6:1215–1228

Suit H, Urie M (1992) Proton beams in radiotherapy. J Natl Cancer Inst 84:155–164

Thames HD, Hendry JH (1987) Fractionation in radiotherapy Taylor and Francis, London

Wheldon TE, Deehan C, Wheldon EG, Barrett A (1998) The linear-quadratic transformation of dose-volume histograms in fractionated therapy. Radiother Oncol 46:285–295

Withers HR, Thames HD, Peters LJ (1982) Differences in the fractionation response of acutely and late responding tissues. In: Karcher, Kogelnik, Reinartz (eds) Progress in radio-oncology, vol 2. Raven Press, New York, pp 287–296

Withers HR (1994) Biology of radiation oncology. In: Tobias JS, Thomas PRM (eds) Current radiation oncology, vol 1. pp 5–23

Yonemoto LT, Slater JD, Friedrichson EJ *et al.* (1996) Phase I/II study of proton beam irradiation for the treatment of subfoveal choroidal neovascularisation in age related macular degeneration: treatment techniques and preliminary results. Int J Radiat Oncol Biol Phys 36:867–871

I Dose-Volume Relationships in Proton Therapy and Radiosurgery for Arteriovenous Malformations, Skull Base Meningiomas and Recurrent Malignant Gliomas

I.1
Introduction

Several dose-volume risk prediction models have been published. The better known models include one for particle therapy, linear accelerator based radiosurgery, several models for the Gamma Knife and a brief recommendation from the RTOG for recurrent malignant brain tumours.

Up to 1997, none of these models predicted the complication rate adequately. Since 1997, several more models, mainly for AVMs treated by Gamma Knife, appeared in the literature which predict the probabilities for AVM obliteration and complication induction.

In this chapter the available models, the importance of the penumbra and the prescription isodose, the volume of brain irradiated to a high dose and the minimum dose delivered to this volume will be discussed.

It seems that a distinction should be drawn between intraparenchymal lesions such as AVMs and skull base lesions such as meningiomas and acoustic neuromas, because the damage to vessels may contribute to the induction of complications, but the relatively avascular consistency of meningiomas may not. Fortunately, the doses required to control meningiomas may be quite low, in the order of 12–15 Gy, considerably lower than may be the case for AVMs.

Recently published implied dose-volume constraints have been used by us to construct dose-volume tables and graphs. These are meant to be used as an additional control in conjunction with all the existing models. The reader is urged not to rely solely on one dose-volume model but rather to consult all of them and err on the safe side, as the brain is in reality exquisitely sensitive to large single doses of irradiation.

Definition of Terms

- PTV is the planning target volume [12].
- CTV is the clinical target volume [12].
- PW is the width of the penumbra, in centimetres, stated from the 90% to the 10% isodose. The PW should in practice be determined from the treatment plan.
- EP is the effective penumbral width, i.e. the part of the total penumbra utilised at each dose level prescribed and it is specific for each treatment plan.
- CI is the critical isodose defining the 10 Gy dose on the surface of a spherical volume of 10 cm^3.
- CV is the critical spherical volume of 10 cm^3 within the dose-volume constraint of [10 Gy, 10 cm^3].
- CVr is the radius of the critical volume and is equal to 1.336 cm.

- PTVr is the complementary radius contributed by the PTV.
- EPr is the complementary radius contributed by the effective penumbra.
- K-index is the minimum single dose times the cube root of the PTV, expressed in Gy-cm.

I.2
Arteriovenous Malformations

The brain is much more sensitive than previously appreciated (Engenhart *et al.* 1994)

Many questions regarding dose-volume relationships are still unclarified (Corm *et al.* 1996).

Karlsson and Lax (1999) pointed out the existing problems of predicting a specific outcome for a specific patient, and to address this problem devised suitable computer software discussed below.

A lesion of 3 cm diameter (14 cm^3) is regarded by Loeffler (1995) as the upper lesion size treatable without complications.

For large AVMs the optimal relationship of dose and volume to obliteration, complications and haemorrhage is not well defined (Miyawaki *et al.* 1999).

The incidence of PRI changes and clinical complications rose with increasing treatment volume. For treatment volumes > 14 cm^3 receiving > 16 Gy the incidence of PRI changes was 72% and the incidence of radiation necrosis requiring resection was 22%. Treatment was by 6 MV linac. A high K-index correlated with complications ($p < 0.001$). For large AVMs the UCSF (University of California at San Francisco) is currently investigating the use of staged radiosurgical procedures separated by six or more months.

I.2.1
Kjellberg's Model for Protons

Kjellberg (1983) published dose-volume curves predicting a 1% risk of cerebral necrosis. The isoeffect risk prediction line relates total dose to beam diameter for proton therapy as shown in Fig. I2.1.

This resulting straight line can be regarded as a reasonable but not infallible guide, since complications occurred below the line, which should have been predicted by the model, but were not. The model has been criticised because of a reasonably small database and because primate data were included in the analysis. The beam diameter is not an accurate reflection of the volume of the planning target volume (PTV), (ICRU Report 50, 1993) which is an important parameter. The PTV is the volume defined by the prescription isodose surrounding the lesion enclosing the clinical target volume (CTV). The Kjellberg-model is unlikely to predict correctly for other radiosurgical modalities like the Gamma Knife, and *vice versa,* Gamma Knife models are unlikely to predict accurately for proton therapy, since the penumbras are not identical, the dose homogeneities are not similar and there may be some RBE (radiobiological effectiveness) variations for protons (RBE = 1.1–1.3) from the RBE = 1 for photons. In addition, the habits of choosing prescription isodoses vary considerably. For proton therapy the 90% prescription isodose (PI) is often used, for the linear accelerator the 80% and for the Gamma Knife the 50% isodose.

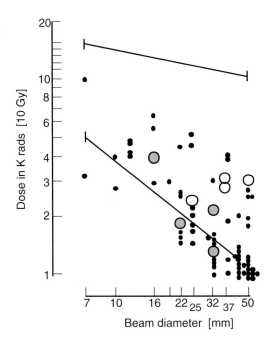

Fig. I2.1
Distribution of post-treatment complications among 74 patients with arteriovenous malformations, according to the determinants of isoeffective doses of proton beam irradiation. Both vertical and horizontal scales are logarithmic. The upper and lower slanted lines represent approximately the 99th percentile and first percentile for isoeffective doses respectively for ionising necrosis of brain.
Open circles indicate the first four, comparatively serious, complications, crosshatched circles the next four complications, which were comparatively mild and solid circles indicate patients without complications. (Redrawn from RN Kjellberg *et al.* 1983, The New England Journal of Medicine 309:269–273)

I.2.2
Dose-volume Observations of Voges *et al.* (1996)

Voges *et al.* (1996) observed, from the data generated by total of 133 patients, that for linear accelerator based radiosurgery, no complications occurred if the volume of the AVM plus surrounding brain did not exceed 10 cm^3 irradiated to a minimum of 10 Gy at the 10 Gy isodose. A very sharp increase in complications occurred as soon as this [10 Gy 10 cm^3] constraint was exceeded. Therefore the [10 Gy 10 cm^3] constraint may represent a base-line dose-volume relationship.

For skull base lesions, they found that the lesion volume *per se* was not important, but that if more than 10 cm^3 of brain outside the lesion received more than 10 Gy, complications were likely to occur. The majority of their patients' complications occurred below the 1% necrosis line of Kjellberg, *so that the Kjellberg model under-predicted the risks for linear accelerator based radiosurgery*. It seems that the integrated logistic model of Flickinger (see below) also underestimates the risk of single dose irradiation in AVM patients (Voges *et al.* 1996), but overestimates the risk for skull base tumours.

I.2.3
Flickinger's Models for the Gamma Knife

Flickinger *et al.* (1991) formulated the logistic regression dose-volume prediction model, with isoeffect lines predicting a 3% risk of brain necrosis. They plotted the average

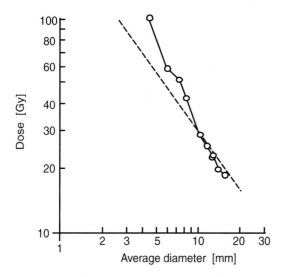

Fig. I2.2 A 3% dose-volume isoeffect curve for brain necrosis from a single-fraction Gamma Knife radiosurgery averaged from predictions by the linear quadratic and exponential versions of the integrated logistic formula. Dose is represented by the minimum dose (Gy) to the treatment volume. The average diameter (mm) is that of the treatment isodose volume treated. For comparison the 1% isoeffect line for brain necrosis from proton beam irradiation described by Kjellberg et al (1983) is included (dotted line).
(Redrawn from JC Flickinger *et al.* 1991, Acta Oncologica 30:363–367)

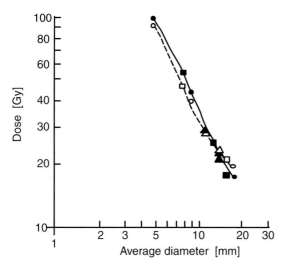

Fig. I2.3 Dose-volume isoeffect curves for a 3% risk of brain necrosis from a single-fraction Gamma Knife radiosurgery predicted by the linear quadratic and exponential versions of the integrated logistic formula. Dose is represented by the minimum dose (Gy) to the treatment volume used. The circles, squares and triangles represent doses prescribed to the 50%, 65% and 80% isodose volumes respectively for a single isocentre radiosurgery with either 4, 8, 14 or 18 mm diameter fields. The average diameter refers to the average diameter (mm) of the treatment isodose volume (50%, 65% or 80%).
(Redrawn from JC Flickinger, 1991, Acta Oncologica 30:363–367)

beam diameter (based on the PTV) *versus* the total dose, shown in Fig(s). I2.2 and I2.3, with permission from the publishers. Kjellberg's line is superimposed on Fig. I2.2 of Flickinger for comparison. They also point out that the limited data available make accurate prediction difficult, and that *"there is no substitute for clinical judgement."*

The above two models have been used widely to guide clinicians but neither the Kjellberg 1% nor the Flickinger logistic regression model predicts postradiosurgery imaging (PRI) changes correctly (Flickinger *et al.* 1997), who found that the complication rate (symptomatic PRI change) is dependent on the volume of tissue receiving 12 Gy, as well as on the region of brain treated. Damage to the target (AVM nidus) may contribute to the observed radiosurgical complications. The same effect was not obvious for skull base lesions (Fig(s). D2.4 and D2.5), corroborating the observations of Voges *et al.* (1996).

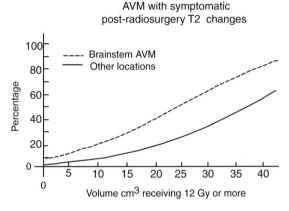

Fig. I2.4
Risk prediction curves derived from multivariate logistic regression analysis that correlate volume receiving 12 Gy to the to probability of developing symptomatic post-radiosurgery imaging changes in patients with brainstem AVM (upper dotted curve) compared to other locations (lower solid line, Gamma Knife). (Redrawn from JC Flickinger *et al.* 1997, Int J Radiat Oncol Biol Phys 38:485–490)

Dose inhomogeneities across the target, e.g. with Gamma Knife radiosurgery, may contribute to the development of complications. There is an increased risk of injury to the normal tissues with significant heterogeneity of dose distribution (Withers 1994). Large fractions damage blood vessels easily, and damaged blood vessels leak protein and will cause oedema and complications. Damaged fibrous material in a meningioma may not cause extravasation and oedema to the same extent.

The onset of vasogenic oedema, symptomatic or asymptomatic, may coincide with the development of an endarteritis associated with thrombosis. The thrombosis may cause severe alterations in the haemodynamics of the area, localised breakdown of the blood-brain barrier, vasogenic oedema and possibly, a mass effect (Lo 1993). For AVMs the high central dose with the inhomogeneity caused by prescribing at, for example the 50% isodose, may be advantageous since it may initiate a process of vascular obliteration which will then spread centrifugally, making AVM obliteration more efficient.

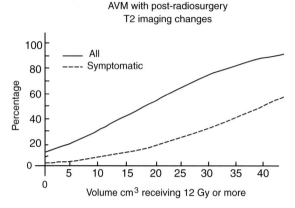

Fig. I2.5
Risk prediction curves derived from multivariate logistic regression analysis that correlate 12 Gy volume to risk for developing all (symptomatic and asymptomatic) post-radiosurgery imaging changes (upper solid curve) and symptomatic post radiosurgery imaging changes (lower dotted curve) for AVM patients (Gamma Knife). (Redrawn from JC Flickinger *et al.* 1997, Int J Radiat Oncol Biol Phys 38:485 490)

From the graph of Flickinger *et al.* (1997), (Fig. I2.4) it can be determined that for a 10 cm^3 volume, the risk of complications (symptomatic post radiosurgery imaging change or PRI) is about 9% for brain lesions and double that (about 18%) for brainstem lesions.

This could be construed as a constraint of [12 Gy 10 cm^3] defining a certain level of complications and appears to be congruent with the observations of Voges *et al.* (1996).

I.2.4
Dose-volume Analysis of Lax and Karlsson (1996)

Lax and Karlsson (1996) based their dose-volume predictions on a large patient database of more than 820 AVMs treated by Gamma Knife. The plot is shown in Fig. I2.6. The average dose to a volume of 20 cm^3 was plotted against the complication rate.

I.2.5
Karlsson and Lax *et al.* (1997)

Karlsson and Lax previously reported on a model predicting the risk for radiation-induced complications following Gamma Knife radiosurgery for AVMs. *No factor other than the dose distribution was related to the risk.* The aim of the study was to define if other parameters are of importance for the risk of complications. Neither age nor gender influenced the risk of complications. Centrally located AVMs had a higher, and peripheral a lower incidence of complications as compared to the calculated risk, and a previous haemorrhage reduced the risk of complications. Flickinger *et al.* (1999) however, found that patients with a history of prior haemorrhage had a lower symptom resolution rate.

Karlsson and Lax concluded that the risk of complications following radiosurgical treatment of AVMs is dependent on the clinical history, AVM location and whether the patient has received radiation earlier.

Karlsson, Lax *et al.* (1999) published graphs predicting the probability of AVM obliteration by Gamma Knife after examining various models and came to the conclusion that the obliteration rate, as well as the complication rate, can be accurately predicted. They have written computer software, which gives the *probabilities for obliteration and complication for a particular clinical situation* as well as for several alternative dose-volume relationships. Provided that the software is available this looks like a very useful model for Gamma Knife users with identical equipment and identical prescription habits, to titrate the risks for individual patients.

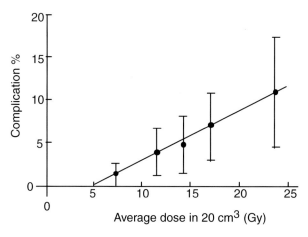

Fig. I2.6 Incidence of complications shown by the point with 95% confidence interval. The line is a fit to the points. Total material includes 862 treatments. (Redrawn from Lax and Karlsson, 1996, Acta Oncologica 35:49–55)

I.3
General Discriminants Influencing Dose-volume Relationships

The concept of a constraint (fixed volume of brain irradiated to a fixed dose) and associated with "zero" complications is attractive, as it appears to provide a much needed clinical reference value.

Figure I3.1 shows a graphic representation of the gross tumour (lesion) volume (GTV), the clinical target volume (CTV) and the planning target volume PTV (ICRU report 50 (1993), for three different penumbral widths (see below).

All three PTVs of largely different volume could be expected to have "zero" complications.

The penumbra of a beam and thus the penumbra on a treatment plan will have a very significant influence on the volume of brain irradiated outside the PTV (planning target volume) and the larger this volume, the greater the risk of complications for any particular radiosurgical dose.

CVr = PTVr + EPr

Radius of 10 cm³ = 1.34 cm (CVr)

(EP = Effective penumbra)

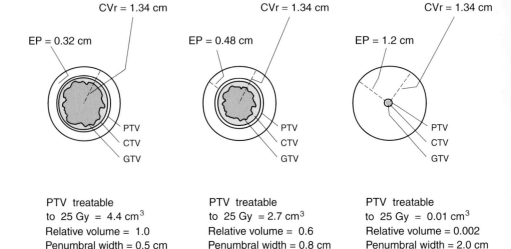

PTV treatable to 25 Gy = 4.4 cm³	PTV treatable to 25 Gy = 2.7 cm³	PTV treatable to 25 Gy = 0.01 cm³
Relative volume = 1.0	Relative volume = 0.6	Relative volume = 0.002
Penumbral width = 0.5 cm	Penumbral width = 0.8 cm	Penumbral width = 2.0 cm
Dose fall-off = 16% per mm	Dose fall-off = 10% per mm	Dose fall-off = 4% per mm

Fig. I3.1 The effect of penumbral width on the volumes treatable for spherical lesions within the [10Gy, 10 cm³] constraint. The figures show that the same risk may apply to lesions (PTVs) differing by a factor of 500 in volume. All three figures were calculated with the prescription isodose = 80%. Also see Fig. M2.2 and P3.1

The optimum dose gradient will allow the dose to decrease from the target dose to 50% of the target dose over a distance of 3 mm. Figure I3.2 shows a drawing from an illustrative proton therapy plan with 3 co-planar beams, and where the beams overlap it is clear that the dose fall-off is especially poor, and this phenomenon may extend the critical volume into the danger zone. It may be wise to arrange the fields wherever possible, in such a way that the dose fall-off in all axes is minimised, and where this is not possible to assess the possible effects very carefully. The dose fall-off on this plan varies from 5-3% per mm dose fall-off, with penumbral widths of 16–26 mm.

According to Voges *et al.* (1996), for intraparenchymal lesions where tissue volumes *more than* 10 cm³ received 10 Gy or more, complications occurred in 23.7% of patients; 37.5% of these in AVM patients.

The prescription isodose has an influence, since the lower the prescription isodose is, the larger the inhomogeneity across the target will be. Perhaps more importantly, the lower the prescription isodose, the smaller the effective penumbra outside the PTV, and the less brain tissue irradiated for a particular prescribed dose. (See calculation on the critical isodose (CI) below.)

The lesion shape has an influence, since the more irregular the shape of the lesion is, the more difficult it is to conform the isodose to the shape. The consequence is that

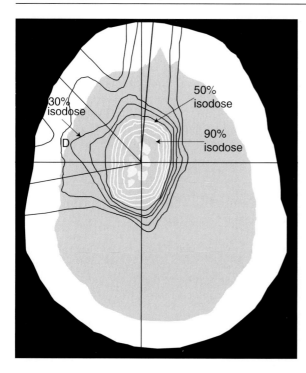

Fig. I3.2 A proton plan for an arteriovenous malformation with central calcifications. Dose fall-off where beams overlap cause relatively large increases in the volume of brain irradiated. All 3 beams are co-planar. At the 50% isodose the dose fall-off is about 4–5% per mm. Point "D marks the shallowest dose fall-off, with about 2% dose fall-off per mm. Non-co-planar arrangement of the beams, with one beam coming from craniad, will improve the plan significantly.

Table I3.1 Dose-volume constraints. LA = Linear accelerator, av = average dose, CGyE = Cobalt Gray Equivalent dose in Gray for protons, K-index [22] = Minimum dose (Gy) multiplied by the cube root (cm) of the volume

Author	Dose Gy	Volume cm³	Complication Rate	K-index Gy-cm
Voges [3] LA	10	10	0	21.5
	> 10	> 10	Sharp increase	> 21.5
Flickinger [6] LA	12	10	8–10% (Brain)* 16–20% (Brainstem)	25.8
Engenhart [9] LA	>20	>4	Sharp increase	31.7
Lax & Karlsson [7]	10 (av)	20	3%	27.1
	12 (av)	20	5%	32.5
	20 (av)	20	9%	54.3
Fabrikant [18]	25 CGyE	>13	50%	58.7
Steinberg [19]	>24 CgyE	>13	All complications in these patients	56.4
Miyawaki [21]	> 16	14	80%	> 38.6
Friedman [24]	25	7	Permanent complications	47.8
	20	14		48.2

* As read from the published tables

an additional volume of normal tissue is irradiated. For many situations, this volume may be 1.5–3 times as large as the lesion volume itself (Verhey *et al.* (1998). However this will not influence the use of the graphs, which are based on the PTV.

The total dose obviously will make the critical volume larger for increasing doses.

Some convergence of data is evident from several divergent publications and the available data point to some dose-volume limit in the general order of magnitude suggested by Voges *et al.* (1996), and Flickinger *et al.* (1997), (Table I3.1). Interestingly, the [10 Gy 10 cm^3] constraint also has the lowest K-index (Karlsson *et al.* 1997). The K-index is the minimum single dose in Gy times the cube root of the PTV and is expressed in Gy-cm.

I.4
Illustration of the Effect of the Penumbra and the Prescription Isodose on a Volume of Brain Tissue Constrained to [10 Gy 10 cm^3]

Figure I3.1 illustrates the effect of a beam or plan with effective penumbrae of 0.32 cm to 1.2 cm for a single radiosurgical dose of 25 Gy. For a generally spherical radiosurgical treatment volume, the radius of the 10 cm^3 volume of the [10 Gy and 12 Gy 10 cm^3] constraint is 1.336 cm. It is assumed that the conformation of PTV to CTV is optimal, but that the PTV will be larger than the CTV.

The radius of 1.34 cm (to 2 decimal points) will consist of the complementary radii due to the residual penumbra (RPr) and the radius of the PTV (PTVr), therefore:

CVr = PTVr + EPr

where:

CVr is the radius of 10 cm^3 volume component of the two constraints mentioned.
PTVr is the complementary radius of the planning target volume and
EPr is the complementary radius of the effective penumbra or fall-off in dose between the PI (prescription isodose) and the CI (critical isodose).

I.5
Methodology for Calculating the Effects of the Prescription Isodose and Penumbra on the Planning Target Volume Treatable to Safe Doses Within the Constraints of [10 Gy 10 cm^3]

I.5.1
The Critical Isodose (CI)

The concept of a constraining dose (10 Gy) necessitates the introduction of the concept of the "critical isodose". The critical isodose (CI) is the isodose defining the 10 Gy limiting or "critical" isodose.

Th CI is determined by dividing the limiting dose (10 Gy) by the single dose prescribed, and multiplying the result by the prescription isodose per cent.

For example, if a single radiosurgical dose of 18 Gy is prescribed to the 90% isodose, the CI will be:

$$CI = \frac{10 \text{ Gy} \times PI\%}{18 \text{ Gy}} = \frac{10}{18} \times 90\% = 50\% \tag{1}$$

The CI therefore will define the 10 Gy isodose on the transverse beam plot (Fig. 13.2) or on the treatment plan.

The "Effective Penumbra" (EP) and how to determine it

The EP represents the portion of the penumbra actually "used", subject to the conditions imposed by the [10 Gy, 10 cm^3] constraint.

$$EP = \frac{(PI - CI)\ \% \times PW}{80\%} \tag{2}$$

Where   EP = the Effective penumbra
         PI = the prescription isodose %
         CI = the critical isodose
         PW = penumbral width (90%–10%)

"80%" is the denominator and is the dose-fall-off over which the PW is stipulated, in this case from the 90% to 10% isodose lines.

Calculation of the PTVr within a constraining spherical volume of 10 cm^3

The PTVr depends on the EPr as follows: The radius of the critical volume (CVr) of 10 cm^3 is 1.336 cm, therefore
$$CVr = EPr + PTVr = 1.336 \text{ cm} \tag{3}$$

Where CVr is the radius of the critical constraining volume EPr is the complementary radius contributed by the "effective penumbra" EP
PTVr is the radius of the planning target volume, which depends on EPr.

Determination of PTVr and the PTV (planning target volume)

If   CVr = 1.336 cm = [PTVr + Epr]

then   PTVr = [1.336 – Epr] $\tag{4}$

Since the formula for the volume of a sphere = $\frac{4}{3} \pi r^3$, then
$$PTV = \frac{4}{3} \pi (PTVr)^3 \tag{5}$$

Construction of the Dose-Volume Tables and Graphs

The above formulae have been used to calculate a series of planning target *volumes* (PTVs) for various prescribed *doses* from 60 Gy down to 10 Gy, for four prescription isodose levels (90%, 80% 65% and 50%) and six penumbral widths (PWs) likely to be encountered on treatment plans.

The penumbra can also be described as the dose fall-off in percent per millimetre. We have chosen representative penumbral widths of 3 cm (2.7% per mm dose fall-off), 2.0 cm (4% per mm fall-off), 1.6 cm (5% per mm fall-off), 1.3 cm (6.2% per mm fall-off), 1.0 cm (8% per mm fall-off), 0.8 cm (10% per mm fall-off) and 0.5 cm (20% per mm fall-off), but not 1.3 cm and 0.5 cm for the skull base graphs. Bova *et al.* (1999) use a simular approach to calculate the "UFX-Index"

Skull Base Lesions

For skull base lesions like meningiomas, it seems that, if the dose to 10 cm^3 of brain *around the lesion* is (10 Gy, the complication rate is likely to be low [3]. In general, the single doses needed to control these lesions have been adjusted downwards as experience was gained by various workers. The recommended doses are in the range of 12–14 Gy, with much reduced risks. Recently Flickinger (1996) indicated that a dose of 13 Gy for acoustic neuromas might suffice.

In order to calculate the volumes of spherical meningiomas, arbitrary volumes from 0.1 cm^3 to 30 cm^3 were used as a point of departure. To these volumes were added a volume of 10 cm^3 (representing the limiting volume of brain that can be irradiated safely to 10 Gy) and the process as outlined above repeated.

$$EPr + PTVr = \text{radius of (lesion volume} + 10 \text{ cm}^3) \tag{6}$$

For example if a PTV of 1.5 cm^3 needs to be irradiated, the PTVr = 0.71 cm, then

$$EPr + PTVr = \text{radius of } (10 \text{ cm}^3 + 1.5 \text{ cm}^3),$$

then   Epr = radius of (11.5 cm^3) – PTVr
i.e.   EPr = 1.40 – 0.71 = 0.69 cm

With the penumbra width known and combining equations (1) and (2) a safe dose value which will conform to specified values of prescription isodose and dose fall-off rate can be calculated using the formula

$$\text{Safe dose, D} = \frac{PI \times D(\text{min})}{[PI - (EPr \times DF \times 10)]} \tag{7}$$

where D(min) = minimum dose to limiting volume (10 Gy)
       PI   = prescription isodose
       DF   = dose fall-off per mm
       EPr   = penumbra width (mm)

I.5.2
Direct (Computer) Determination of the PTV

The PTV can be obtained directly from the planning computer. The CI can be calculated as shown above.

PTVr + Epr can the be measured directly by the computer, and if PTVr + Epr (average) > 1.34 cm (13.4 mm), then there is by definition an increased risk for complication induction.

In such a case, if PTVr + Epr exceeds 1.34 cm, then the radiosurgeon may be well advised to be very cautious. Clinical judgement and experience will have to supervene.

I.6
Dose-volume Graphs Based on Voges (1996)

As an additional guide to the clinician, supplemental to existing guidelines discussed above, we have prepared graphs to facilitate the determination of the dose volume relationships for AVMs to individualise dose volume options for specific clinical situations. The graphs for AVMs are shown in Fig. I6.1.

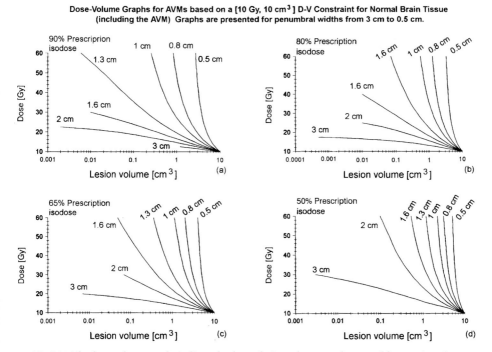

Fig. I6.1 The dose-volume graphs indicate that larger lesion volumes can be treated for any given dose, the smaller the penumbra and/or the prescription isodose is.

For example, if for a small lesion, the PTV is 2.0 cm^3, the tables (Appendix P.3.1) suggest several dose-volume options. (Fig. I6.1)

The result obtained from dose-volume combinations read off from the graphs will then have to be compared with all the available risk prediction models. In this way all possible precautions can be taken to ensure an adequate dose with minimal risks to the patient.

The corresponding graphs for skull base lesions are represented in Fig. I6.2 and tables in P3.2.

Dose-volume graphs for skull base lesions based on a [10 Gy, 10 cm³] D-V constraint for normal brain tissue (excluding the skull base). Graphs are presented for penumbral widths from 3 cm to 0.8cm.

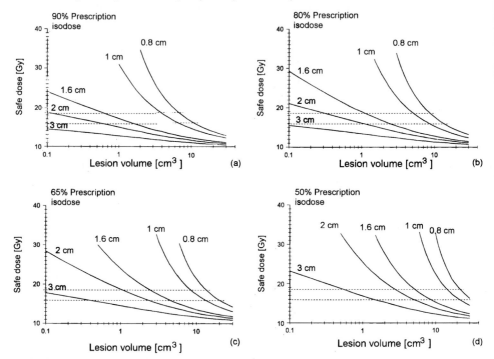

Fig. I6.2 The zone between the dotted lines indicate the probably effective single dose range of 13–16 Gy for the control of meningiomas and acoustic neuromas.

I.7

Practical Implementation of the Various Dose-volume Relationships Available Presently for AVM Radiosurgery

Table I7.1 illustrates how the diverse dose-volume relationships from Table I3.1 may be reconciled by the dose-volume relationships based on the [10 Gy 10 cm³] constraint.

The K-index is also a single, generalised index, and our dose-volume tables and graphs can accommodate various K-indices, depending upon the penumbra and prescription isodose.

1. After obtaining the several available dose volume options based on the constraints from the tables (Appendix P3) or graphs (Fig(s). I6.1 a–d, I6.2 a–d) for a PTV calculated by the planning computer, for protons, firstly compare the result to Kjellberg *et al*.'s (1983) dose volume isoeffect graph (Fig I2.1 above).

2. Control the results against the logistic regression dose-volume models of Flickinger *et al*. (1989). (Fig I2.2, I2.3 above)

Table I7.1 A comparison of the Kjellberg (1983) Flickinger (1989) Engenhart (19949 and Fabrikant (1992) dose-volume data with the [10 Gy, 10 cm³] constraint prescribed at the 80%, 65% and 50% iso-doses for 5 different penumbral widths as obtainable from the treatment plans (30 mm, 20 mm, 16 mm, 10 mm and 8 mm).

Radiosurgical Dose (Gy)	Kjellberg (1983)	Flickinger (1989)	Engenhart (1994)	Fabrikant (1992)	PI	[10 Gy, 10 cm³] Penumbral Widths (cm) Percent dose fall-off per millimetre				
						3 cm 2.7%	2 cm 4.0%	1.6 cm 5.0%	1.0 cm 8.0%	0.8 cm 10%
60 Gy										
Beam diam	Na	6-7 mm	Na	Na						
PTV	Na	0.1 cm³	Na	Na	80%	0	0	0	0.3	1.3
					65%	0	0	0.1	1.2	2.0
					50%	0	0.1	0.5	0.54	3.19
30 Gy										
Beam diam	13 mm	11 mm								
PTV		0.7 cm³	Na	Na	80%	0	0.01	0.22	1.2	2.6
			Na	Na	65%	0	0.1	0.43	2.1	3.1
			Na	Na	50%	0	0.5	1.26	3.2	4.2
25 Gy										
Beam diam	16 mm	12 mm	Na	Na						
PTV	Na	0.9 cm³	Na	13 cm³	80%	0	0.01	0.2	**0.7**	1.7
					65%	0	0.20	**0.7**	2.5	3.6
					50%	0	**0.84**	1.7	3.7	4.7
20 Gy										
Beam diam	22 mm	14 mm								
PTV		1.4 cm³	4 cm³	Na	80%	0	0.2	0.6	0.7	3.3
					65%	0	0.6	**1.4**	3.4	**4.3**
					50%	0.3	**1.5**	2.5	**4.5**	5.4
15 Gy										
Beam diam	27 mm	18 mm								
PTV	Na	3.1 cm³	Na	Na	80%	0.16	1.3	2.2	4.3	5.1
					65%	0.60	2.1	**3.1**	5.1	5.6
					50%	1.51	**3.3**	4.2	6.0	6.7
12 Gy										
Beam diam	Na	Na								
PTV	Na	10 cm³ (1997)*	Na	Na	80%	3.0	4.8	5.5	6.6	7.7
					65%	3.8	4.9	6.0	7.0	7.8
					50%	4.0	6.0	7.0	8.0	8.5

3. Compare the result also to the graphs of Lax and Karlsson and their computer predictions, if the software is available, before finally deciding on a dose for a particular lesion. (Fig I2.6 above)

4. Also consult the Spetzler-Martin grading system and its suggested alternative (Appendix P1 and P2), keeping in mind that extremely sensitive areas like for example the brain stem should be approached with extreme caution.

5. Determine directly from the planning computer whether PTVr + Epr > 1.34 cm. If so the [10 Gy 10 cm³] constraint is violated, and extreme caution should be exercised.

6. A new tool for dose conformity evaluation of radiosurgery treatment plans have recently been described by Leung *et al.* (1999) and it is described as a useful tool for evaluating rival plans. The proposed method has demonstrated the effectiveness in conformity evaluation and supplements the integral dose-volume histogram.

I.8
Recurrent Previously Irradiated Brain Tumours

For recurrent, previously irradiated brain tumours, the RTOG found the maximally tolerable radiosurgical doses (MTDs) for various tumour diameters as shown in Table I8.1. (Shaw *et al.* 1996)

Obviously these patients are not expected to live for more than about 10 months, and the doses are higher than those recommended for benign lesions.

Table I8.1 The maximum tolerable radiosurgical doses for various tumour diameters for recurrent previously irradiated brain tumours

Lesion diameter	Approximate volume	Gy (cm^3)
< 20 mm	4.3	27
21–30	4.4–14	21
31–40	14.1–33.5	15

I.9
The Effects of Imperfect Conformation

Hamilton *et al.* (1995) compared static conformal fields with multiple non-coplanar arcs to a single isocentre based on linear accelerator technology. The volume receiving the prescription isodose (the PTV) was found to be more than 3.5 times larger than the target volume for all the plans investigated. This means that for irregularly shaped targets, the PTV volumes calculated at each dose level for the idealised spherical lesions, should be divided by 3.5 to obtain the "safe *lesion* volume" for linear accelerator radiosurgery.

Verhey *et al.* (1998) compared radiosurgery treatment modalities (linear accelerator, Gamma Knife and protons) based on the physical dose distributions for lesions of irregular shape for volumes of 1 cm^3 to 26 cm^3. The average conformity index for a small 1 cm^3 lesions was 1.45, for a 6.0 cm^3 lesion 1.56, for a 6.5 cm^3 lesion 1.62, for a 14,5 cm^3 lesion 1.60 and for a 26 cm^3 lesion 1.37. The conformity index is defined as the ratio of the prescription isodose contour to the volume of the target. It seems safe to assume that for non-spherical lesions, the PTV volumes should be divided by 1.5 to get an idea of the lesion volumes likely to fit into the PTVs.

More specifically, the mean conformity index for protons was 1.32, for linac single isocentre 1.79, complex linac 1.39, and for the Gamma Knife 1.44. This does not effect the use of the dose-volume tables and graphs, since the PTV has been used to calculate them. Also see G2.1.

Shaw *et al.* (1996) found that for *brain tumours,* the use of multiple isocentres gave a much better maximum dose/peripheral dose ratio (MD/PD), than using single isocentres. For example, the volume of target contained by the 60% and 90% isodose lines is for a target of 11.5 cm^3, 19.2 cm^3 *versus* 14.6 cm^3, and 10.8 cm^3 *versus* 1.4 cm^3 for single and multiple isocentres respectively. Comment: Multiple isocentres prescribed at the 50% isodose may therefore be an optimal approach to large lesions.

Multivariate analysis identified a target volume ≥ 8.2 cm^3 and a MD/PD ≥ 2 as risk factors, but that the toxicity appeared rather to be a function of the volume contained within the higher isodose lines than the ratio MD/PD, as shown above.

I.10
Retreatment

If an AVM is treated in a very sensitive area, it may be wise to treat to a low dose, e.g. 15 Gy single dose and rather retreat a year later after assessment by MRA or angiography for obliteration, if the lesion is not obliterated. This may be a better approach than to risk serious complications, for instance in a young patient with a largish lesion in a sensitive area. Delivering the dose of each treatment lesion in 1–2 fractions may lower the risk of acute reactions. Sequential treatment of sections of a large AVM is a promising approach. (Miyawaki *et al.* 1999)

I.11
Summary

Several dose-volume prediction models in the form of dose-volume graphs have appeared in the literature, one for proton therapy, others for Gamma Knife users. None of these are entirely reliable.

Recently computer software has been written for Gamma Knife users that predict the obliteration probability for AVMs, as well as the risk for complications for individual patients. These results can probably not be extrapolated to the users of particles or linear accelerators.

There is a need to predict specific risks for individual patients. This is partly addressed by the above mentioned computer software.

We have prepared dose-volume tables and graphs to help the clinician to obtain further dose-volume reference points that should predict a low complication rate for individual parameters. These should not be used in isolation, but should be checked against all other models, and finally clinical judgement should be the final arbiter, keeping in mind that there is a trend towards lower doses, fractionation of treatment and perhaps retreatment of lesions if low doses fail to control the lesion.

The K-index is a single generalised index, and is not likely to predict the response for any specific patient for a particular dose dose-volume relationship. The "UFX Index" is another new tool to assess stereotactic treatment plans (Bova *et al.* 1999)

I.12
References

Bova FJ, Meeks SA, Friedman WA *et al.* (1999). Stereotactic plan evaluation tool "The UFX Index". Int J Radiat Oncol Biol Phys 45 (supplement):188

Corm BW, Currin WJ (1996) Can we disentangle dose from volume in the radiosurgical management of arteriovenous malformations? Int J Radiat Oncol Biol Phys 36:965–967

Engenhart R, Wowra B, Debus J *et al.* (1994) The role of high dose single-fraction irradiation in small and large intracranial arteriovenous malformations. Int J Oncol Biol Phys 30:521–529

Fabrikant JI, Levey RP, Steinberg GK *et al.* (1992) Charged particle radiosurgery for intracranial vascular malformations. Neurosurgery Clinics of North America 3:99–139

Flickinger JC (1989) The integrated logistic formula and predictions of complications from radio-surgery. Int J Radiat Oncol Biol Phys 17:879–885

Flickinger JC Lunsford LD, Wu A *et al.* (1991) Predicted dose-volume isoeffect curves for stereotactic radiosurgey with the ^{60}Co Gamma unit. Acta Oncologica 30:363–367

Flickinger JC, Kondziolka D, Pollock BE *et al.* (1997) Complications from arteriovenous malformation radiosurgery: Multivariate analysis and risk modelling. Int J Radiat Oncol Biol Phys 38:485–490

Flickinger JC, Kondziolka D, Pollock BE, Lunsford LD (1996) Evolution in technique for vestibular schwannoma radiosurgery and effect on outcome. Int J Radiat Oncol Biol Phys 36:275–280

Flickinger JC, Kondziolka D, Lunsford D et al (1999). A multi-institutional analysis of complication out-comes after arteriovenous malformation radiosurgery. Int J Radiat Oncol Biol Phys 44:67–74

Hamilton RJ, Kuchnir FT, Sweeney P, Rubin SJ *et al.* (1995) Comparison of static conformal field with multiple non-coplanar arc techniques for stereotactic radiotherapy. Int J Radiat Onc Biol Phys 33:1221–1228

ICRU Report-50 (1993) Prescribing, recording and reporting photon beam therapy, International Com-mission on Radiation Units and Measurements.

Karlsson B, Lax I, Söderman M (1997) Factors influencing the risk for complications following Gamma Knife radiosurgery of cerebral arteriovenous malformations. Radiother Oncol 43:275–280

Karlsson B, Lindquist C, Steiner L (1997) Prediction of obliteration after Gamma Knife radiosurgery for cerebral arteriovenous malformations. Neurosurgery 40:425–431

Karlsson B, Lax I, Söderman M (1999) Can the probability for obliteration after radiosurgery for arte-riovenous malformations be accurately predicted? Int J Radiat Oncol Biol Phys 43:313–319

Kjellberg R, Hanamura T, Davis K *et al.* (1983) Bragg peak proton beam therapy for arteriovenous mal-formations of the brain. N Engl J Med 309:269–274

Lax I, Karlsson B (1996) Prediction of complications in Gamma Knife radiosurgery of arteriovenous malformation. Acta Oncologica 35:49–55

Lee M, Nahum AE, Webb S (1993) An empirical method to build up a model of proton dose distribu-tion for radiotherapy treatment planning package. Phys Med Biol 38:989–998

Leung LHT, Chua DTT, Wu PM (1999) A new tool for dose conformity evaluation of radiosurgery treat-ment plans. Int J Radiat Oncol Biol Phys 45:233–241

Lo EH (1993) A theoretical analysis of haemodynamic and biomechanical alterations in intracranial AVMs after radiosurgery. Int J Radiat Oncol Biol Phys 27:353–361

Luxton G, Petrovich Z, Jozsef G, Nedzi LA, Apuzzo MLJ (1993) Stereotactic radiosurgery: Principles and Comparisons of treatment methods. Neurosurgery 12:241–260

Miyawaki L, Dowed C, Wara W *et al.* (1999) Five year results of linac radiosurgery for arteriovenous malformations: outcome for large AVMs. Int J Radiat Oncol Biol Phys 44:1089–1106

Shaw W, Scott C, Souhami L *et al.* (1996) Radiosurgery for the treatment of previously irradiated recur-rent primary brain tumours and brain metastases: initial report of Radiation Therapy Oncology Group Protocol

Smith A, Goitein M, Durlacher S *et al.* (1994) The Massachusetts General Hospital Northeast Proton Therapy Centre. In: Amaldi U, Larsson B (eds) Hadron Therapy in Oncology. Excerpta Medica, International Congress Series 1077, 1994

Verhey LJ, Smith V, Serago F (1998) Comparison of radiosurgery treatment modalities based on phys-ical dose distributions. Int J Radiat Oncol Biol Phys 40:497–505

Voges J, Treuer H, Sturm V *et al.* (1996) Risk analysis of linear accelerator radiosurgery. Int J Radiat Oncol Biol Phys 36:1055–1063

Withers HR (1994) Biology of Radiation Oncology. In: Tobias JS. Thomas PRM (eds) Current Radiation Oncology Vol 1 pp 5–23

J Low Energy Proton Beam Therapy for Eye Lesions

J.1
Introduction

Proton therapy has been found very useful for the treatment of uveal melanomas, and may be useful for other tumours in or around the eye. A possible new indication for proton radiotherapy of the eye is age related macular degeneration (ARMD), but this should be regarded as experimental. Protons may have an advantage over photon therapy for this condition, and relevant clinical trials are under way.

For uveal melanoma, it is likely that a larger number of fractions than 4 or 5 and lower doses may reduce the complication rate without compromising the control rate.

Using two proton fields, instead of the usual single field, may also reduce complications by improved sparing of the normal anterior tissues of the eye.

Plaque therapy is widely available at present but in general protons seem to give better results.

Gamma Knife therapy for uveal melanoma includes amongst others, a treatment report of an enormous single dose of 70 Gy with a predictably high complication rate. (See Chapter H.3 on BED)

Many peri-orbital lesions have extremely complex shapes. Protons may help to spare the very sensitive eye structures and may make radiation therapy more useful for these lesions.

Children are particularly vulnerable to the negative effects of radiation therapy and may benefit from the tissue sparing potential of proton therapy for lesions like retinoblastoma.

J.2
Benign Lesions

J.2.1
Peri-orbital Lesions

Protons, especially in spot scanning mode, may avoid treating substantial parts of a normal eye and orbit especially in children, where radiotherapy should be avoided if possible because of dystrophic and cancer risks.

The management of angiomata is usually by corticosteroid injection into the lesion, or if that fails surgical excision. Where this is not feasible, low-dose irradiation, 3 Gy × 5, may suffice. Despite this low dose, proton therapy offers superior plans with better sparing of normal tissues.

Other similar planning problems include conditions like pseudo-tumour or pseudo-lymphoma of the orbit. These lesions can be controlled with 20 Gy to 24 Gy photons in 10 to 14 fractions (Freire *et al.* 1998).

For tumours of peri-orbital structures like the ethmoid sinus, lacrimal gland, the nasal vestibule and similar difficult-to-treat tumour sites, protons offer superior comparative plans to photons.

Coltrera *et al.* (1996) described the treatment with protons of 13 chondrosarcomas of the temporal bone, with good result.

For basal cell carcinomas recurring after excision on the temple, careful planning with protons may help to avoid irradiating the lacrimal gland.

J.2.2
Age Related Macular Degeneration

Synonyms for age related macular degeneration ARMD:
CNVM: – choroidal neovascular membrane, SRN: – Subretinal neovascularisation, CNV: – choroidal neovascularisation.

This may be a new fruitful field of application for proton therapy. Contradictory articles are still appearing whether radiotherapy should be used at all and for the moment *radiotherapy for this condition must be regarded as experimental.*

Incidence: This disease occurs in almost 30 per cent of people older than 75 years in the USA. Macular degeneration may be responsible for 90 per cent of the cases of legal blindness in industrialised nations.

Pathology and natural history: Untreated choroidal neovascularisation causes progressive loss of vision, with more than 60% of untreated patients losing more than six lines of vision within 2 to 3 years.

ARMD is characterised by degenerative changes in the retinal pigment epithelium and Bruch's membrane, especially of the macular region of the eye. In many patients the degenerative lesions are followed by subretinal neovascularisation. The new vessels grow from the choriopapillaris into the sub-pigment epithelial space and subretinal space causing a serous detachment of the macula, which later heals with scar formation and with the resultant irreversible loss of visual acuity. ARMD may occur away from the fovea, abutting the fovea or sub-foveally, with the latter understandably leading to the more severe visual impairment. ARMD occurs in two forms: an atrophic "dry" form and an exudative "wet" form. The "wet" type of ARMD, where radiotherapy may help, accounts for 15 per cent of the cases.

Treatment so far is not satisfactory.

Interferon: This is experimental and not promising (Williford and King 1996).

Argon Laser Therapy of foveal lesions leads to an immediate decrease in vision, but with a longer time of residual visual function as benefit.

Extra-foveal ARMD is amenable to laser treatment, but sub-foveal lesions do poorly. At 2 years post laser treatment, patients with sub-foveal neovascularisation had better visual acuity by about 1-and-a-half lines than patients who were not treated. Unfortunately for 3 to 6 months after treatment, laser treated eyes will have worse visual acuity than untreated eyes.

Radiotherapy promotes inactivation of the neo-vasculature, and the re-absorption of blood and fluid from the eye. This reduces the risk of further leakage and subretinal bleeding as well as subsequent subretinal fibrosis. The proliferative vascular cells of the neovascularisation process are reasonably radiosensitive.

Radiotherapy was first reported to be effective by Chackravarthy et al. (1993). The results were encouraging: (Chisholm et al. 1993, Bergink et al. 1994, Berson et al. 1995, Freire et al. 1996 and Valmaggia et al. 1995.)

Yonemoto et al. (1996) reported good results from their *proton therapy based experience*. They assessed both the response of the neovascularisation (CNV) to *proton beam irradiation* as well as treatment-related morbidity to a dose of 8 Cobalt Gray Equivalent (CGy). Twenty-one patients received proton irradiation of which 19 were eligible for evaluation. Fluorescein angiography was performed; visual acuity, contrast sensitivity, and reading speed were measured at study entry and at 3-month intervals after treatment. Follow-up ranged from 6 to 15 months.

No measurable treatment-related morbidity was seen during or after treatment. Of 19 patients evaluated at 6 months, fluorescein angiography demonstrated treatment response in 10/19; 14/19 patients had improved or stable visual acuity. With a mean follow-up of 11.6 months, 11/19 patients have demonstrated improved or stable visual acuity.

Similar results have been reported by Freire et al. (1996), Berson et al. (1996) and Sasai et al. (1997). The authors concluded that irradiation seems to be useful for CNV.

There are potential advantages in using protons instead of photons. Protons enable the radiotherapist to reduce the dose to the normal tissues, compared to photon techniques, by a factor of 2–5, making it possible to spare not only the lens, but also all the brain tissue and the sinuses. (Moyers et al. 1999)

Brady (1996) concludes in an editorial that: "Age related macular degeneration represents an exciting new area of potential application of radiation therapy technology in the treatment of a significant and important problem in the United States".

Some representative results are given in Table J2.1.

Table J2.1 Representative results of radiotherapy for age related macular degeneration. For a comparison of the dosage schedules, see Chapter H.3.13. *Sas* Sasai, *Bers* Berson, *Frei* Freire, *Berg* Bergink, *Yon* Yonemoto. Bergink et al. produced some evidence for a dose-response of ARMD lesions. The single dose tolerance for the optic nerve seems to be 8 Gy.

Author	Date	Pt no.	Total dose	Fraction number	Stable vision (%)
Yon[a]	1996	21	8	1	74
Bers[b]	1996	52	15	8	79
Sas[b]	1997	18	10	5	66
Frei[b]	1996	18	20	10	61
Berg[b]	1994	41	15	8	71
Berg[b]	1994	10	8	1	50
Berg[b]	1994	10	12	2	70
Berg[b]	1994	10	18	3	60
Berg[b]	1994	10	24	4	80

[a] Proton therapy
[b] Photon therapy

J.3
Malignant Lesions: Uveal Melanoma

J.3.1
Introduction

Uveal melanoma is an uncommon tumour, but a fairly common eye tumour in Caucasians, and of the about 1800 new cases of primary malignant tumours of the eye seen in the USA in 1989, about 75% were malignant melanoma. Melanomas of the anterior uvea are usually detected earlier than those located posteriorly (Winter 1963, 1974).

Enucleation may worsen the prognosis of patients with ocular melanoma. (Zimmerman 1975). An overall death rate of 50% for ocular melanoma in 1974 led to the formation of the Collaborative Ocular Melanoma Study Group (COMS), which has led to some refinement in the selection of patients for photocoagulation, radiotherapy, local resection, enucleation, orbital exenteration and immunotherapy.

Protons were first used for the treatment of uveal melanomas at the Massachusetts General Hospital and the Harvard Cyclotron Laboratory in 1975.

J.3.2
Proton Therapy

J.3.2.1
General

Uveal melanoma is one of the recognised indications for proton therapy. Proton therapy results in a very good coverage of the irregularly shaped lesions by a homogeneous dose and could be employed for tumours located posteriorly and close to the disc or macula, or even if the macula is involved. The low energy beams needed (70 MeV) for the treatment of uveal melanomas have very sharp dose fall-off characteristics, which are ideal for eye tumours.

Suit and Urie (1992) state that 2822 patients have been treated by proton beam techniques up to that date with protons. To date an estimated 3000 patients have been so treated.

The goals of treatment are to eradicate the malignant melanoma and to preserve a cosmetically intact eye. These goals have largely been met. Table J3.1 summarises the results. Also see page 80 and Fig. E2.6 and Table H3.8.

Table J3.1 Results of proton therapy for uveal melanoma. *HCL* Harvard Cyclotron Laboratory, *PSI* Paul Scherrer Institute, *LBL* Lawrence Berkeley Laboratories. Table adapted from Suit and Urie (1992) and Courdi *et al.* (1999)

Institute	Year	Total dose (CGyE)	Fraction number	Local control (%)	5-Year survival %
HCL	1991	70	5	96	80
PSI	1991	60	4	97	88
LBL	1991	70	5	96	80
Nice	1999	57.2	4	89	82

J.3.2.2
Results of Proton Therapy

The actuarial control rate of uveal melanoma within the globe at the three most active centres globally is around 96%, and the control of tumour within the treated volume 99% with 14 CGyE × 5. Vision has been retained at 20/200 or better in 66% of patients with lesions located more than 3 mm from the fovea and/or disc but in only 33% with lesions less than 3 mm from the fovea and/or disc (Suit and Urie 1992).

Most of the local failures occurred at tumour margins, or at other, more distant parts of the globe due either to second tumours or unexpected seedings.

Five year survival figures of 80% – 88% have been achieved at the Paul Scherrer Institute (PSI) with protons at 60 GyE in four fractions (Egger and Zographos 1994) on 1229 patients with uveal melanoma treated by proton beam irradiation.

Failure of local control occurred in 18 of the 263 cases (6.84%) treated before 1988, and in 15 of 966 (1.55%) treated after 1988. Actuarial survival was 85% at 5 and 80% at nine years. Of the patients' lesions, 44.6% were located < 3 mm to the macula. Even in this unfavourable group, about 50% of the patients retained useful vision 5 years after irradiation.

Large intraocular melanomas: It is generally agreed that very large ocular melanomas and patients with extra-scleral extension of the tumour at diagnosis should not be treated with radiation. Irradiation to 8 Gy in a single dose prior to enucleation made no difference to the post-operative survival statistics (Luyten *et al.* 1995, Courdi *et al.* 1999).

Melanomas of the ciliary body: These are associated with a higher enucleation rate after helium particle therapy than posterior tumours. Decker *et al.* (1990) found that out of 54 patients treated with helium ions the 5-year specific survival rate was only 59% despite a 5-year local control rate of 98%. The incidence of neovascular glaucoma (NVG) was 43% at 5 years, and the actuarial 5-year enucleation rate 26%, and 70% of the NVG occurred in patients with tumour volumes > 5.5 cm^3. The volume of the globe is about 8.5 cm^3.

J.3.2.3
Techniques of Proton Irradiation

Single track technique of Gragoudas (1980) and Saunders (1985): Routine evaluation includes B-scan and quantitative A-scan ultrasonography, wide-angle photography, fluorescein angiography, wide-angle photography, and trans-illumination.

For planning, a combined team approach of ophthalmic surgeon, radiation oncologist, physicist and radiologist is needed. The tumour needs to be localised, measured for north south and east west diameter, height of the tumour (base to apex) and tumour volume needs to be calculated. The volumes are obtained by fitting an oval over the base dimensions of the tumour and a paraboloid from the base to the height of the tumour (Decker *et al.* 1990).

Some form of marking the perimeter of the tumour is needed, and one approach is to suture or glue small tantalum rings to the perimeter of the tumour. The base of the tumour is shown up to the surgeon by trans-illumination of the globe.

Some of these techniques have been described for helium ions (Char *et al.* 1982, 1983; Saunders *et al.* 1985; Lindstadt *et al.* 1988) and for proton beams by Gragoudas *et al.* (1980).

Patients must be able to remain immobile in a sitting position fitted with a customised immobilisation mask of plastic material as commonly used in radiation oncology departments. They must also be able to maintain a fixed stare (gaze) at a particular angle for a minute or two, which is a typical time needed to deliver the dose.

Figure J3.1 shows a fairly typical treatment set-up:

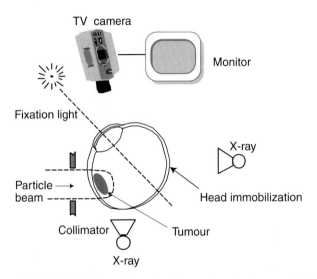

Fig. J3.1 A typical set-up for proton therapy of uveal melanoma. The *dotted line* is the "gaze line" and the angle to direction of the proton beam, the "gaze angle". Patients must be capable to co-operate and to maintain the gaze angle for 1–3 minutes at a time. An operator monitors the patient and will switch off the beam if the patient breaks the gaze. (Also see Fig. E2.6)

Following recovery from the surgery, the patients have their custom moulded polystyrene head holders made for immobilisation. They are then taken through a "practice run" with the beam turned off, for a "treatment simulation".

In this procedure, the patient must fix his/her gaze on a small target light, usually a light emitting diode (LED) set at a known, suitable and convenient angle.

Sets of orthogonal films (at right angles to each other) are then taken. The position of the tantalum rings are identified and measured on the two X-ray films.

A specially developed planning computer is needed to model the eye and the position of the tumour, optic disc and nerve, as well as the lens (to avoid cataract formation), and macula. The program presents an anatomically correct-to-scale line drawing of the patients eye on a video display unit. (Gragoudas 1980; Goitein and Miller 1983). Workers at Clatterbridge have developed their own planning system.

The diameter of the eye, height of the tumour, ring positions, shape and position of the base of the tumour, defined by the tantalum rings and the position of the tumour relative to the photographs and a drawing of the tumour relative to other retinal structures and photo's are all correlated. The radiation oncologist in collaboration with the ophthalmic surgeon can then choose the optimal angle for the beam to enter. The aim is to avoid the cornea, lens, optic disc and macula. Figure J3.2 shows an illustration of a treatment plan for uveal melanoma for the 2 beam technique, compare fig J3.3.

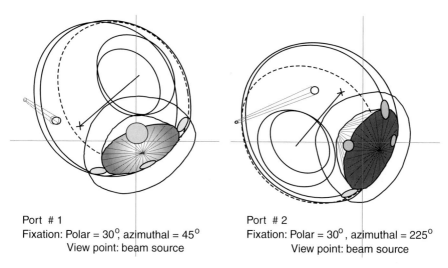

Port # 1
Fixation: Polar = 30^0, azimuthal = 45^0
View point: beam source

Port # 2
Fixation: Polar = 30^0, azimuthal = 225^0
View point: beam source

Fig. J3.2 The illustration of the treatment plan of uveal melanoma of the left eye in beam's-eye-view using (a) port 1 (gaze direction 1) having polar and azimuth angle of $(30^0, 45^0)$. The patient is looking towards the upper right-hand corner of the box (up and out), (b) port 2, having polar and azimuth angle of $(30^0, 225^0)$. The patient is looking towards the lower left-hand corner of the box (down and in). The contour around the tumour represents the 50% isodose line. The optic nerve and macula are outside the 50% isodose in both ports, while a portion of the lens is in the field. (Redrawn from Daftari IK et al., 1997, Int J Radiat Oncol Biol Phys 39:997–1010) (Also see Fig. E2.6)

The program calculates the beam energy required. The basic beam energy should be about 60–70 MeV to ensure sharp dose fall-off. The energy determines the depth that the proton beam will penetrate. The amount that the Bragg peak must be spread and the collimator (aperture) size and shape down the "beam's eye view" is also calculated.

The collimator is custom made and designed to leave a safety margin around the tumour base of about 2 mm. This margin is specified by the 90% isodose. The distal fall-off of the Bragg peak is placed 3 mm beyond the tumour outside the sclera, and 2 mm in front of the maximal height of the tumour, leaving a margin of at least 2 mm around the tumour in all dimensions.

The patient is placed in the specially designed treatment chair, and the polystyrene head mask is fixed to the chair's headrest. The patient is approximately positioned using a laser pointer and previously marked external landmarks. The eyelids are pulled out of the way as far as possible, to get them out of the beam path, with a suitable eyelid retractor.

Modifications to the "Eyeplan" software to include modelling of the lids have been made by the Clatterbridge Group. (Also see Section E.2.3b)

A simulation X-ray film is taken with the patient gazing at the "gaze-fixing" light source.

The X-ray tube is aligned with the beam axis and a film is taken from behind the patient's head, with the film cassette positioned between the patient's eye and the tumour shape-defining collimator. Radio-opaque crosshairs are placed on the cassette, these mark the beam axis. The film is exposed by the X-ray tube, and a second exposure is made with a low dose of irradiation from the proton (or helium ion) beam. This outlines the collimator on the film, and will indicate its position relative to the tantalum rings marking the tumour base recorded on the film by the exposure from the X-ray tube. It may be necessary to adjust the position of the rings relative to the magnification induced by the divergence of the X-ray beam. A photo of a technique used by Saunders *et al.* (1985) shows the marks in position (Fig. J3.3)

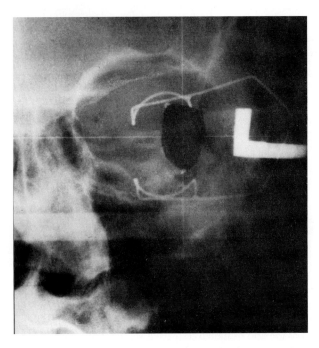

Fig. J3.3 Pre-treatment port film used for uveal melanoma treatment. The film shows the markers defining the tumour plus a 2 mm margin. (From W Saunders *et al.*, 1985, Int J Radiat Oncol Biol Phys 11:227–233)

During the positioning X-ray and during the treatment itself, the patient's eye is closely monitored using a close-up television camera. Any change in the gaze angle will cause the physicist doing the monitoring to switch off the beam immediately. Automation of this process is being investigated.

Double Track Technique of Daftari

Recently, Daftari *et al.* (1997) described a modification to the usual treatment approach. Instead of one beam, two beams were used from different gaze angles. This *reduces the biological effect per track relative to the biological effects of a single track* and this approach is expected to reduce the incidence of neovascular glaucoma (NVG), which sometimes necessitates enucleation of the eye. In his series, using a single helium ion field, NVG developed in 121/347 (35%) of patients. A multivariate analysis showed that the amount of lens in the irradiation track strongly correlated with the development of NVG. Dose-Volume histograms showed that for patients in the medium to large tumour groups, the two port technique could result in a significant decrease in the dose to the structures in the anterior segment of the eye.

Figure J3.4 illustrate the two treatment methods, and illustrate that the dose to the lens could be reduced to 40% for the double beam method *versus* 80% for the single-track method. The biologically effective dose (BED) will be reduced, not 100%, but for a 14 Gy fraction from 73.9 Gy to 19.8 Gy, by 273% for an α/β ratio = 2 Gy.

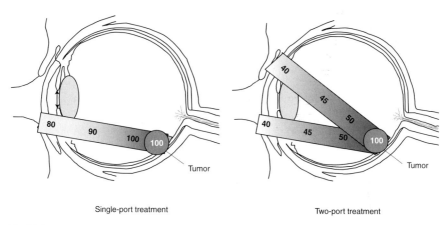

Single-port treatment   Two-port treatment

Fig. J3.4
Schematic illustration of the treatment of uveal melanoma (a) with single port and (b) with two ports. The percentage of dose levels in the techniques are labelled. The two-port treatment will reduce the dose to the lens from about 85% to about 42.5% as shown. For a dose of 14 Gy x 5 to the tumour, the BED_2 for a single beam at the lens will give 88 Gy per fraction for a single beam *versus* 23.7 Gy per fraction. That means that the biological reduction in dose is not 100% but 271%. (Redrawn from IK Daftari *et al.* 1997, Int J Radiat Oncol Biol Phys 39:997–1010) (Compare Fig J3.2)

J.3.3
Treatment of Uveal Melanoma by Gamma Knife

Rennie *et al.* (1996) reported on 14 patients with posterior uveal melanoma. These patients received 70 Gy as a single fraction to the periphery of the tumour. Regression was seen in 13, lesion unchanged in 1 patient. The visual acuity deteriorated in all 14 patients. Significant radiation induced adverse events have been observed in 13/14 patients and include retinopathy, optic neuropathy, rubeosis iridis and secondary glaucoma. Two patients required enucleation because of intractable rubeotic glaucoma. One patient died from proven metastases. Although stereotactic radiosurgery appears to be a practical and effective method of treating uveal melanomas, its usefulness is limited by a high incidence of radiation induced adverse reactions. They conclude that further work is necessary to refine the current protocol and to establish an optimal dose.

If the dose is examined, it is found that the BED_2 values are very high ($BED_2 = 2520$ Gy equal to 630 conventional fractions of 2 Gy) and for late effects this dose is likely to be nine times more damaging than 70 GyE in five fractions. The dose in the centre of the lesion would have been much higher still.

Marchini et al. (1996) reported on 36 cases of uveal melanoma treated by Gamma Knife between March 1993 and September 1995. The choroid was affected in 35 patients and the ciliary-body in 1. The same preoperative and follow-up protocol was adopted for all cases. The procedure included fixation and positioning of the eye with retrobulbar injection of long-lasting anaesthetic and two extraocular muscle sutures, application of a frame, computed tomography scan localisation, dose planning and treatment with the Gamma Knife. The patients were divided into three groups.

Group A: ten patients with a follow-up of ± 4 months, treated with a high dose (surface dose 58 ± 9 Gy, maximum dose 81 ± 15 Gy, mean dose 66 ± 11 Gy).

Group B: nine patients with a follow-up of 16 ± 2 months, treated with a lower dose (surface dose 41 ± 3 Gy, maximum dose 76 ± 10 Gy, mean dose 53 ± 11 Gy).

Group C: 17 patients with follow-up of 6 ± 3 months, treated with a lower dose (surface dose 42 ± 3 Gy, maximum dose 72 ± 16 Gy, mean dose 54 ± 6 Gy).

In Group A they observed marked tumour regression in nine cases, tumour recurrence in one case and severe complications in five cases (neovascular glaucoma and/or radiation retinopathy and/or radiation optic neuropathy). In Group B significant local control of tumour was obtained with minor complications (cotton wool spots hard exudates, intraretinal haemorrhages). In Group C a regression of the tumour in seven cases and one severe complication (neovascular glaucoma) occurred.

Zehetmayer et al. (1995) described a plastic suction cup to fix the eyeball for radiosurgery with the Leksell Gamma Knife. This seems to have the potential of making fractionation for these lesions feasible for the Gamma Knife, and may reduce complications.

J.3.4
Plaque Techniques

Proton therapy requires surgical placement and removal of tumour markers, plaque therapy requires the surgical placement and removal of the plaque.

The dose with protons across the tumour is homogeneous, that of the plaque very inhomogeneous. For example, Shields et al. (1995) treated 14 such patients with ^{125}I plaques delivering a dose of 293 Gy to the lesion base trans-scleral, with 106 Gy at the apex. Thirteen out of the 14 patients had tumour control and retained the eye. The sclera tolerated this dose without "melting". Plaques are useful for countries where proton facilities are not available.

Figure J3.5 shows a fairly typical modern plaque dose distribution.

The indications for plaque therapy are for (1) selected small melanomas that are documented to be growing, or are showing clear-cut signs of activity at the first visit, (2) most medium sized and some large choroidal and ciliary body melanomas in an

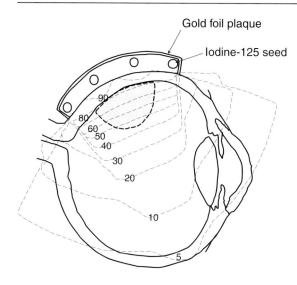

Gold foil plaque

Iodine-125 seed

Fig. J3.5 Dose distribution to a retinoblastoma treated with an I-125 plaque showing a dose of 45 Gy to the apex of the tumour and 90 Gy to the base. The edge of the plaque reduces the dose to the lens to 10 Gy with 20 Gy to the optic nerve. (Redrawn from C Stannard, 1998, Specialist Medicine 3:33–36)

eye with potential salvageable vision, and (3) almost all actively growing melanomas growing in the patients only useful eye. If a melanoma exceeds 15 mm in diameter, and 10 mm in thickness morbidity from radiotherapy is likely to be the result and enucleation should be advised (Freire *et al.* 1998).

Stallard started in the 1950s with radioactive cobalt 60 plaques sutured to the sclera opposite the tumour base. Other isotopes give better dose distributions, e.g. ^{125}I, ^{192}Ir, ^{106}Ru/^{106}Rh, with better tumour coverage and better sparing of the normal tissues. The normal tissues were also more easily protected, for example by thin gold foil. The plaque techniques are more suitable for the more anteriorly located lesions, away from the optic nerve and optic disc and the macula. Proton beams can be shaped better to avoid these posterior structures, although specially notched plaques are available so that the notch can accommodate the nerve.

There does not appear to be major differences in the local control between the various type of plaques. The relapse rate after plaque therapy is about 16%, *versus* 4% for protons.

More than 85% of patients who obtain local control with plaque therapy will retain useful vision for prolonged periods (Packer 1987). In patients where the plaque touches the optic disc, patients experienced a decrement of at least three lines of vision for up to 20 months, progressively increasing to 72% by 50 to 60 months (De Potter *et al.* 1996)

J.4
Metastatic Lesions in the Eye

Metastatic lesions in the eye are probably the most common malignant condition of the eye. The majority of metastatic lesions are from breast and lung carcinoma in the female, and from the lung and gastro-intestinal tract in men (Brady *et al.* 1982; Ferry and Font 1975; Stephens and Shields 1979).

The aim of therapy is to restore vision to the eye. The majority of these patients will have systemic metastatic disease with a short life expectancy of 3–6 months after the diagnosis of an ocular secondary.

Systemic chemotherapy appropriate to the individual tumour type may help to resolve the ocular lesions.

If this is not helpful focal radiotherapy may be useful, and about 90% of patients will resolve satisfactorily (Brady *et al.* 1984). The dose required is usually about 35 Gy in 3 weeks to 50 Gy in 4 to 5 weeks. The time to deliver this dose, represents a large fraction of the patient's remaining life, and plaque therapy (86 hours) has been used. (Shields *et al.* 1995). There may be a place for a few fractions of proton therapy in this setting in the new hospital based proton therapy facilities.

J.5
Complications

J.5.1
Neovascular Glaucoma

Neovascular glaucoma (NVG) is a significant complication of charged particle irradiation of uveal melanomas and it occurs in 42% of patients treated with helium ions after a mean interval of 14 months, which correlated with tumour volume ($p = 0.0017$), distance to the fovea ($p = 0.0005$), initial tumour height ($p = 0.011$) and dose ($p = 0.035$). The actuarial probability of developing NVG was 43% at 5 years (Decker *et al.* 1990).

Daftari *et al.* (1997) found that the intensity of the dose to the lens, as well as the percentage of the lens and anterior chamber structures irradiated, correlated with the development of NVG besides the other factors mentioned above, and suggest a double beam path approach (Fig. J3.4).

J.5.2
Retinopathy, Optic Neuropathy, Rubeosis Iridis

A single fraction of 70 Gy developed by Gamma Knife caused *retinopathy, optic neuropathy, rubeosis iridis, secondary glaucoma and intractable rubeotic glaucoma*, which necessitated enucleation (Rennie *et al.* 1996).

Out of 59 patients treated by protons for para-papillary choroidal melanoma who had visual field testing prior to therapy and again at least 18 months after therapy, progressive visual field loss was seen in 73%. The visual field loss correlated with the area of retina predicted to be exposed to irradiation (Park *et al.* 1997). They concluded that progressive visual field loss is common after proton irradiation for para-papillary choroidal melanoma. The scotoma usually correlates with the retinal area exposed to irradiation. The development of *radiation induced papillopathy* does not appear to be associated with additional visual field defects in most cases.

Gragoudas *et al.* (1993) reported that the histopathological changes in irradiated melanomas vary according to the time elapsed since the irradiation. *Inflammatory changes* diminished with time whereas *fibrosis* became more prevalent with time after irradiation. Among controlled tumours, mitotic figures only appear in recently irradiated tumours.

Visual preservation down to 20/200 or better occurred in 66% of the patients with lesions located more than 3 mm from the fovea and or disc, but vision was preserved in only 33% of the patients with lesions less than 3 mm from the fovea and or disc (Suit and Urie 1992).

A clinical trial is under way testing 50 GyE in five fractions over 8–10 days. The aim is to see whether this will lead to a similar good local control rate, but a decreased incidence of choroidal and optical nerve atrophy. (See Chapter H.3.12 for a comparison using the BED of various dose levels)

Cataract formation may be inhibited by Verapamil administration, since it blocks ca^{++} entry into the lens, in Wistar rats (Cengiz *et al.* 1999)

J.6
Comparison of the Various Dose Levels Used to Treat Uveal Melanoma Using the BED

This comparison is discussed in the chapter especially devoted to the BED, and the reader is referred to section H.3.12, Table H3.8.

J.7
Tolerance of the Optic Nerve and Retina

Please refer to Chapter H.3.11 (BED)

J.8
Summary

Protons may find good application in peri-orbital lesions which often have very complicated shapes, even if fairly low doses are required. This may be especially useful in children.

Protons remain the best way of treating uveal melanomas with a local control rate of about 96% but lower doses and a larger number of fractions may improve results further by lowering the complication rate. A double beam technique recently described may help to lower the complication rates especially with the larger lesions. Lower doses or smaller doses per fraction may help to preserve vision and to avoid other complications.

Protons may be better than photons for the treatment of age related macular degeneration (ARMD), the radio-therapeutic treatment of which should only be undertaken only within prospective, randomised clinical trials.

Plaque therapy is cheaper than proton therapy is more widely available presently, and technical improvements are made regularly. It is a good alternative therapy where proton beams are not available.

Therapy with stereotactic radiosurgery by Gamma Knife should be approached with caution, as single large doses proved to be excessively toxic.

J.9
References

Bergink GJ, Deutman AF, Broek JE van den *et al.* (1995) Radiation therapy for age related subfoveal choroidal neovascular membranes. Doc Ophthalmol 90:67–74

Berson AM, Finger PT, Sher DL *et al.* (1996) Radiotherapy for age related macular degeneration: preliminary results of a potentially new treatment. Int J Radiat Oncol Biol Phys 36:861–865

Brady LW (1996) Radiotherapy in macular degeneration. (editorial) Int J Radiat Oncol Biol Phys 36:936

Brady LW, Shields JA, Augsburger JJ *et al.* (1982) Malignant intra-ocular tumours. Cancer 49:578–585

Cengiz M, Gürkaynak M, Atahan IL *et al.* (1999) The effect of Verapamil in the prevention of radiation-induced cataract. Int J Radiat Oncol Biol Phys 43:623–626

Chakravarthy U, Houston Rand Archer D (1993) Treatment of age related subfoveal membranes: a pilot study. Br J Ophthalmol 77:265–273

Char DH, Castro JR (1982) Helium ion therapy for choroidal melanoma. Arch Ophthalmol 100:935–938

Char DH, Saunders WM, Castro *et al.* (1983) A charged particle therapy for choroidal melanoma. Ophthalmology 90:1219–1225

Chisholm IH (1993) The prospects of the new treatments in age related macular degeneration. Br J Ophthalmol 77:757–758

Coltrera MD, Googe PB, Harrist TJ *et al.* (1996) Chondrosarcoma of the temporal bone. Diagnosis and treatment of 13 cases and review of the literature. Cancer 58:2689–2696

Courdi A, Caujolle J-P, Grange J-D *et al.* (1999) Results of proton therapy of uveal melanomas treated in Nice. Int J Radiat Oncol Biol Phys 45:5–11

Daftari IK, Char DH, Verhey LJ *et al.* (1997) Anterior segment sparing to reduce charged particle radiotherapy complications in uveal melanoma. Int J Radiat Oncol Biol Phys 39:997–1010

Decker M, Castro JR, Lindstadt DE *et al.* (1990) Ciliary body melanoma treated with helium particle therapy irradiation. Int J Radiat Oncol Biol Phys 19:243–247

De Potter P, Shields CL, Shields JA *et al.* (1996) Plaque radiotherapy for juxtapapillary choroidal melanoma. Visual acuity and survival outcome. Arch Ophthalmol 114:1357–1365

Egger E, Zographos I (1994) Proton beam irradiation of uveal melanoma at PSI: latest results. Int Congr Ser 1077:145–164

Ferry AP, Font RL (1975) Carcinoma metastatic to the eye and orbit. A clinicopathologic study of 26 cases. Arch Ophthalmol 93:472–482

Freire JE, Brady LW, De Potter P *et al.* (1998) Eye. In: Perez C, Brady L (eds) Principles and practice of radiation oncology, third edition. Lippincott-Raven, Philadelphia, pp 867–888

Freire JE, Longton WA, Miyamoto CTS *et al.* (1996) External radiotherapy in macular degeneration: technique and preliminary subjective response. Int J Radiat Oncol Biol Phys 36:857–860

Goitein M, Miller T (1983) Planning proton therapy of the eye. Med Phys 10:275–283

Gragoudas ES, Egan KM, Saornil *et al.* (1993) The time course of irradiation changes in proton beam treated uveal melanomas. Ophthalmology 100:1555–1559

Gragoudas ES, Goitein M, Verhey L, Munzenrider J, Suit HD, Koehkler A (1993) Proton beam irradiation, an alternative to enucleation for intra-ocular melanomas. Ophthalmology 87:571–581

Harbour JW, Murray TG, Byrne SF *et al.* (1996) Intra-operative echographic localisation of iodine-125 episcleral radioactive plaques for posterior uveal melanoma. Retina 16:129–134

Lindstadt D, Char DH, Castro JR *et al.* (1988) Vision following helium ion therapy of uveal melanoma: a Northern California Oncology Group study. Int J Radiat Oncol Biol Phys 15:347–352

Luyten GP, Mooy CM, Eijkenboom WMH *et al.* (1995) No demonstrated effect of pre-enucleation irradiation on survival of patients with uveal melanoma. Am J Ophthalmol 119:786–791

Marchini G, Gerosa M, Piovan E *et al.* (1996) Gamma Knife stereotactic radiosurgery for uveal melanoma: clinical results after 2 years. Stereotact Funct Neurosurg 66 [Suppl 1]:208–213

Moyers MF, Galindo, Yonemoto LT, Loredo L (1999) Treatment of macular degeneration with proton beams. Med Phys 26: 777–782.

Packer S (1987) Iodine-125 radiation of posterior uveal melanoma. Ophthalmology 94:1621–1626

Park SS, Walsh SM, Gragoudas ES (1996) Visual field deficits associated with proton beam irradiation for para-papillary choroidal melanoma. Ophthalmology 103:110–116

Petrovich Z, McDonnell JM, Palmer D *et al.* (1994) Histopathologic changes following irradiation for uveal tract melanoma. Am J Clin Oncol 17:289–306

Rennie I, Foster D, Kemeny A *et al.* (1996) The use of single fraction Leksell stereotactic radiosurgery in the treatment of uveal melanoma. Acta Ophthalmol Scand 74:558–562

Sasai K, Murata RM, Mandai M *et al.* (1997) Radiation therapy for ocular neovascularisation (phase I/II study): preliminary report. Int J Radiat Oncol Biol Phys 39:173–178

Saunders WM, Char DH, Quivey JM *et al.* (1985) Precision high dose radiotherapy: Helium ion treatment of uveal melanoma. Int J Radiat Oncol Biol Phys 11:227–233

Shields CL, Shields JA, De Potter P *et al.* (1995) Short-term plaque radiotherapy for the treatment of choroidal metastases. Proceedings of the 99th Annual Meeting of the American Academy of Ophthalmology, Atlanta, Georgia

Shields CL, Shields JA, De Potter P *et al.* (1995) Treatment of non-resectable malignant iris tumours with custom designed plaque radiotherapy. Br J Ophthalmol 79:306–312

Stannard C (1998) Iodine-25 brachytherapy in the management of retinoblastoma. Specialist Medicine Sept:33–36

Stephens RF, Shields JA (1979) Diagnosis and management of cancer metastatic to the uvea: a study of 70 cases. Ophthalmology 86:1336–1349

Suit H, Urie M (1992) Proton beams in radiotherapy. J Natl Cancer Inst 84:155–164

Valmaggia C, Bischoff P, Ries G (1995) Low dose radiotherapy of subfovceal neo-vascularisation in age related macular degeneration. Preliminary results. Klin Monatsblatt Augenheilkunde 206:343–346

Williford SL, King T (1996) Interferon alpha for macular degeneration. Ann Pharmacother 36:378–379

Winter FC (1963) Surgical excision of tumours of the ciliary body and iris. Arch Ophthalmol 70:19

Winter FC (1964) Iridocyclectomy for malignant melanoma of the iris and ciliary body. In: Boniuk M (ed) Ocular and adnexal tumours: new and controversial aspects. Mosby, St Louis, pp 341–352

Yonemoto LT, Slater JD, Friedrichson EJ *et al.* (1996) Phase I/II study of proton beam irradiation for the treatment of subfoveal choroidal neovascularisation in age related macular degeneration: treatment techniques and preliminary results. Int J Radiat Oncol Biol Phys 36:867–871

Zehetmayer M, Menapace R, Kitz K *et al.* (1995) Experience with a suction fixation cup for stereotactic radiosurgery of intra-ocular malignancies. Stereotact Funct Neurosurg 64 [Suppl 1]:80–86

Zimmerman LE (1975) Changing concepts concerning the malignancy of ocular tumours. Arch Ophthalmol 78:166–173

K High Energy Proton Therapy for Tumours in Body Sites Other than the Brain

K.1
Introduction

The success with proton therapy for uveal melanoma, and the advantages of its superior dose localising potential, encouraged interested physicians and physicists to develop hospital based proton therapy centres that could also be used, like the versatile isocentric linear accelerators, for a variety of other cancer sites in the body. The conviction that superior dose distributions will translate to superior local control and survival for cancer patients, keeping the complication rate constant or even lowering it, remained an attraction perpetuating enthusiasm for protons over four decades.

Two proton therapy groups have been formed to aid the initiation and conduct of clinical trials, which should serve to affirm the intuitive superiority of proton therapy *versus* photon therapy for extracranial sites.

K.2
Co-operative Proton Therapy Groups

K.2.1
The Proton Therapy Co-operative Oncology Group

The Proton Therapy Co-operative Oncology Group (PTCOG) is an informal organisation which provides an open forum to all interested persons for the discussion, status of progress in and future directions for proton radiation therapy.

This group advocates that the specification for a proton radiotherapy centre should demand that (1) The facility be hospital based, (2) the energy needs to be 230 MeV or higher, (3) there be two or more treatment rooms, with the capacity to increase to three or four bays, and (4) isocentric gantry systems need to be provided in one or more of the treatment rooms. Plans for co-operative studies have been made at PTCOG meetings (Suit and Urie 1992).

K.2.2
The Proton Radiation Oncology Group

This group was formed at the XIVth PTCOG meeting in May 1991. It is sponsored by the U.S. National Cancer Institute and the American College of Radiology. It is charged to: (1) stimulate co-operative clinical trials by the various proton therapy centres in the USA and abroad, (2) organise and manage clinical trials, (3) provide the data management system, and (4) encourage the prompt reporting of results from the trials (Suit and Urie 1992).

K.3
Protons for Superficial Tumours

K.3.1
Skin and Chest Wall

There is no strong case to be made for treating *skin* lesions with protons; the cost factor is likely to prove prohibitive. Despite this statement, Umebayashi *et al.* (1994) reported on 12 skin cancers treated with protons, 4 with Bowen's disease, 5 with verrucous carcinoma and 3 with squamous cell carcinoma. Of these 4/4 Bowen's, 3/5 verrucous carcinomas and 3/3 squamous cell carcinomas completely regressed. Proton therapy produces good local control without morbidity to the surrounding tissues and it may be a useful therapeutic modality for the treatment of skin carcinoma.

For the *chest wall*: In breast cancer, the tumour bed following lumpectomy can present many problems of geometry and dose delivery, and 3-D proton dose distributions may be useful. For the chest wall, Sandison *et al.* (1997) made measurements in a phantom comparing electron "chest wall irradiation" to proton arc therapy to compare the resultant lung doses. A 200 MeV proton beam from the Indiana University Cyclotron was range shifted (energy degraded) and modulated to provide a spread out Bragg peak (SOBP) extending from the surface to a depth of 4 cm in water. The chest wall of an Alderson Rando phantom was irradiated by this beam collimated to a 20 × 4 cm field size, while it rotated on a platform at approximately 1 rpm. For comparison, electron arc therapy of the Rando phantom chest wall was similarly performed with 12 MeV electrons and the resultant lung dose measured in each case.

Dose-Volume histograms for the Rando phantom's left lung indicated a *reduced volume of irradiated lung for protons at all dose levels and an integral lung dose that is half that for electron arc therapy in the case studied. In addition more uniform dose coverage of the target volume was achieved with the proton therapy.*

Some other clinical situations may benefit from proton therapy, especially if spot scanning and fully 3-dimensional techniques were available.

Many articles have appeared in the literature about the potential advantages of protons in many clinical settings, so many of these are semi-speculative and therefore some speculation may be useful to focus the attention to the possibilities for 3-D, especially spot scanning of proton beams.

K.3.2
Ethmoid Sinus Tumours

Any site with a plethora of sensitive structures around, like the ethmoid sinus with the eyes, optic tract, lacrimal gland, the brain etc. is a logical choice for protons if a beam is available for 4 or 5 fractions per day, and non-coplanar planning and positioning is available. Tumours of the lacrimal gland itself may be a useful target for proton therapy.

K.3.3
Chordomas, Chondromas and Chondrosarcomas

Chordomas are rare tumours and arise form the remnant of the primitive notochord. About 35% arise intracranially, where they usually involve the clivus and 15% arise along the path of the notochord, where they usually involve the cervical spine. The remainder, 50%, arises in the sacrococcygeal area.

They can occur in any age group, but are more common in patients in their 50s and 60s. The prognosis is better in younger patients than in older patients, and they occur 2–3 times more often in males.

Chordomas are usually slow growing, but they are locally invasive and with a tendency to destroy bone.

Chondromas of the basisphenoid cause symptoms early and may resemble chondrochondromas and chondrosarcomas histologically. Radiologically, they may be difficult to differentiate from craniopharyngiomas, pineal tumours, hypophyseal and pontine gliomas.

They can be lethal because of their proximity to critical structures, aggressive local behaviour and high local recurrence rate. About 25% or higher of these will metastasise, usually to the lung, liver or bone (Perez and Chao 1998).

Sarcomas of the skull base can lie immediately adjacent to the brain, brain stem, cranial nerves, blood vessels, eyes and middle ear, which makes surgical resection difficult or impossible.

Table K3.1 summarises proton- and X-ray therapy results.

Table K3.1 Results of X-ray and proton therapy for chordomas, chondromas an chondrosarcomas near spinal cord and brain

Modality	Author	Dose (Gy)	Pt no. (%)	Local control (%)
X-ray	Austen-Seymour (1985)	55	36	36.0
X-ray	Catton (1986)	50	48	2.1
Proton	Suit and Urie (1992)	60–75	215	91 (chondrosarcomas) 65 (chondroma)
Proton	Nowakovski (1992)	70	36	58.3
Surgery + photon/proton	al-Mefty (1995)	–	25	64

K.3.3.1
Photon Therapy for Chondromas and Chordomas

Austin-Seymour (1985) noted that the intricate anatomical relationships limit the dose deliverable by conventional photon therapy to about 55 Gy, which resulted in a *local control rate in 8 patients of 36% at 3.5 years.*

Catton *et al.* (1996) retrospectively analysed the long-term results of treatment and the patterns of failure for patients with chordoma of the sacrum, base of skull and spine treated predominantly with postoperative photon irradiation. Forty-eight adult patients with chordoma of the sacrum (23), base of skull (20) or mobile spine (5), were seen between 1958–1992. Forty-four were referred postoperatively with overt disease and 31 of these were irradiated with conventionally fractionated radiation to a median dose of 50 Gy / 25 fractions / 5 weeks (range 25–60 Gy). Eight received a hyperfractionation protocol of 1 Gy, 4 hourly, four times a day (median 40 Gy / 44 fractions / 14 days), two sacral patients were treated with a hypofractionation protocol and three cases with skull base tumours were referred elsewhere for proton therapy. End points measured were survival time from diagnosis, objective response rate, symptomatic response rate and clinical or radiological progression-free survival from radiotherapy. They found that the median survival was 62 months (range 4–240 months) from diagnosis with no difference between clival and non-clival presentations. *One complete and no partial responses were identified in 23 assessable patients with photon therapy.* A subjective response was recorded for 12/14 with pain and 10/23 with neurological signs or symptoms, and the median time to progression for those with overt disease was 35 months (range 5–220 months). There was no survival advantage to patients receiving radiation doses > 50 Gy (median 60 Gy) compared to doses < 50 Gy (median 40 Gy). There was no difference between the conventional or hyperfractionation regimens with respect to the degree or duration of symptomatic response, or in progression-free survival. *The authors concluded that overt residual chordoma is rarely cured with conventional external beam irradiation, but treatment does provide useful and prolonged palliation of pain for most patients.*

Chordoma is a disease with low metastatic potential, and better local control may improve survival. Because radiation therapy may prove to be more successful in controlling microscopic disease, it should be considered as a pre- or postoperative adjuvant to a macroscopically complete resection. These patients will not obtain local control with conventional photon irradiation, and *suitable patients should be considered for irradiation with stereotactic photon or particle beam therapy.* For patients who progress after irradiation, there is limited symptomatic benefit to re-treatment with surgery or re-irradiation, and this should be limited to treating life-threatening complications.

K.3.3.2
Proton Therapy

Suit and Urie (1992) found that the dose with proton therapy could be escalated to 65–75 CGyE in 1.8 CGyE fractions, which amply confirmed the expectation of improved local control probability. At MGH/HCL *the actuarial local control rates at 5 years in 215 patients, 85 with chondrosarcoma and 130 with chordomas of the skull base and cervical spine, was 91% and 65%, respectively – a vast improvement on photon therapy.*

Nowakowski *et al.* (1992) treated 52 patients with tumours adjacent to and/or involving the cervical, thoracic or lumbar spinal cord at the University of California Lawrence Berkeley Laboratory (UCLBL). The histologies included chordoma and chondrosarcoma (24 pts) and other bone and soft tissue sarcoma (14 pts). Radiation doses varied from 29–80 CGyE with a median fractionated dose of 70 CGyE

For 36 previously untreated patients, local control was achieved in 21/36 patients and the 3 year actuarial survival was 51%.

For patients with chordoma and chondrosarcoma the probability of local control was influenced by tumour volume ($< 100 \text{ cm}^3 > 150 \text{ cm}^3$) and whether disease was recurrent or previously treated.

Complications occurred in 6/52 patients including one spinal cord injury one cauda equina and one brachial plexus injury, and three cases of skin or subcutaneous fibrosis.

They concluded that charged particle therapy could often be used to deliver higher tumour doses to paraspinal tumours than photons, with sparing of adjacent critical tissues, that *local control of paraspinal tumours appears higher with charged particle radiotherapy compared to historical (photon) data.* Smaller tumour volumes at the start of radiotherapy correlated with improved local control of chondroma and chondrosarcoma. The authors recommend debulking surgery prior to radiotherapy and observed that the control of chordoma and chondrosarcoma appears to be better when radiotherapy is used at the time of initial diagnosis rather than at the time of recurrence, and they recommend immediate postoperative radiotherapy rather than observation after surgery.

K.3.3.3
Surgery plus Radiotherapy

al-Mefty and Borba (1996) recognise that, because of their critical location, invasive nature, and aggressive recurrence, skull base chordomas are challenging and, at times, frustrating tumours to treat. *These tumours are best treated with sequentially combined radical surgery and proton-photon beam therapy.* During the last 5 years, they treated 25 patients (15 females and 10 males) who harboured pathologically diagnosed skull base chordomas. The mean age of the patients was 38.4 years (range 8–61 years). Previous surgery or radiation therapy was performed at other institutions in seven and two patients, respectively. The authors performed 33 surgical procedures on 23 patients. Radical removal (defined as absence of residual tumour on operative inspection and postoperative imaging) was achieved in 10 patients; subtotal resection (defined as resection of > 90% of the tumour) was achieved in 11 patients; and partial resection (defined as resection of < 90% of the tumour) was achieved in two patients. *Radical surgical removal included not only the excision of soft-tumour tissue, but also extensive drilling of the adjacent bone. Adjuvant therapy consisted of postoperative combined proton-photon beam therapy* (given to 17 patients) and conventional radiation therapy (two patients); three patients received no adjunct therapy. To date, four patients have died. One patient who had undergone previous surgery and sacrifice of the internal carotid artery died postoperatively from a stroke; one patient died from adenocarcinoma of the pancreas without evidence of recurrence; and two patients died at 25 and 39 months of recurrent tumour. Permanent neurological complications included third cranial nerve palsy (one patient) and hemi-anopsia (one patient); radiation necrosis occurred in three patients. *Of the 21 patients followed-up for more than 3 months after surgery, 16 have had no evidence of recurrence and five (including the two mortalities noted above) have had recurrent tumours* (four diagnosed clinically and one radiologically). The mean disease-free interval was 14.4 months.

K.3.4
Esthesioneuroblastoma and Chemo-Proton Radiation

Bhattacharyya *et al.* (1996) studied the efficacy of chemo-radiotherapy in nine consecutive patients with newly diagnosed esthesioneuroblastoma or neuroendocrine carcinoma of the paranasal sinuses from June 1992 to October 1995. After histological diagnosis and detailed imaging, two cycles of cisplatin and etoposide chemotherapy were instituted. *Chemotherapy responders were treated with combined photon and stereotaxic fractionated proton radiation therapy totalling approximately 68 Gy to the primary site*, whereas poor responders were treated with surgical resection followed by postoperative radiation. In both cases, therapy was then concluded with two additional cycles of cisplatin and etoposide chemotherapy. Nine patients with a median Dulguerov T stage of T3 (range T2–T4) completed the treatment protocol, with mean follow-up after diagnosis of 20.5 months. *Eight of nine patients exhibited a dramatic response to therapy with remission of their tumour, and resection was not required.* One patient failed to respond to induction chemotherapy and received surgical therapy to be followed by postoperative radiotherapy. There have been *no recurrences* (mean disease-free interval of 14.0 months). Complications were limited and generally transient. *The use of combined cisplatin and etoposide chemotherapy with proton radiation has demonstrated initial success in treatment of these tumours.* Dramatic response from chemotherapy is possible even in bulky or irresectable disease. This protocol has an acceptable complication rate. Further follow-up will be required to determine the long-term success rate of this therapeutic protocol.

K.4
Protons for Deep-Seated Body Tumours

K.4.1
Large Field Therapy with Horizontal Beams

K.4.1.1
Prostate Carcinoma (also see Fig G5.1)

Table K4.1 summarises the results for proton therapy for prostate carcinoma.

Table K4.1 Proton therapy for prostate carcinoma (see text)

Author	Regimen dose Gy (Ph) CGyE (Pr) T3 – T4	Pt no.	Local control at 5 y (%)	PSA	Rectal bleed (%)
Shipley (1995)	Ph (16.8+50.4)	93	92	–	9
	Pr (25.2+50.4)	96	80	–	27
	Ph Gleason 4–5	–	10	–	–
	Pr Gleason 4–5	–	94	–	–
Yonemoto (1997)	T2b – T3	106	FU <5y	(>4–10)	12
	Pr 30+Ph 45		96	(>10–20)	
			97	(>20)	
			63		

Shipley *et al.* (1995) reported on their experience in 189 patients in a phase III clinical trial with carcinoma of the prostate with proton therapy. All patients with T3–T4, Nx N0–2, M0 carcinoma of the prostate were treated with "conventional" external therapy to a dose of 50.4 Gy by four field photons and then randomised to receive either 16.8 Gy (total 62.2 Gy) photons or *25.2 CGyE with a perineal conformal proton plan to a total dose of 75.6 CGyE.*

With a median follow-up of 61 months (range 3 months to 139 months) 135 patients were alive and 67 have died from causes other than prostate cancer.

No differences were found between actuarial overall survival, disease specific survival, total recurrence free survival and local control. Among 93 patients in the proton arm (arm 1)) and 96 patients in the photon arm (arm 2), the local control at 5 and 8 years for the proton arm is 92% and 77%, respectively, and 80% and 60%, respectively, in the photon only arm (p = 0.89).

The local control in the proton arm was better in 57 patients with a Gleason Score of 4 or 5, at 94% and 64% at 5 and 8 years than in the photon only arm at 19% and 16% (p=0.0014). The authors conclude that a proton boost only improves local control in a subset of patients with an unfavourable Gleason Score. The complication rate with protons have been higher than in the photon arm, so it is obvious that the 12.5% escalation in dose from 67.2 Gy to 75.6 Gy could not be delivered harmlessly by a proton boost.

Comments: Modern day conformal 3-D photon therapy will also allow doses of 75 Gy to be given. This, in general, has been the dilemma with proton therapy: the technical advances in X-ray therapy have been so fast, that the majority of historical controls are no longer applicable.

With modern hospital based proton therapy centres, the question should be asked again: will isocentric conformal well-fractionated proton therapy for the whole course be better than either well fractionated conformal photons or than a brachytherapeutic prostatic implant?

This proton therapy trial was a single institute trial and it took so long (10 years from 1982–1992) that Hanks (1995) pointed out that it crossed the development of the cat scan (CT) magnetic resonance imaging (MRI) transrectal ultrasound and the introduction of the prostate specific antigen (PSA) test.

The rectal and bladder complications were more severe in the proton arm. Rectal bleeding was seen in 27% of the proton patients *versus* 9% in the photon arm; urethral stricture in 12% *versus* 5% and hematuria in 14% *versus* 6%.

This trial shows that single institutional trials are unlikely to find answers, and co-operative prospective proton therapy trials for rapid patient accrual will be essential. It was probably difficult with a single perineal field to avoid the rectum adequately.

K.4.2
Large Field Therapy with Isocentric Beams

K.4.2.1
Prostate Carcinoma

Yonemoto *et al.* (1997) reported on the preliminary results of a phase I/II study of combined proton and photon study of conformal radiation therapy for locally advanced carcinoma of the prostate. The study was developed to evaluate the use of combined photons and protons for the treatment of locally advanced carcinoma of the prostate. One hundred and six patients in stages T2b (B2), T2c (B2), and T3 (C) were treated with 45 Gy photon-beam irradiation to the pelvis and an additional 30 Cobalt Gray Equivalent (CGyE) to the prostate with 250 MeV protons, yielding a total prostate dose of 75 CGyE in 40 fractions. Median follow-up time was 20.2 months (range 10–30 months). Toxicity was scored according to the Radiation Therapy Oncology Group (RTOG) grading system; local control was evaluated by serial digital rectal examination (DRE) and prostate specific antigen (PSA) measurements.

Morbidity evaluation was available on 104 patients. *The actuarial 2-year rate of Grade 1 or 2 late morbidity was 12% (8% rectal, 4% urinary).* No patients demonstrated Grade 3 or 4 late morbidity. Treatment response was evaluated on 100 patients with elevated pre-treatment serum PSA levels. The actuarial 2-year rate of PSA normalisation was 96%, 97%, and 63% for pre-treatment PSAs of > 4–10, > 10–20, and > 20, respectively. The 13 patients with rising PSA demonstrated local recurrence (3 patients), distant metastasis (8 patients), or no evidence of disease except increasing PSA (2 patients). *The authors concluded that a low incidence of side effects, despite the tumour dose of 75 CGyE, demonstrates that conformal protons can deliver higher doses of radiation to target tissues without increasing complications to surrounding normal tissues.* The initial tumour response, as assessed by the high actuarial rate of normalisation with pre-treatment PSA < or = 20, and the low rate of recurrence within the treatment field (2.8%), were considered encouraging.

Many other questions relative to prostate carcinoma are now probably of greater importance than dose escalation studies, such as hormonal cyto-reduction prior to radiotherapy. It is unlikely that dose escalations over 71–72 Gy will lead to further improvements in local control (Cox 1995).

K.4.2.2
Potential Improvement in the Results of Proton Irradiation for Prostate Cancer

Sandler *et al.* (1992) state that nearly 33% of patients with Stage C carcinoma of the prostate fails locally after radiotherapy. They devised a 3-D treatment plan, which was in fact the currently in vogue 6 field technique for conformal photon therapy. This CT based, 3-D planning technique, is now, 6 years later in 1998, probably standard practice in the majority of academic and leading private hospitals, and serves to illustrate the enormous progress in photon therapy over the last 5 years. It has become the norm to give photon doses in excess of 64 Gy in 2 Gy fractions, and patients tolerate 3-D conformal therapy to doses of up to 75 Gy in 2 Gy fractions.

This article by Sandler *et al.* (1992) signifies a turning point in the radiotherapy of prostate cancer.

Can one improve on the present results with proton therapy?

A relatively simple prostate boost plan is depicted in Fig. G5.1. It is simply made up of two lateral 200 MeV fields but well collimated. This field arrangement was necessitated by the constraint imposed by the single horizontal beam available.

Modern intensity modulation can give comparable photon plans. Spot scanning can give very good conformity with fewer proton than photon fields (Schreuder *et al.* 1998).

K.4.2.3
Brachytherapy for Prostate Carcinoma

A newcomer with potential for prostate carcinoma is the perineal prostate implant with radioactive seeds.

Which of these modalities will prevail?

External beam therapy takes 6–8 weeks, but the modern linear accelerators are very reliable. Prostate implants are unlikely to incapacitate the patient for more than 7 days. Proton therapy may take 6–8 weeks as well, or more, unless faster fractionation schedules can be worked out, and tested by clinical trial.

K.4.3
Oesophageal Carcinoma

Koyama *et al.* (1994) reported on 15 patients with oesophageal carcinoma, six cases with superficial tumours who were treated with a 250 MeV proton beam with or without external photon irradiation with a 12 MV linear accelerator. Eleven patients were initially treated with doses of 16.2–50.4 Gy (mean 42.8 Gy) followed by proton beam at doses from 30.0–50.9 Gy (mean 37.6 Gy). Four patients were treated with proton beams alone to doses of 75.0–88.5 (mean 81.4 Gy). The mean total dose for the 15 patients was 80.4 Gy, and all the primary tumour lesions of all 15 patients disappeared. Approximately 4–5 months later 9/15 patients developed ulcers in the oesophagus at the site of the primary lesions. The ulcers healed with conservative management.

K.4.4
Brain Metastases

Advantage for radiosurgery *versus* neurosurgery could be shown for single brain metastases, with median survival of 40 weeks for surgery and 40–49 weeks for radiosurgery, and 20% local failure for surgery *versus* 11% local failure for radiosurgery. Neurological deaths in the surgery group was 29% *versus* 17% – 18% for radiosurgery (Loeffler *et al.* 1995)

The annual incidence of brain metastases in the United States may be in excess of 100,000 cases (Mehta 1995). The median survival time may only be 1 month.

Recent RTOG studies using 1.6 Gy twice daily to total doses of 48–70.4 Gy showed a significant survival advantage and symptomatic improvement at the higher doses. The MTD was found to be 54.4 Gy, providing clear evidence that intracranial disease control is dose dependent and that control translates to a survival advantage (Curren *et al.* 1991). This topic is further discussed in Chapter L.5.

K.5
Potential Gains with Protons in Various Anatomical Sites

An entire volume of the International Journal of Radiation Oncology Biology and Physics (vol. 122,1992) was devoted to this topic.

According to Suit (1992) there are two classes of failure in radiation therapy: (1) local control not achieved and (2) radiation induced morbidity. Closer approximation of target to volume may well address these problems and the superior dose distributions of proton therapy may realise these objectives. Urtasun (1992) showed that, for conventional external beam irradiation over a period of decades, in every instance where there has been a major advance in physical delivery of radiation dose to the tumour, there has been a corresponding major improvement in the treatment results.

K.5.1
Glioblastoma

Superior dose distribution of protons *versus* photons could be shown for glioblastoma multiforme, which has (1) a highly radioresistant macroscopic tumour mass and (2) extensive microscopic invasion. Tatsusaki *et al.* (1992) showed by means of comparative planning, that 90 CGyE could be delivered with fractionated external proton radiation to some gioblastomas located in the cerebral hemisphere with a minimal volume of normal brain receiving > 70 CGyE.

The advantage of proton beams over radioactive implants is the elimination of the trauma of surgery, better conformity, and a likely reduction in the incidence of brain necrosis.

K.5.2
Brain Tumours in Children

Wambersie *et al.* (1992) found that if protons were available for brain tumour treatment for children, then about 50% of all these patients would have been chosen for proton therapy.

Medulloblastoma: One of the components of radiotherapy (RT) in medulloblastoma/primitive neuroectodermal tumours is the prophylactic irradiation of the whole brain (WBI). Miralbell *et al.* (1997) undertook a CT-scan-based dosimetric study with the aim of reducing late neuropsychologic morbidity in which treatment was confined mainly or exclusively to supratentorial sites considered at high risk for disease recurrence. They employed a three field (two laterals and one posterior) proton plan (spot scanning method) which was compared with a two-field conventional whole brain irradiation (WBI) 6 MV X-ray plan, to a 6-field "hand-made" 6 MV X-ray plan, and to a computer-optimised 9-field "inverse" 15 MV X-ray plan. For favourable patients, 30 Gy was delivered to the ventricles and main cisterns, the subfrontal and subtemporal regions, and the posterior fossa. For the unfavourable patients, 10 Gy WBI preceded a boost to 30 Gy to the same treatment volume chosen for favourable patients. The dose distribution was evaluated by means of dose-volume histograms to examine the coverage of the targets as well as the dose to the non-target brain and optical structures.

Proton beams succeeded better in reducing the dose to the brain hemispheres and eye than any of the photon plans. A 25.1% risk of an IQ score <90 was predicted after 30 Gy WBI. Almost a 10% drop in the predicted risk was observed when using proton beams in both favourable and unfavourable patients. However, predicted normal tissue complication probabilities (NTCPs) for "hand made" and "inverse" photon plans were only slightly higher (0.3% – 2.5%) than those of proton beams. Children between 4 years to 8 years of age benefited most from the dose reduction in this exercise with similar NTCP predictions for both proton and "inverse" plans. *A decrease in morbidity can be expected from protons and both optimised photon plans compared to whole brain irradiation.*

Spinal irradiation in medulloblastoma: Miralbel *et al.* (1997) compared proton plans to photon plans because conventional postoperative photon-beam radiotherapy to the spine in children with medulloblastoma/primitive neuroectodermal tumours (PNET) is associated with severe late effects, which are related to the exit dose of the beams and is particularly severe in young children. A posterior modulated 100 MeV proton beam (spot scanning method) was compared with that of a standard set of posterior 6 MV X-ray fields. The potential improvements with protons were evaluated, using dose-volume histograms to examine the coverage of the target as well as the dose to the vertebral bodies (growth plates), lungs, heart, and liver. They found that the spinal dural sac received the full prescribed dose in both treatment plans. However, *the proportions of the vertebral body volume receiving > or = 50% of the prescribed dose were 100% and 20% for 6 MV X-rays and protons, respectively. For 6 MV X-rays > 60% of the dose prescribed to the target was delivered to 44% of the heart volume, while the proton beam was able to completely avoid the heart, the liver, and in all likelihood the thyroid and gonads as well. This study demonstrates a potential role of proton therapy in decreasing the dose (and toxicity) to the critical structures in the irradiation of the spinal neuraxis in medulloblastoma/primitive neuroectordermal tumours (PNET).* The potential bone marrow and growth arrest sparing effects make this approach specially attractive for intensive chemotherapy protocols and for very young children. Sparing the thyroid gland, the posterior heart wall, and the gonads may be additional advantages in assuring a long-term post-treatment morbidity-free survival.

Thalamic astrocytoma: Archambeau *et al.* (1992) found that it was possible to deliver a simulated tumour dose of 74 Gy for a thalamic astrocytoma. This plan was compared to an X-ray plan, which showed that a decreased integral dose to normal brain and a decreased dose to the volume of normal brain were achieved, despite the 20 Gy "boost".

K.5.3
Maxillary Sinus

Miralbell *et al.* (1992) showed that there are challenging technical problems for radiotherapists for planning treatment for maxillary sinus tumours. This is due to the complexity of the regional anatomy and the close relations of the dose limiting structures like the eyes, the optic nerve, optic chiasm and brain stem. Although tumour coverage was the same for a 3-D X-ray plan, compared to X-rays plus a proton boost, the critical structures received less dose in the X-ray plus proton beam plan. They conclude that because a superior dose distribution should yield an improved local control and reduced morbidity, a benefit in survival could be expected.

K.5.4
Cervical Carcinoma

Slater *et al.* (1992) cited a local failure rate of 40% – 45% for advanced cervical carcinoma when treated with a combination of external beam irradiation and intracavitary implants, and approximately 60% – 65% when treated by external beam alone. Computer modelled examples showed a therapeutic advantage for proton therapy in local control and morbidity. The use of protons plus intracavitary implants offer larger tumour doses with protons than with photons, while the dose-volume to normal structures is decreased.

Smit (1992) determined by CT scanning, the likely minimal volume that would be required for the adequate coverage of patients with cervical carcinoma, stage IB–IIIB. The mean uterine volume was found to be 152 cm^3, the volume enclosing the major blood vessels and parametria 754 cm^3 with a total target volume (uterus, parametria, lymph node) of 906 cm^3. The volumes for a four field unleaded "box" varies from 2016–3220 cm^3 for stage IB. Suitably collimated proton beams therapy could reduce the target volume from a mean of > 2000 cm^3 to < 1000 cm^3.

The volume irradiated could be reduced by 60% with protons compared to photons.

It was thought unlikely that proton therapy will render intracavitary therapy unnecessary.

K.5.5
Para-aortic Lymph Nodes

Levin (1992) showed that carcinoma of the cervix managed with surgery and conventional radiotherapy (about 55 Gy) is associated with an unacceptably high incidence of major morbidity. He could show that the addition of a proton boost to photon treatment would permit the delivery of 60–70 Gy to the nodes with a morbidity expected to be equal to that of 45 Gy photons (13%). *The potential for improved control rates may be of the order of 10% – 20% depending on the initial stage of disease.* (Fig. K5.1)

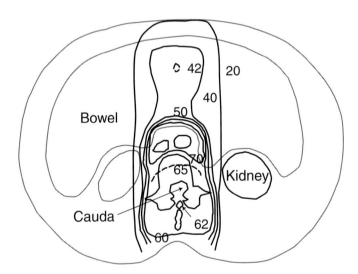

Fig. K5.1 CT Schematic of a transverse plane within the treatment volume. Composite isodoses for 40 Gy delivered by parallel opposed 20 MeV X-rays plus 30 Gy SOBP 5 cm protons from the posterior. This arrangement will limit the dose to (62% of 70 Gy to the cord) for 70 Gy to the para-aortic lymph nodes. (Redrawn from CV Levin et al., 1991, Int J Radiat Oncol Biol Phys 22:355–359)

K.5.6
Retroperitoneal Cancer in a Child with Wilm's Tumour

Gademan and Wannenmacher (1992) showed superior comparative plans for protons. It is very clear from the plans that for some such situations, a vertical proton beam, or isocentric proton gantry has very distinct advantages, and this sort of improvement may signal a return to radiotherapy in the management of at least some paediatric tumours.

K.5.7
Rectal Cancer

Isacson *et al.* (1996) studied conformal treatment planning with megavoltage X-rays and protons for medically inoperable patients with a large rectal tumour in an attempt to determine if there are advantages of using protons instead of X-rays. Three dose plans were made for each of six patients: one proton plan, including three beams covering the primary tumour and adjacent lymph nodes and three boost beams covering the primary tumour: one X-ray plan, eight beams including a boost with four beams and one mixed plan with four X-ray beams and a boost with three proton beams. A three-dimensional treatment-planning system called TMS was used. Evaluation of the different plans was by dose-volume histograms. *Protons showed an advantage for all six patients compared to X-rays, but in half of them the advantage was found to be only marginal.* The dose-limiting organ at risk is the small bowel, but the proton plan and the mixed plan also spare the bladder and the femoral heads better. The authors concluded that proton beam therapy has potential advantages for treating medically inoperable patients with a large rectal cancer to conventional X-ray therapy. Since the benefits are comparatively small, although clinically worthwhile, large randomised studies are needed.

New comparative plans and potential gains should be undertaken by comparing spot scanning isocentric proton plans with conformal photon or in some cases, even brachytherapy plans.

K.6
Summary

Horizontal protons beam therapy has proved its value indisputably for chondromas and chondrosarcomas near the spinal cord and brainstem.

Horizontal beams, if of sufficient energy (200 MeV and more) can offer acceptable plans, but prostate carcinomas should perhaps not be treated by horizontal beams with less than the energy needed to pass 4–6 cm beyond the sagittal mid plane of the body.

Protons are valuable in areas where it is very difficult to avoid a host of sensitive structures like the ethmoid and maxillary sinuses although comparative data with photons are lacking. Chemo-proton therapy for esthesioneuroblastomas is very promising, and this concept should perhaps be tested for other sites.

The results for prostate carcinoma treated by isocentric beam delivery proton therapy are promising, but protons may have to be tested against conformal photon therapy as well as radioactive implants (brachytherapy).

Potential gains for protons have been published for many sites, including paediatric tumours. These potential gains will only become science if proven by randomised clinical trials, although some of the dosimetric arguments are so strong that where suitable proton therapy facilities are available, the ethics of controlled trials for some situations may well be questioned. Such situations may be for the paediatric tumours mentioned, and for the irradiation of the para-aortic lymph nodes, to mention two examples.

New comparative plans and potential gains should be undertaken by comparing spot scanning isocentric proton plans with conformal photon or in some cases, brachytherapy plans.

K.7
References

al-Mefty O, Borba LA (1997) Skull base chordomas: a management challenge. J Neurosurg 86:182–189

Archambeau JO, Slater JD, Slater JM, Tangeman R (1992) Role for proton beam irradiation in treatment of paediatric CNS malignancies. Int J Radiat Oncol Biol Phys 22:287–295

Archambeau JO, Schulte RW, Miller DW, Teichman SL, Slater JM (1997) Int J Radiat Oncol Biol Phys 37:21–29

Austin-Seymour M, Munzerider JE, Goitein M et al. (1989) Progress in low LET heavy particle therapy: intracranial, paracranial tumours and uveal melanomas. Radiat Res Suppl 8:S219–S226

Bhattacharya N, Thornton AF, Joseph MP, Goodman ML, Amrein PC (1997) Successful treatment of esthesioneuroblastoma and neuroendocrine carcinoma with combined chemotherapy and proton irradiation: results in 9 cases. Arch Otolaryngol Head Neck Surg 123:34–40

Blomgren H, Lax I, Naslund I, Svanstrom R (1995) Stereotactic high dose fraction radiation therapy of extracranial tumours using an accelerator. Clinical experience of the first thirty-one patients. Acta Oncol 34:861–870

Catton C, O'Sullivan B, Bell R, Laperriere N, Cummings B, Fornasier V, Wunder J (1996) Chordoma: long-term follow-up after radical photon irradiation. Radiother Oncol 41:67–72

Cox JD (1995) Dose escalation by proton irradiation for adenocarcinoma of the prostate. (editorial) Int J Radiat Oncol Biol Phys 32:265–266

Curran W, Scott C, Nelson D et al. (1991) Results from the RTOG Phase I/II twice daily RT dose escalation trials for malignant glioma (83-02) and brain metastases (85-28). Ninth International Conference on Brain Tumour Research and Therapy, Asilomar, California

Hanks GE (1995) A question filled future for dose escalation in prostate cancer. Editorial, Int J Radiat Oncol Biol Phys 32:267–271

Henkelman M (1992) New imaging technologies: prospects for target definition. Int J Radiat Oncol Biol Phys 22:251–257

Isacsson U, Montelius A, Jung B, Glimelius B (1996) Comparative treatment planning between proton and X-ray therapy in locally advance rectal cancer. Radiother Oncol 41:263–272

Koyama S, Tsujii H, Yokota H et al. (1994) Proton beam therapy for patients with oesophageal carcinoma. JPN J Clin Oncol 24:144–153

Levin CV (1992) Potential for gain in the use of proton beam boost to the para-aortic lymph nods in carcinoma of the cervix. Int J Radiat Oncol Biol Phys 22:355–361

Loeffler JS, Larson A, Shrieve DC et al. (1995) In: DeVita V, Hellmann S, Rosenberg SA (eds). Lippincott, Philadelphia pp 141–156

Miralbell R, Lomax A, Bortfeld T, Rouzaud M, Carrie C (1997) Potential role of proton therapy in the treatment of paediatric medulloblastoma/primitive neuroectodermal tumours: reduction of the supratentorial target volume. Int J Radiat Oncol Biol Phys 38:477–484

Miralbell R, Lomax A, Russo M (1997) Potential role of proton therapy in the treatment of paediatric medulloblastoma/primitive neuroectodermal tumours: spinal theca irradiation. Int J Radiat Oncol Biol Phys 38:805–811

Miralbell R, Crowell C, Suit H (1992) Potential improvement in of 3-dimension treatment planning and proton therapy in the outcome of maxillary sinus cancer. Int J Radiat Oncol Biol Phys 22:305–311

Nowakowski VA, Castro JR, Petti Pl et al. (1992) Charged particle radiotherapy of paraspinal tumours. Int J Radiat Oncol Biol Phys 22:295–303

Perez CA, Chao KSC (1998). Unusual non-epithelial tumours of the head and neck. In: Perez CA, Brady L (eds) Principles and practice of radiation oncology. Lippincott-Raven, pp 1095–1134

Sandison GA, Papiez E, Bloch C, Morphis J (1995) Phantom assessment of lung dose from proton arc therapy. Int J Radiat Oncol Biol Phys 38:891–897

Sandler HM, Perez-Tomayo C, Ten Haka RK (1992) Dose escalation for stage C(T3) prostate cancer. Minimal toxicity observed using conformal therapy. Radiother Oncol 23:53–54

Schreuder AN, Jones DTL, Conradie JL et al. (1998) The non-orthogonal fixed beam arrangement for the second proton therapy facility at the National Accelerator Centre. 15th Conference on the application of accelerators in commerce and industry. American Institute of Physics

Shipley WU, Verhey LJ, Munzerider JE et al. (1995) Advanced prostate cancer: the results of a randomised comparative trial of high dose irradiation boosting with conformal protons compared with conventional dose irradiation using photons alone. Int J Radiat Oncol Biol Phys 32:3–13

Slater JD, Slater JM, Wahlen S (1992) The potential for proton beam therapy in the locally advanced carcinoma of the cervix. Int J Radiat Oncol Biol Phys 22:343–347

Smit BJ (1992) Prospects for proton therapy in carcinoma of the cervix. Int J Radiat Oncol Biol Phys l22:349–355

Suit H (1992) Editors note. Proton workshop: potential clinical gains by use of superior dose distribution. Int J Radiat Oncol Biol Phys 22:233–234

Suit H, Urie M (1992) Proton beams in radiation therapy: Review. J Natl Cancer Inst 84:155–164

Tatsusaki H, Urie M, Linggood R (1992) Comparative treatment planning: proton *versus* X-ray beams against glioblastoma multiforme. Int J Radiat Oncol Biol Phys 22:265–275

Umebayoshi Y, Uyeno K, Tsujii H et al. (1994) Proton radiotherapy of skin carcinomas. Br J Dermatol 130:88–91

Urtasun (1992) Does improved depth dose characteristics and treatment planning correlate with gain in therapeutic results? Evidence from past clinical experience using conventional radiation sources. Int J Radiat Oncol Biol Phys 22:235–239

Wambersie A, Gregoire V, Brucher JM (1992) Potential clinical gain of proton (and heavy ion) beams for brain tumours in children. Int J Radiat Oncol Biol Phys 22:275–287

Yonemoto LT, Slater JD, Rossi CJ Jr. et al. (1996) Phase I/II study of proton beam irradiation for the treatment of subfoveal choroidal neovascularisation in age-related macular degeneration: treatment techniques and preliminary results. Int J Radiat Oncol Biol Phys 36:867–871

L Radiosurgical Applications of Protons and Photons

L.1
Vascular Malformations

L.1.1
Introduction

Vascular malformations are congenital lesions comprising different pathologies, all with a tendency to bleed, often with disastrous consequences for the patient either on the first or subsequent bleeding episodes. Surgical removal is curative, and immediately removes the risk of bleeding.

Radiosurgery offers an alternate treatment method, especially for inoperable patients and patients with large AVMs. The drawback with radiosurgery for these lesions is the latent period before occlusion occurs.

This latent period can be 2–3 years and re-bleed can occur following radiosurgery, although at a reduced rate.

There is evidence that the probability for AVM obliteration is related to the dose to the AVM periphery (only for Gamma Knife treatment of AVMs). The AVM volume seems to have no independent impact on the probability of obliteration.

Cavernous malformations (cavernous angiomas and angiographically occult venous malformation, AOVMs) are congenital vascular anomalies of the vasculature of the brain. They can be located in any brain region and are characterised by dilated thin-walled vascular channels lined by a single endothelium and thin fibrous adventia: typically no brain parenchyma is found within the lesion.

AOVMs should probably only be treated *if they are symptomatic*, as they appear to be more liable to cause radiation related complications, and young people and children are especially prone to complications.

Nonetheless, for many patients radiosurgery is a modality with a strong curative potential and it is a useful addition to the armamentarium for the treatment of AVMs.

The results with proton therapy produced contradictory conclusions, which will be discussed.

L.1.2
Arteriovenous Malformations

Mehta (1995), in an excellent overview on radiosurgery, gives the following information: John Hunter first described AVMs in 1775, Rudolph Virchov gave the first pathology reports 1863, Olivecrona did the first angiogram in 1940, the first surgical removal in 1948 and Steiner reported the first radiosurgical treatment in the 1970s.

Fabrikant *et al.* (1992) summarised their clinical experience with protons and helium ions, in an excellent review from work done at the University of California, Berkeley, Lawrence Berkeley Laboratory (UCB-LBL).

L.1.2.1
Clinical Features of AVMs

Vascular malformations are classified into arteriovenous malformations (AVMs), venous angiomata, cavernous angiomata and capillary telangiectases. Of these, only AVMs and AOVMs will be discussed.

Signs and Symptoms
1. Haemorrhage and its consequences in about 50 per cent.
2. Seizures in 30 per cent.
3. Paresis in 15 per cent.
4. Migraine in 5 per cent of patients.

Some of these features can occur in combination.

For example, one of our patient recently presented at the uncommon age of 74, with a combination of migraine and focal epilepsy.

Haemorrhage: Most haemorrhages from an AVM is parenchymal but blood may enter the subarachnoid space or the ventricles. The ongoing risk of intracranial haemorrhage from an untreated AVM is 3% – 4% per year, and the risk of recurrent haemorrhage is higher than this after an AVM has bled before. The risk of death of an AVM rupture is approximately 10%, and the mortality rate increases with each subsequent haemorrhage.

Epilepsy may be focal, or may manifest with very incapacitating grand mal attacks. The epilepsy may be difficult to control with the usual anti-convulsants, since the stimulus may be haemosiderin, which is deposited as a result of a prior bleeding episode.

Paresis: Focal ischaemic neurological deficits of a variety of types may occur, depending on the lesion site and side due to the phenomenon of "vascular steal", sometimes leading to progressive neurological deficit. One young patient presented with an irresistible urge to eat, probably due to ishaemia of the hypothalamus caused by AVM steal.

Migraine-like headaches, sometimes of chronic type, and somewhat resistant to the usual painkillers is a frequent manifestation.

L.1.2.2
Pathology and Prognostic Factors

Histopathology: These congenital lesions seem to arise from a failure to form a capillary bed during embryogenesis. Thus AVMs consist of high flow, direct connections between arterioles and venules. Although they are congenital lesions, they usually manifest in the second or third decade of life. They may enlarge slowly with age.

The long-term prognosis for patients with an untreated AVM is poor, because as much as 23 per cent of patients, if not treated, will die as a result of bleeding from their AVM at some point in the future. The bleeding risk may in fact be slightly higher for small than for large lesions (Spetzler 1992).

The incidence of neurological deficit is approximately 50% for each episode of haemorrhage, and the risk of death is about 30% for such a lesion and about 66% for posterior fossa AVMs (Lunsford 1990).

Children are at special risk since they will have to live through the period with the highest risk for AVM rupture, i.e. 15 to 40 years of age.

Patients suffering from AVMs are also likely to develop neurological deficits as a result of shunted blood flow, or "steal", not only from bleeding. This "steal" may be evident on the angiograms and may manifest as an area of reduced perfusion.

Cerebral arterial aneurysms occur simultaneously in 3%–9% of reported series, and all the angiograms of patients with AVMs should therefore be scrutinised for arterial aneurysms.

If such aneurysms are found in the circle of Willis or in the vessels feeding the AVM they should be treated before or immediately after radiosurgery for the AVM (Fabrikant 1992).

Radiopathology: Radiotherapy induces thrombosis in small blood vessels and causes reproductive cell death, with sclerosis of the vessels. The consequence is obliteration of the AVM. A concomitant danger is radionecrosis of the surrounding brain, which can be avoided by careful planning and choice of dose. Radionecrosis mimics the symptoms of a brain tumour with mass effect, therefore the production of radionecrosis should not be the primary aim of treatment and should be avoided as it often needs neuro-surgical intervention to correct the problem.

L.1.2.3
Evaluation Methods for AVMs

For an excellent description of the radiology, the reader is referred to the textbook by Haaga *et al.* 1994.

The diagnostic methods available include angiography, computerised tomography, magnetic resonance angiography (MRA) and 3-dimensional "time of flight" angiography. Figure L1.1 shows the beautiful picture that can be obtained with modern MRA, which may replace conventional angiograms.

Where available positron emission tomography (PET scanning) may be of use.

Computerised tomography (CT): On non-contrast scans, AVMs are slightly denser than grey matter. Areas of calcification may be present within the malformation, and areas of low density may surround the malformation. These areas of low density may represent areas of gliosis or encephalomalacia caused by previous haemorrhage or by ischaemia. On contrast, AVMs manifest as hyperdense, serpiginous, dilated efferent and afferent vessels (Haaga 1994).

The larger vessels are usually the draining veins.

Magnetic resonance imaging (MRI): The majority of the vessels are seen as black areas (areas of "signal void"). At times, an intermediate or high signal may be visualised in some of the vessels. This signal may reflect thrombosis or may be secondary to slow turbulent blood flow. MRI is superior to CT in determining the relationship of the AVM to parenchymal structures. MRI can also pick up ischaemic and gliotic changes in the brain (TE/long TR spin echo sequences), (Haaga 1994).

Because of the sensitivity of MRI to the paramagnetic effect of haemosiderin, MRI is highly sensitive to areas of previous bleeding in the vicinity of the lesion.

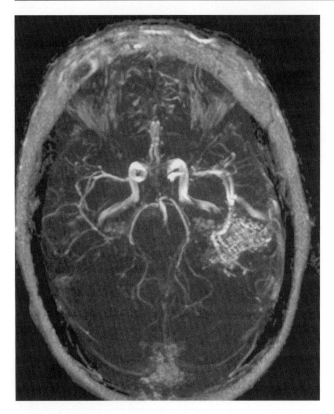

Fig. L1.1 MRA (magnetic resonance angiogram) next to a conventional CT (computerised tomography) picture with contrast. (Courtesy Dr Fred Vernimmen, Radiation Oncologist, Tygerberg Hospital and Dr Leon van Rensburg, Radiologist, Durbanville, Cape Province, South Africa)

MRA (magnetic resonance angiography) is capable of providing information about the arterial supply and venous drainage.

It is also possible to say which part of an AVM nidus a particular artery supplies, by applying saturation pulses.

It is possible to determine blood flow velocities in arteries and veins involved with the AVM.

Magnetic Resonance Scanning Parameters for pre-and postoperative imaging for AVMs: With regard to pre-treatment MRI, Morikawa *et al.* (1996) found that spin echo (SE) images showed up the nidus in 19/20 patients. Feeding arteries and draining veins were seen in 18/20 of the patients studied.

Signal changes due to previous haemorrhage were detected in 13/20 of the patients.

Eight out of nine of the patients imaged showed contrast enhancement in the nidus with gadolinium DTPA (Gd.MRI) before treatment.

MRA demonstrated the feeding arteries and veins clearly in 100%, i.e. in all ten patients studied.

These results with a 1.5 Tesla unit with MRA capability should greatly aid the radiosurgical team where a 1.5 Tesla MRI unit is available. The diagnostic parameters are given in detail in Morikawa (1996)

Angiography is a standard procedure and will not be discussed further. Orthogonal stereotactic angiograms are considered essential for radiosurgical planning.

Positron emission tomography (PET): This may be of some value in some cases but the spatial resolution is poor.

L.1.2.4
Treatment Options for Ateriovenous Malformations

The treatment options available include surgery, embolisation and radiosurgery or a combination of these.

Radiosurgery is characterised by the rapid dose fall-off at the target boundary; this fall off is much sharper than can be achieved with conventional radiotherapy techniques. However, not all beams are of equal quality, and the radiosurgeon is advised to take cognisance of the effects of the fall-off characteristics of beams *and* the treatment plans. (See chapter I on Dose-Volume Relationships, Appendix P.4 and the Introduction in Chapter G)

For 3, 5 and 10 cm diameter circular proton beams (Jones *et al.* 1995) with a 5 cm spread-out Bragg peak (SOBP) the following data may be of interest (Table L1.1).

Table L1.2 shows that for a prescribed dose of 16 CGyE, the prescription isodose dictates the lesion volumes that can be irradiated for a constraint of 10 Gy to 10 cm^3 (Voges 1996). This table illustrates that if homogeneity is sacrificed for an improved

Table L1.1 A representative ratio of penumbral widths to the prescription isodose diameter for beams of circular diameter 3, 5 and 10 cm for proton beam profiles at 11.5 cm depth

Prescription isodose	3 cm	5 cm	10 cm
100%	0.14	0.44	0.55
90%	0.33	0.55	0.73
80%	0.44	0.66	0.78
50%	0.64	0.76	0.94

penumbra, protons may have a much greater utility for radiosurgery for small lesions. (See Chapter L on Dose-Volume Relationships)

Surgery: Successful surgical removal immediately removes the risk of re-bleeding and is preferable to the other treatment options where feasible.

Contra-indications to surgery are: Localisation of the lesion in sensitive and critically delicate areas of the brain, large lesions, and lesions with drainage to the deep venous system. These vessels are friable, inclined to retract and to result in uncontrollable bleeding. This type of drainage is fortunately not an obstacle to the radiation oncologist.

Embolisation is effective, but the results are not necessarily permanent as these lesions are prone to re-canalise after embolisation. Embolisation does not help to

Table L1.2 The influence of prescribing at the 100%, 90%, 80%, 70% and 60% isodoses on the lesion volume assuming a constraint of 10 Gy to 10 cm3 as the smallest dose-volume likely to cause zero complications, that can be irradiated with a representative 30 mm diameter proton beam with 11.5 cm residual range using the data from Table L1.1 *(first column)*. (See Chapter F on Dose-Volume Relationships) Also see Appendix P3

Prescription isodose	Lesion volume cm^3 (spherical lesion assumed)	Total volume receiving 10 Gy minimum
100%	0.11	10
90%	1.77	10
80%	2.57	10
70%	4.19	10
60%	7.24	10

reduce the volume of the AVM for subsequent radiosurgery, since small patent vessels, which later enlarge, may remain behind and may later re-bleed or re-expand.

Radiosurgery for AVMs

Indications include patients who are not fit for surgical removal or who have inoperable lesions. Angiographically occult arteriovenous malformations (AOVMs) are only considered for treatment if there is clinical and radiological evidence of a prior haemorrhage – totally asymptomatic patients should probably not be treated. Patients should have a good performance status and should be able to co-operate during the planning and treatment procedures.

L.1.2.5
Multidisciplinary Teams

A very important principle is that a multidisciplinary team, which should include the neurosurgeon, neuroradiologist, neuropathologist, the radiation oncologist, medical physicist and experienced radiographer, should assess each patient, and should be involved in defining the target.

L.1.2.6
Proton Radiosurgery for AVMs and Other Methods

General: Radiosurgery is effective and non-invasive, but the draw-backs are a latent period of 1–3 years before the obliteration of the AVM is likely to be complete, and the treatment of large lesions is likely to cause radiation associated complications.

The latent period may be shorter with larger total doses, but the risk of complications will also be higher with the larger doses. This is so because the larger the dose, the larger the volume of brain tissue or brain containing tissue to receive a critical dose, is likely to be. (See also Chapter I on Dose-Volume Relationships)

During the latent period there seems to be a progressive reduction in the risk for a re-bleed per year, on average about a 1%–2% after radiosurgery, as compared to untreated patients, where the risk of an untreated AVM to bleed is about 3%–4% per annum. If complete obliteration is achieved, the risk for a re-bleed should vanish.

Planning: Determination of the volume of the lesion can be done by drawing the outline of the lesion on each of about 50 or more CT slices. The total area of all slices can then be calculated, and since the slice thickness is known, the volume can be calculated. The shape of the lesion is important, since more brain tissue will be included in the planning target volume than with regular or spherical lesions.

Unfortunately, the AVM is not always visible on the CT scan. CT scans are therefore done with and without contrast.

Other methods of delineating the nidus include stereotactic angiography, MRI and MRA (magnetic resonance imaging and magnetic resonance angiography). Scanning with the immobilisation frame or mask in situ is essential to achieve the required degree of accuracy.

It is imperative that planning systems for radiosurgery should have image registration or image fusion capabilities, otherwise it is easy to misplan and miss the target.

The reader is also referred to the sections on planning procedures and requirement (F.1.4) and the section on planning in part 1 of the book.

L.1.2.7
Quality Control

The Proton Therapy Co-operative Oncology Group (PTCOG) is working on a quality assurance program specifically for protons. Proper quality control is essential at all institutions practising radiosurgery.

In this regard, the Radiation Therapy Oncology Group (RTOG) has published radiosurgery quality assurance guidelines. (Shaw *et al.* 1993). The aims of the guidelines are to:

- Reduce the variability among RTOG protocol participants by defining basic technical quality assurance and clinical guidelines for participation on RTOG Stereotactic Radiosurgery Protocols.
- Establish criteria for facility participation in stereotactic multi-institutional trials.
- Develop a mechanism for participant procedure reporting.
- Define a quality assurance (QA) program for the purpose of procedure review and verification.

Prior to participation, facilities intending to participate must submit a radiosurgery facility questionnaire comprising a description of the equipment, a radiosurgery treatment prescription form and treatment **planning data,** which include:

- *Coverage:* (does the 90% isodose line cover the target?).
- *Homogeneity Index:* maximum dose in the treatment volume divided by the prescription dose (MD/PD ratio, 2 or <2).
- *Conformity Index:* The volume of the prescription isodose surface is determined from the dose volume histogram and divided by the target volume. This gives the PI/TV ratio, which should be between 1.0 and 2.0. (See Chapter G on Rationale)

Clinical requirements should include:

– Baseline clinical information data, neurological signs and symptoms, steroid dose, baseline and follow-up tumour measurements and assessment of oedema. The follow-up scans should be the same as the baseline study (CT or MRI with contrast).
– Failure patterns: (a) infield , i.e. within the isodose line in Gy corresponding to 80% of the prescription isodose, (b) "marginal, i.e. outside "infield" as defined above, but within the isodose line corresponding to 50% of the prescription isodose, (c) distant, but within the brain. (d) Distant i.e. metastases, or spinal axis seeding.
– Cause of Death classified as (a) tumour, (b) treatment toxicity, (c) other.

Comment: Coverage, homogeneity- and conformity indexes may not be totally adequate. The observations of Voges (1996) and Flickinger (1997) strongly suggest that the actual volume of normal brain tissue receiving 10 Gy is a critical factor determining the complication rate. (See Chapter I on Dose-Volume Relationships). The calculation of the conformity index however, may be very useful in helping to determine safe doses for specific volumes. (See Chapter I on Dose-Volume Relationships)

L.1.2.8
Grading the AVM

The Spetzler Martin Classification (1986) for Neurosurgeons
This classification system takes into account the major risk factors of interest to the surgeon.
Spetzler and Martin (1986) classified these lesions into six categories. The degree of difficulty of a resection depends on lesion size, the number of feeding arteries, the amount of blood flow through the lesion, the degree of steal from the surrounding vessels supplying the normal brain tissue, the location, the surgical accessibility, the "eloquence" of the adjacent brain and the pattern of venous drainage.
Spetzler and Martin narrowed the parameters to the three considered most important:

1. The size of the AVM
2. The pattern of venous drainage
3. Neurological eloquence of the brain regions adjacent to the AVM.

The pattern of venous drainage is not a major consideration for radiosurgeons. The size of the lesion and the eloquence are, but of possible greater importance are the dose-volume relationships as discussed in Chapter I.
The Spetzler-Martin grading system, with comments, and a suggested alternative grading system that may be more useful to radiosurgeons, are given in Appendix P.1 and P.2.

L.1.2.9
Assessing Treatment Outcome – The Scale of Drake

The Scale of Drake (1979), (Table L1.3) is used to assess the clinical (surgical) treatment outcome of AVMs. Perhaps the aim with radiosurgery should be to avoid category 3.

L.1.2.10
Assessing the Radiological Outcome of Radiosurgery

Table L1.4 gives a classification of radiological response.

Table L1.3 The scale (of Drake) for assessing the neurological status of patients treated surgically

1. Excellent	Able to work with no neurological handicaps
2. Good	Some neurological deficit, but patient can work and live independently
3. Poor	Dependent on nursing or family aid because of disabling deficit

Table L1.4 A classification of angiographic response

Complete obliteration	No evidence of any demonstrable shunt
Partial obliteration	Ten to 90 per cent reduction in volume, but with persisting shunting
No change	Less than 10 per cent reduction in volume with persistent shunting

L.1.2.11
Treatment Related Risks

The mortality risk with embolisation is 1%–3%, the morbidity risk is 5%–10% *versus* a morbidity risk of 5%–15% for neurosurgery.

The risk with radiosurgery depends on the volume of tissue treated to a high dose.

The risk of radiosurgery also depends on the situation of the AVM, i.e. "silent" *versus* "eloquent" areas, the age of the patient and the absence or presence of other medical conditions like diabetes mellitus. (See Chapter I on Dose-Volume Relationships and M on complications)

L.1.2.12
Post-Treatment Observation, Follow-up and Medication

Serial angiographic volume determination gives a good indication of the response to treatment, but since this is an invasive procedure, many patients are not agreeable to re-examination by angiogram.

Follow-up examinations should be frequent, at six monthly intervals and should include the clinical neurological status, change in AVM grade, evidence of haemorrhage and complications, MRI, CT scans with conventional angiograms every 12 months, or as suggested in the quality control procedures above.

It is necessary, post-radiosurgically, to follow-up patients with regard to post-radiosurgical imaging (PRI) changes.

These can give information with regard to radiation induced change or damage, which can be symptomatic or asymptomatic, or lesion obliteration (Flickinger *et al.* 1997).

Angiography is still the gold standard for the assessment of residual AVM, but MRI is used increasingly as a non-invasive alternative following treatment (Morikawa *et al.* 1996).

Early follow-up: In the immediate post-operative period, the patients should be observed one day in hospital – there is a risk of post-therapeutic seizures, which can largely be prevented by giving 10–20 milligrams of dexamethasone orally 2 hours before and 8 hours after the radiosurgery and tegretol (carbamazepine).

For fractionated therapy, especially for larger lesions, this dose is repeated before each of the 2, 3 or 4 fractions. It is important, where patients are already on medication for seizures because of the AVM, that anticonvulsant medication should be continued during and after treatment, probably for 2 years.

Late follow-up: If symptomatic vasogenic oedema manifests, prompt treatment with corticosteroids is indicated. (See Chapter M on complications and their management)

L.1.2.13
Radiosurgical Prescription and Dose – CGyE for Protons

A word of caution about dose prescription: Proton doses are reported in CGyE (Cobalt Gray Equivalent)

All doses prescribed must be corrected by the RBE of the proton beam where protons are used.

Where fractionation is intended, the single fraction equivalent must be determined (see Appendix P.5 and P.7) and it should be entered on the prescription sheet, as well as the RBE corrected dose for protons. This is essential in order to avoid confusion and possible unintended overdosage. The fractionated total dose will depend on the α/β ratio chosen of the lesions to be treated. Fractionation does not appear to have any specific benefit for AVM management, except to reduce the acute effects. (See Chapter H.3.2 on Radiobiology of Radiosurgery)

L.1.2.14
Recommended Doses for AVMs

There seems to be a threshold dose for the successful treatment of AVMs. Below 15 Gy, linear accelerator, (Engenhart *et al.* 1994) or 10 Gy to 13 Gy single dose equivalent, Gamma Knife, (Flickinger 1996), AVMs won't be obliterated, or only partially. The latent period is also apparently longer with lower doses than with higher doses.

The recommended dose to obliterate AVMs is not completely settled, and dose-volume relationships have not been clarified sufficiently (Corm *et al.* 1996). The pitfalls with the penumbral width/prescription isodose zone with proton beams have been discussed above.

Karlsson and Lax (1999) developed models based on 838 AVMs treated by Gamma Knife, for predicting the obliteration probability accurately. Karlsson and Lax (1997) produced computer software to predict the probability of AVM obliteration and complications. Their articles should be consulted as space prohibits an extensive discussion here.

Table L1.5 reflects the doses prescribed in the literature.

Table L1.5 Doses used for AVM obliteration. *GK* Gamma Knife, *LA* Linear accelerator, *min.* minimum

Obliteration (%)	Dose (Gy, CGyE)	Author
Threshold dose	13.0 Gy	Flickinger 1996 (GK)
	15.0 Gy	Engenhart 1994 (LA)
	15.0 CGyE	Steinberg 1991 (He^{++})
42% at 2 years (at best)	10.5–50.0 Gy	Kjellberg 1986
50%	16.0 Gy	Engenhart 1994 (LA)
70%	15.8 Gy	Flickinger 1996 (GK)
80%	17.4 Gy*	Flickinger 1996
80%	20.0 Gy$^+$	Engenhart 1994 (LA)
83% at 2 years	20.0 Gy	Steiner 1992
88% (< 1 cm3)	20.0 Gy min.	Lunsford 1993 (GK)
81% (1 cm^3–3.7 cm^3)		
46% (> 4 cm^3)		
81% (1 cm^3–4 cm^3)	10–25 Gy	Friedman 1995 (LA)
89% (4 cm^3–10 cm^3)	med. 15.6 Gy	
69% (10 cm^3)		
90%–95%	20.0 Gy$^+$	Flickinger 1996 (GK)
70%–100%	24 GyE**	Steinberg 1991 (He^{++})

$^+$ 20 Gy and upwards
* If the entire lesion is covered (Gamma Knife)
** Due to the high complication rate, the maximal prescribed dose was reduced to 19.2 Gy
N.B. The choice of a dose is the individual physician's sole responsibility.

Older literature suggest 20 to 25 Gy single dose equivalent as safe and adequate, with the lower dose reserved for the larger lesions, although Flickinger *et al.* (1996) came to the conclusion that *the rate of occlusion (of AVMs) depends on the minimum dose and not on the volume of the AVM.* Their dose inhomogeneity with the Gamma Knife is large, so that part of the lesions receive a dose, which can be 100% higher than the prescribed dose. The BED centrally will be even larger (see Chapter H.3). There is evidence that the probability for AVM obliteration is related to the dose to the AVM periphery for Gamma Knife treatment of AVMs. The AVM volume seems to have no independent impact on the probability of obliteration. This finding is corroborated by Karlsson and Lax (1999).

Engenhart *et al.* (1994) used, for AVMs, a range from 12.5 to 36 Gy, with a mean single dose of 23.6 Gy. With 20 Gy or more, 80% obliteration can be achieved and according to Flickinger (1996), 90%–95% obliteration can be achieved, with the proviso that the *entire* nidus should get the minimum prescribed dose.

These data suggest that the Gamma Knife with its inhomogeneous dose distribution and small penumbra for compact nidus AVMs may have an advantage. A prescription isodose of 65% or lower for protons should be investigated, in order to reduce the penumbra, and spare more normal brain. (See Appendix P.4.)

There appears to be significant differences in the control rates for AVMs treated with protons and helium ions, as can be seen from Table L1.6, discussed below, possibly due to smaller amounts of brain irradiated with helium ions.

L.1.2.15
Proton and Helium Ion Bragg Peak Therapy for AVMs

Protons: Kjellberg (1986) obtained a 2-year obliteration rate of 15%, in 1000 patients treated between 1965 and 1986. Patients who had lesions < 30 mm (14.14 cm^3) (already large for radiosurgery) in size had a complete obliteration rate of 42% compared to about 6% for larger lesions. Radiation related complications occurred in 1.7% from 6 months to 6 years after therapy. Seifert *et al.* (1994) reported on 68 patients with AVMs, treated between October 1980 and May 1990, with stereotactic Bragg peak proton irradiation. Radiosurgery was indicated because the patients were considered at high risk for surgery due to size or location, or because the patients refused surgery. Complete follow-ups were available in 63/68 patients. Obliteration was only obtained in 10/68 patients, all with lesions smaller than 3 cm diameter (14.14 cm^3). Almost 85% of the patients treated with proton therapy showed no angiographic change of the AVM. The authors concluded that proton therapy should not be used for patients with AVMs larger than 3 cm (14.14 cm^3), Only 4.4% (three patients) of the lesions were in Grade I (Spetzler and Martin 1986) and 5.9% (four patients) in Grade II. Nine patients had an AVM larger than 6 cm (113 cm^3)

Comparisons of dose distribution suggest that lesions smaller than 5 cm^3 can be treated equally well by Gamma Knife, linear accelerator and protons, but that larger lesions should be treated by protons. In the chapter on dose-volume relationships it is already evident that Kjellberg's (1984) maximum beam diameter is 5 cm, so that the maximum volume could not have been larger than about 65 cm^3. Of 74 patients 14 had lesions needing a 5 cm diameter beam, and about half the patients (39) had lesions needing beam diameters from 0.7 cm to 3.2 cm; which may represent volumes of from 0.18 cm^3 to 17.2 cm^3.

In Chapter I on Dose-Volume Relationships, the maximum AVM lesion diameter of Flickinger (1997) is only about 25 mm (8.18 cm^3) of the *treatment isodose volume,* which means that maximal lesion volumes would have been much smaller (< 8 cm^3).

In interpreting the data therefore, the lesion volumes should be taken into account carefully, as with any radiosurgical modality. The complication rate increases rapidly with lesion size, therefore lower (possibly ineffective doses if less than 15 Gy) are prescribed for many of the large lesions to avoid complications. Lesions < 5 cm^3 can probably be treated equally well with anyone of the radiosurgical modalities, lesions > 5 cm^3 will probably benefit from the better conformal and localising qualities of proton beams. On the other hand, Mehta (1995) states that the common themes emerging from the Bragg peak trials are that lesions > 4 cm^3 are not treated well with this modality. This confusion may be due to the fact that proton beams have relatively large penumbras for small beams, helium ion beam penumbras are more favourable and Gamma Knife and linear accelerator beams have a very sharp dose fall-off (small penumbra) for lesions < 1 cm^3. A dose fall-off of 26.7% per mm can be achieved with a linear accelerator (Mehta 1995; Appendix P.4.). the physical evidence suggests that proton beams should be good for large lesions since the larger the proton beam, the better the ratio penumbra to 90% isodose area (Table F1.4). Helium ions are likely to give better results than protons for small beams, merely on physical considerations – and also linear accelerator systems with sharp dose fall-off. Plateau therapy with protons may solve this problem, or sacrificing dose homogeneity and prescribing at a lower (smaller) isodose, for example 50%. This should not be done outside of carefully constructed clinical trials.

The penumbra may be an important factor, as the penumbra for a proton beam is virtually as wide for a 3 cm diameter beam as for a 10 cm diameter beam.

Helium ions: In contrast to protons, Steinberg's Group in UCLA, Berkeley, treated 426 patients with AVMs with helium ions, at the 90% prescription isodose. A subset of 89 patients with good follow-up of 2 and 3 years obtained complete obliteration rates of 70% and 90%. The obliteration rate at 2 years for lesions < 4 cm^3 (2 cm diameter) was 94%. This reduced to 75% for lesions 4 cm^3 to 25 cm^3 and 39% for lesions > 25 cm^3 (3.7 cm diameter). At 3 years, the corresponding complete obliteration rates were 100%, 95% and 70%. Doses < 15 GyE were not effective, and clinically significant complications occurred in ten (12%) of patients between 3 and 21 months, all in patients receiving > 24 GyE for volumes > 13 cm^3.

All the complications occurred before the maximal dose was reduced to 19.2 Gy.

The above figures suggest that Voges *et al.* (1996) and Flickinger *et al.* (1997) were correct with regard to the dose-volume limits. (See Chapter I)

L.1.2.16
The Obliteration Rate of AVMs with Particles

Table L1.6 elaborates on the results for AVM obliteration with protons and helium ions.

The existing data up to 1995 suggest that doses of < 15 CGyE result in low rates of obliteration and that doses > 24 CGyE produce unacceptably high complications. Lesions > 5 cm^3 should preferably be treated by protons or other charged particles, as suggested by Table L1.6.

The total re-bleed rate after treatment is 7%–14% (about 3%–4% per annum) and serious neurologic sequelae occur in 2%–11% of the patients, which together with bleeding, results in a mortality of 2%–4% of treated patients.

Table L1.6 Obliteration rate of AVMs with protons and He^{++} ions

PROTONS

Author	Pt no.	Per cent obliteration	Interval (years)	Complication (%)
Kjellberg (1986)	1000	15 (overall)	2	1.7
		42 ($<$ 30 mm diam)	2	
		6 ($>$ 30 mm diam)	2	
Seifert (1994)	68	16 ($<$ 30 mm diam)	–	–
		0 ($>$ 30 mm diam)		

Helium beams

Steinberg (1991)	89	94 ($<$ 20 mm diam)	2	12
		75 (20–26 mm diam)		
		39 ($>$ 27 mm diam)		

After 36 months no further obliteration of the lesions should be expected.

The differences in outcome between< proton therapy and helium therapy are surprising and need an explanation, which may eventually only be settled by a clinical trial.

Gamma Knife Results

Lunsford *et al.* (1993) evaluated 111/348 patients angiographically, at 2 or 3 years and noted an overall obliteration rate of 70%. Of the lesions < 1 cm³ (diameter < 1.24 cm), 88% were obliterated *versus* 81% of lesions between 1 cm³–3.7 cm³ (1.24 cm–1.96 cm diameter) and 46% for lesions > 4 cm³ (about 2.0 cm diameter). Re-bleeding occurred in 16% of patients over the period. Patients who received a peripheral dose < 20 Gy were excluded from this analysis. It needs to be noted that the central lesion would get a much higher nominal dose, and a still higher biologically relevant dose.

Flickinger (1996) upgraded these results. Figure(s) L1.2 and L1.3 summarise the data.

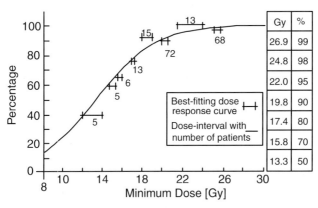

Patients with in-field AVM obliteration (Gamma Knife)

Gy	%
26.9	99
24.8	98
22.0	95
19.8	90
17.4	80
15.8	70
13.3	50

Fig. L1.2 Dose-response curve for in-field obliteration of AVM nidus according to minimum dose (D_{min}) within the target (treatment) volume. The *numbers* identify the numbers of patients within each adjacent dose-interval bar. The position of each dose-interval bar reflects the percentage of patients in the group with in-field obliteration. A *table* on the right side lists the D_{min} for different in-field obliteration rates predicted by the logistic dose-response curve. (Redrawn from JC Flickinger, 1996, Int J Radiat Oncol Biol Phys 36:873–879)

Obliteration rates of AVMs by linear accelerator: Friedman (1995) reported an 81% obliteration rate for lesions of 1 cm³–< 4 cm³ (1.24–1.96 cm diameter) 89% for lesions 4 cm³–10 cm3 (1.96–2.68 cm diameter) and 69% for lesions >10 cm³. Two of 158 patients experienced permanent radiation related complications. Doses were prescribed at the 80% isodose line and varied from 10 to 25 Gy with a median of 15.6 Gy.

Engenhart (1994) reported on a large series of 212 patients, of whom 120 had a follow-up of more than 2 years. No patient who received 14 Gy or less achieved obliteration. At 15–16 Gy the obliteration rate reached 50%; above 20 Gy it exceeded 80%. Lesions < 4.2 cm³ obtained the best results.

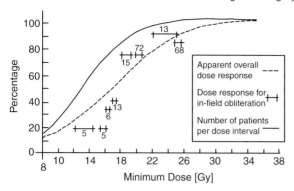

Fig. L1.3 Apparent dose-response curve for overall obliteration of AVM nidus *(dotted curve)* according to minimum dose (D_{min}) within the target (treatment) volume. The *numbers* show the numbers of patients within each adjacent dose-interval bar. The position of each dose-interval bar reflects the percentage of patients in the group with complete in-field obliteration of their AVM. The dose-response curve for in-field obliteration *(solid curve)* from Fig. L1.1 (with no corresponding dose-interval bars) is also included for reference. (Redrawn from JC Flickinger, 1996, Int J Radiat Oncol Biol Phys 36:873–879)

L.1.2.17
The Obliteration Rate of AVMs by Gamma Knife and Linear Accelerator
This is discussed above and summarised in Table L1.7.

Table L1.7 Obliteration rate of AVMs by Gamma Knife and linear accelerator

Author	Pt no.	Per cent Obliteration	Dose (Gy)	Interval (years)
Gamma Knife				
Lunsford (1993)	111	70 (overall) 88 (< 10 mm diam) 81 (12.4–19.8 mm diam) 46 (> 20 mm diam)	18–25	2–3
Steiner (1992)	573	82	10–30	> 2
Forster (1992)	96	59	25	≥ 2
Linear accelerator				
Friedman (1995)	158	81 (overall) 89 (19.6–26.8 mm diam) 69 (> 26.8 mm diam) 46 (> 20 mm diam)		2–3
Engenhart (1994)	120	80 (< 20 mm diam)		
Columbo (1989)	67	75	19–40	2

The results with the Gamma Knife and linear accelerator are very similar, and similar to helium ion therapy results, and all three of these are apparently much better than proton therapy. The possible reasons for this were discussed above.

L.1.2.18
Reducing the Risk of Radionecrosis

For a more complete discussion, see Chapter I on Dose-Volume Relationships but the
following factors should be considered:

Volume: Cerebral necrosis correlates very strongly with the treatment volume and
total dose, but minimal problems were encountered in large lesions if the dose was kept
below 20 Gy. Large doses (> 20 Gy) to large volumes (> 4 cm^3) are not safe (Engenhart
1994).

Field arrangement: In order to minimise risk to normal brain tissue, 3–4 or more
fields should be used with particles like protons to reduce the dose to below 5–6 Gy in
the plateau area of each field, and to keep the skin dose low.

Grade of lesion: Brain necrosis is related to grade – 4% for Grade 4 AVMs and 10%
for Grade 5 Spetzler and Martin (1986) within 4 years (Engenhart 1994).

L.1.2.19
Side Effects of Treatment

The side effects of treatment are summarised in Table L1.8. (See also Chapter M.)

Table L1.8 Summary of the
side effects of treatment

Author	Early effects		Late effects	
	Nausea and vomiting	Seizures	Oedema asymptomatic	Oedema symptomatic
Engenhart (1994)	0.5%	3.3%	10%	7.5%
Flickinger (1997)			37%	43%
Voges (1996)			37.5%	

The complications are discussed below, and in Chapter M.

Early effects: Nausea and vomiting are seen in about 0.5%, seizures 0.5% and
headaches in 3.3% of patients treated by linear accelerator (Engenhart 1994).

Late effects: Engenhart (1994) reported asymptomatic oedema in about 10% of
patients. Symptomatic oedema, which respond well to dexamethasone, was observed
in 7.5%; this may be as high as 80% if more than 40 cm^3 receives 12 Gy by Gamma Knife
(Flickinger *et al.* 1997).

For patients who had more than 10 cm^3 of tissue irradiated to more than 10 Gy,
Voges *et al.* (1996) found radiation induced changes in 37.1% of patients with intraparenchymal lesions and in 37.5% of patients with AVMs (linear accelerator based
radiosurgery). This is in contrast to no radiation induced tissue changes in patients
who received less than 10 Gy to less than 10 cm^3 of brain tissue. Serious neurological
dysfunction has been observed in 2.8% of patients, thought to be due to Wallerian

degeneration of the pyramidal tract in one patient, and to radionecrosis of brain tissue in four patients.

L.1.2.20
Causes for Recurrence of AVMs

According to some analyses, 18% of the patients had non-obliteration of the AVMs because of residual untargeted nidus ("geographical miss"). Of these patients, the causes for residual untargeted nidus included incomplete definition of the AVM nidus margins and/or shape with bi-planar 2-D angiography in 66%. Inadequate angiographic technique was to blame in 14% of the non-obliterated AVMs.

Re-appearance of a nidus temporarily compressed by a haematoma inside the nidus was thought to be responsible for 11% of the failures. Re-canalisation of an embolised nidus contributed to 9% of the failures.

Flickinger *et al.* (1996) found that the *success rate for complete occlusion of an AVM depends on the minimum peripheral dose* and that the obliteration rate does not appear to change with volume or maximum dose.

A plateau may occur over 22 Gy, as the curve by these authors suggest no further benefit from doses up to 35 Gy (Fig. L1.2).

This finding is entirely in tune with the modern trend to use lower doses, and it is difficult to justify, on the basis of these findings, single doses over 22 Gy for AVMs; doses lower than 15 Gy on the other hand are unlikely to be effective. AVM obliteration lies in a narrow window of 7 Gy (BED$_2$ 127.5–264 Gy). Keep in mind that 35# of 2 Gy each has a BED$_2$ of 140.

Cerebral cavernous malformations: Kondziolka *et al.* (1995) reviewed these lesions and their treatment. The annual bleed rate varies from 0.21%–0.7% with up to 1.1% for familial history. Out of 122 patients in their series, 80% of lesions were solitary and multiple in 20%. Fifty per cent of the patients never had a haemorrhage. Thirty five per cent of the lesions occurred in the brain stem. Patients with a brain stem lesion and a previous haemorrhage had a subsequent annual haemorrhage rate of 5%.

Treatment was conservative in the majority of the patients, but 14/122 had microsurgery in the follow-up interval, two after they developed a new haemorrhage and five for a persistent seizure disorder. The remaining seven had surgery for progressive neurological deterioration. Five additional patients with recurrent haemorrhage had stereotactic radiosurgery. The role of stereotactic radiosurgery in the management of haemorrhagic intraparenchymal critically located malformations is currently being defined (Kondziolka *et al.* 1995).

L.1.2.21
A Critique on Radiosurgical Techniques

Corn and Curren (1996) state in an editorial that there is no consensus as to the ideal margin around the nidus for delineating the target volume. Most investigators rely on angiographic criteria to define the target itself, once considered the standard. It is now, however, recommended that anteroposterior and lateral stereotactic angiography is done, since ordinary angiograms are fraught with errors in determining the target size and shape. *Despite the fact that nearly 10,000 patients have been treated with radio-surgery for AVMs, few RT dose response relationship data have been generated for AVM obliteration, the available data lack information on the volume of the lesions treated, assorted conventions to quote dose at varying isodose lines are used, and there is failure to standardise target definitions because of the inconsistent interpretation of imaging studies.*

With radiosurgical units proliferating, clinical trials may provide answers to some of these problems. Before such trials can be done, a uniform method of prescribing, recording and reporting stereotactic irradiation of AVMs is needed.

The RTOG protocols should help to achieve standardisation. The chapter on dose-volume relationships may prove to be of use in this regard.

Targeting the feeding vessels in the past was difficult, but with ever improving imaging and localisation techniques, this may become feasible and fashionable again.

L.1.3
Summary

Radiosurgery is particularly effective for small AVMs (<4 cm^3–5 cm^3 in volume) situated in insensitive areas of the brain. Radiosurgery for the larger lesions should be fairly effective, but care should be taken to limit the normal brain tissue including the lesions so that no more than 10 cm^3 receives 10 Gy to 12 Gy, if possible.

Radiosurgery by Gamma Knife and linear accelerator proton beam are equally effective for small lesions, but protons have superior conformity for the larger AVMs, a lower integral dose and an excellent homogeneity of the dose over the target lesion and may be better for larger lesions, although some people interpret the data to indicate that lesions larger than 4 cm^3 should not be treated by protons. However proton beams appear to be less effective for the <u>smaller</u> lesions (< 5 cm^3) and the physics certainly suggest that they should be better for AVMs > 5 cm^3 than photon techniques.

For smaller lesions the penumbra for proton beams is relatively large and it may be useful to prescribe at the 60% isodose line; increased inhomogeneity "designed in" for proton beams may improve the results for proton beams.

The Gamma Knife is less suitable for lesions of over 3 cm^3 (about 30 mm in diameter), because of the inferior dose localising and conformal qualities due to collimator constraints. For larger lesions multiple isocentres are needed which increase dose inhomogeneity across the target, which may be undesirable, but not necessarily so, as the "hot spot" may initiate the obliteration process.

The results for proton therapy appear to be much worse than that for helium ions, Gamma Knife or linear accelerator, but this is largely due to the fact that much larger lesions have been treated with protons than with the Gamma Knife or linear accelerator.

Only controlled trials will be able to sort out apparently contradictory results.

The main drawback of radiosurgery for the treatment of AVMs is the long, 2 year latency period before obliteration is achieved.

Proper imaging of the lesions is of cardinal importance for accurate planning. Stereotactic angiograms are essential, as well as CT scans with and without contrast. MRI is capable of excellent imaging and PET, if available, may be useful. Planning systems must have image fusion (image registration) capabilities to ensure optimal localisation of the lesions.

The minimal dose delivered to the AVM seems to be the factor determining the obliteration rate, and not the volume of the lesion. The problem with large lesion therapy may be more related to the volume of normal brain irradiated rather than to a volume effect itself. Evidence is accumulating that the dose should be such that no more than 10 cm^3 of normal brain receives a dose greater than 10 Gy in order to avoid complications, prescribing the dose at 50% may help to limit the amount of normal tissue irradiated outside the target volume.

Doses in excess of 22 Gy are unlikely to add to the control rate of AVMs; such doses are simply likely to elevate the complication rate.

The entire nidus should be included in the treatment volume, otherwise obliteration will not be achieved and this tends to enlarge the rim of normal brain and hence the risk for complications.

Targeting the feeding vessels in the past was difficult, but with ever improving imaging and localisation techniques, this may become feasible and fashionable again.

The Spetzler Martin grading system is probably not the optimal grading system for the radiosurgical management of AVMs, and a possibly more useful system is proposed.

The doses employed for AVM obliteration have been down-scaled with experience, because of too many complications experienced with the larger doses. The beams with the sharpest fall-off in dose seem to achieve the best results, for example helium ion beams which seem to do better than protons.

Quality control measures have been identified for the photon modalities, but may be equally applicable to proton (or other particle therapy). These measures may have to be revised e.g. with regard to the recommended prescription isodoses.

There seems to be is a threshold dose of 12 Gy–15 Gy for AVM obliteration.

Fractionated therapy is unlikely to be of any real benefit, except to reduce possible acute reactions. A few fractions, in the order of 2 to 3 will help to eliminate unwanted acute effects.

Finally, the clinical results are not easy to interpret because of the difficulty of interpreting dose-volume relationships, and lesions of the same size that received the same dose probably were not treated with the same prescription isodose or were located in different regions of the brain. Adhering to the suggested RTOG Quality Assurance Programme may help to make the results more comparable and interpretable.

The best indicator of lesion obliteration status is by means of a repeat angiogram. Obliteration results are often reported in terms of CT, MRI and MRA, so that only a selected number of patients in fact have had follow-up angiograms. In order to compare "apples with apples" the MRA and conventional angiographs obliteration rates should be reported separately.

Co-operative, prospective randomised clinical trials are needed to answer the many questions presenting themselves.

The optimal management for cavernous malformations (cavernous angiomas and angiographically occult vascular malformations or AOVMs) is still under investigation. Radiosurgery may have a role, but only in symptomatic patients.

L.1.4
References

Columbo F, Benedetti A, Casentini L *et al.* (1989) Linear accelerator radiosurgery of cerebral arteriovenous malformations. Neurosurgery 29:833–840

Corm BW, Curran WJ (1996) Can we disentangle dose from volume in the radiosurgical management of arteriovenous malformations? Int J Radiat Oncol Biol Phys 36:965–967

Drake CG (1979) Cerebral arteriovenous malformations. Considerations for and experiences with surgical treatment in 166 cases. Clin Neurosurg 26:145–208

Ebershold M, Harner S, Beatty C *et al.* (1992) Current results of the retrosigmoid approach to acoustic neurinoma. J Neurosurg 76:901–909

Engenhart R, Wowra B, Debus J, Kimmig B, Hover KH, Lorenz W, Wannenmacher M (1994) The role of high dose single fraction irradiation in small and large intracranial arteriovenous malformations. Int J Radiat Oncol Biol Phys 30:521–529

Fabrikant JI, Levy RP, Steinberg GK, Phillips MH, Frankel KA, Lyman JT, Marks MP, Silverberg GD (1992) Charged particle radiosurgery for intracranial vascular malformations. Neurosur Clin North Am 3:99–139

Flickinger JC (1989) The integrated logistic formula and prediction of complications from radiosurgery. Int J Radiat Oncol Biol Phys 17:879–885

Flickinger JC, Pollock BE, Kondziolka D, Lunsford LD (1996) A dose-response analysis of arteriovenous malformation obliteration after radiosurgery. Int J Radiat Oncol Biol Phys 36:873–879

Flickinger JC, Kondziolka D, Pollock BE, Maitz A, Lunsford LD (1997) Complications from arteriovenous malformation radiosurgery: multivariate analysis and risk modelling. Int J Radiat Oncol Biol Phys 38:485–490

Friedman WA, Bova FJ, Mendelhall WM (1995) Linear accelerator radiosurgery for arteriovenous malformations: the relationship of size to outcome. J Neurosurg 82:180–189

Foster DF (1992) The Sheffield "Gamma Knife" experience: results in arteriovenous malformation radiosurgery in 507 patients. In: Lunsford LD (ed) Stereotactic radiosurgery. Update. Elsevier, New York, pp 113–116

Hall EJ, Brenner DJ (1993) The radiobiology of radiosurgery: rationale for different treatment regimes for AVMs and malignancies. Int J Radiat Oncol Biol Phys 25:381–385

Haaga J, Lanzieri CF, Artorius DJ, Zerhoun EA (1994) Computed tomography and magnetic resonance imaging of the whole body, 3rd edn. Mosby, St. Louis

Hall EJ, Brenner DJ (1993) The radiobiology of radiosurgery: rationale for different treatment regimes for AVM's and malignancies. Int J Radiat Oncol Biol Phys 25:381–385

Karlsson B, Lax I (1999) Can the probability for obliteration after radiosurgery for arteriovenous malformations be accurately predicted? Int J Radiat Oncol Biol Phys 43:313–319

Kjellberg RN, Hanamura T, Davis KR *et al.* (1983) Bragg peak proton therapy for arteriovenous malformations of the brain. N Engl J Med 309:269–274

Kondziolka D, Lunsford MD, Kestle JRM (1995) The natural history of cerebral cavernous malformations. J Neurosurg 83:820–824

Larson DA, Flickinger JC, Loeffler JS (1993) The radiobiology of radiosurgery. Int J Radiat Oncol Biol Phys 25:557–561

Lunsford LD (1990) Stereotactic radiosurgery of intracranial arteriovenous malformations. In: Wilkins RH (ed) Neurosurgery update. McGraw-Hill, New York, pp 175–185

Lunsford LD (1993) Current radiosurgical strategies for brain arteriovenous malformations. J Neurosurg 78:366A

Mehta M (1995) The physical, biologic and clinical basis of radiosurgery. Curr Problems Cancer pp 269–329

Morikawa M, Numagichi Y, Rigamonti D, Kuroiwa T, Rothman MI, Zoarski GH, Simard JM, Eisenberg H, Amin PP (1996) Radiosurgery for cerebral artereovenous malformations: assessment of early phase magnetic resonance imaging and significance of gadolinium DTPA enhancement. Int J Radiat Oncol Biol Phys 3:663–675

Seifert V, Stolke D, Mehdorn HM *et al.* (1994) Clinical and radiological evaluation of long-term results of stereotactic proton beam radiosurgery in patients with cerebral arteriovenous malformations. J Neurosurg 81:683–689

Shaw E, Kline R, Gillen M *et al.* (1993) Radiation Therapy Oncology Group: radiosurgery quality assurance guidelines.

Int J Radiat Oncol Biol Phys 27:1231–1239

Spetzler RF, Martin NA (1986) A proposed grading system for arteriovenous malformations. J Neurosurg 65:476–483

Spetzler RF, Hargraves RW, McCormick PW (1992) Relationship of perfusion, pressure and size to risk of haemorrhage from arteriovenous malformations of the brain. J Neurosurg 76:918–923

Steinberg GK, Fabrikant JI, Marks MP et al. (1991) Stereotactic helium ion Bragg peak radiosurgery for intracranial arteriovenous malformations. Sterotact Funct Neurosurg 57:36–49

Steiner L, Lindquist C, Adler JR, Torner JC, Alves W, Steiner M (1992) Clinical outcome of radiosurgery for cerebral arteriovenous malformations. J Neurosurg 77:1–8

Voges J, Treuer H, Sturm V, Buchner C, Lehrke R, Kocher M, Staar S, Kuchta J, Müller RP (1996) Risk analysis of linear accelerator radiosurgery. Int J Radiat Oncol Biol Phys 36:1055–1063

L.2
Acoustic and Non-acoustic Neuromas

L.2.1
Introduction

Synonyms: acoustic schwannoma, acoustic nerve sheath tumour.

Radiosurgery has proven to be very useful as a primary or adjunctive treatment of benign intracranial lesions.

So far, the preferred treatment is surgery. Microsurgical techniques have made the operations precise and less dangerous. However, some patients are not suitable candidates for surgery, or the tumour may recur after surgery. In such patients radiosurgery offers an excellent alternative treatment.

Radiosurgery can be done by means of protons or other particles like helium ions, the Gamma Knife or the linear accelerator.

The finding that single doses of 10–15 Gy may be sufficient to achieve local growth arrest, rather than 20–35 Gy, has impressively reduced the complication rate associated with radiosurgery, and may boost this modality as the treatment method of choice, if these results can be corroborated.

The goal with radiosurgery is to arrest growth of the tumour, preserve cranial nerve function, and to prevent further neurological deficits, *not* to cause necrosis of the lesion or its immediate surrounds like nearby cranial nerves.

L.2.2
Incidence and Symptoms

The annual incidence of these tumours is 1 per 1,000,000 of the population. Acoustic neuromas grow slowly, mostly on one side only, and they manifest with progressive loss of hearing, although in 6% there may be a sudden loss of hearing. Other primary symptoms include tinnitus or vertigo.

Bilateral acoustic neuromas is strongly associated with an uncommon genetic disorder, neurofibromatosis type 2 (Kondziolka *et al.* 1993).

L.2.3
Radiation and Growth Arrest of Neuromas

Because acoustic neuromas grow slowly, the question is often raised whether radiosurgery achieves anything at all, because often the tumour does not shrink after radiotherapy.

Linskey *et al.* (1992) and Flickinger *et al.* (1993) evaluated patients with bilateral acoustic neuromas who underwent unilateral radiosurgery, the untreated side serving as a control and found that change in tumour size with time as well as tumour growth rate all significantly *(p = 0.003)* favoured the treated side. This provided convincing evidence that growth arrest and control could be achieved. Hearing was well preserved in the tumours of bilateral nature associated with neurofibromatosis Type 2, and hearing was preserved in 33.3% of patients who had pre-operative hearing.

Protons may have an advantage due to the greater homogeneity of dose possible, but against this must be weighed the possibly larger penumbra with Bragg peak proton therapy if the dose is prescribed at 90% or 100%, it would seem logical to prescribe at the 50% isodose for these lesions with protons. (See Chapter L.1.2.6)

There is controversy whether radiosurgery should be the primary modality for some of these lesions (Sekhar *et al.* 1996). This issue is debated well (Sekhar 1996) with comments by Thomsen (1996), Brackmann (1996), Lunsford (1996), Norén (1996) and Steiner (1996).

The recommendations from the National Institutes of Health Consensus Conference on Acoustic Neuroma are that microsurgical removal should be the standard of therapy with radiosurgery limited to cases in which the surgical risks are considered excessive.

According to a report by the Committee of Brain Tumour Registry of Japan, the 10-year survival rate of patients with benign brain tumours (meningioma, neurinoma and pituitary adenoma) is more than 95% (Yoshida 1996).

L.2.4
Indications for Radiosurgery

Indications for radiosurgery:
- Patients who have only one ear with hearing and the tumour is on that side.
- Elderly patients where the operation may be too strenuous.
- Patients with medical contra-indications.
- Recurrent tumours after surgery are also an indication (Goldsmith *et al.* 1994).
- Patients who refuse surgery, in which case radiosurgery is the only reasonable option.

Eligibility criteria:
- Tumour location consistent with that of an acoustic neuroma and a diameter less than 40 mm. (See Fig. I6.2)

L.2.5
Strategies for Hearing Preservation

According to Loeffler *et al.* (1995) 30 mm represents an approximate target dimension beyond which a clinically unacceptable volume of normal tissue may be damaged if the target receives a curative dose. (Also see Fig. I6.2)

Radiosurgery: *Fractionation:* Andrews *et al.* (1995) reported improved conservation of cranial nerve function by radiosurgical therapy for acoustic nerve tumours if the stereotactic treatment was fractionated. On purely radiobiological grounds fractionation may not be essential. (See Chapter H.2)

In patients with bilateral neuromas, the ear with the best hearing should be treated with radiosurgery preferentially. One could speculate that protons might be the best option because of the homogeneity of dose possible with protons; this may avoid nerve damage due to "hot spots" such as may occur with other radiosurgical systems. However, the bone and air cavities bring reasonably large uncertainties in dose distribution to bear, and the penumbra of the Bragg peak of the particular beam needs to be kept in mind. A major factor with radiosurgery however, is that volumes of normal brain larger than 10–13 cm^3 receiving more than 10–< 24 Gy may also lead to complications (Voges *et al.* 1996), therefore this aspect needs very careful assessment. (See Chapter I on Dose-Volume Relationships)

When the tumours are still small: *Early treatment;* Ogunrinde *et al.* (1995) showed that for intracanalicular (small) acoustic tumours, which constitute roughly 4.7% of all acoustic tumours, tumour volume stabilisation could be achieved in 80%, preservation of preoperative hearing could be preserved in all patients postoperatively and in 80% at 1 year. No patient developed facial or trigeminal nerve dysfunction in from 3–36 months. All patients returned to their pre-treatment functional status within 3–5 days after radiosurgery with the Gamma Knife, emphasising the good results and rapid return to function in contrast to microsurgery.

The doses were low and varied from 12–20 Gy with a median of about 17 Gy.

Linskey *et al.* (1993) also showed that the length of the cranial nerves irradiated predicts prognosis. It is therefore unwise to "observe" acoustic tumours, since they will get bigger, and the length of nerve that will have to be irradiated, longer. It is therefore better to treat while the tumours are as small as possible.

Conventional radiotherapy: Although radiosurgery has obvious advantages in terms of dose distribution, many of these lesions can be controlled with conventionally fractionated radiotherapy, with few complications, due to the relatively gentle effects of well fractionated therapy. The advantage is, however lost due to large volumes irradiated. Because of the limitations in the dose deliverable conventional radiotherapy is inclined to give inconsistent results.

Microsurgery: Hearing loss preservation with microsurgery:

For intracanalicular lesions can apparently be further improved by the retrosigmoid approach (Rowed *et al.* 1997). Ebershold *et al.* (1992) indicated that progress has been made in preserving auditory and facial nerve function with microsurgery.

L.2.6
Complications Other than Hearing Loss with Microsurgery

Postoperative meningitis	5%
Cerebrospinal fluid leakage	15%
Cranial nerve palsies	2%–4%
Post operative haematomas	2%
Mortality	0%–1%
Hydrocephalus	Occasionally, 10% of these need a shunt (Thompsen 1996)
Stroke	

Microsurgery may result in postoperative meningitis in 5% of patients, cerebrospinal fluid leakage in 15% of patients, with 2% of these requiring re-operation.

Cranial nerve palsy in each of V, IX, X and XI occurs in 2%–4% of patients. Post-operative haematomas can be a problem. Mortality rates are low: between 0% and 1%. Hydrocephalus occurs in a significant number of microsurgically treated patients (Kondziolka *et al.* 1993). Ten percent (10%) of these patients need a shunt (Thompsen 1996).

Stroke has been observed following these operations.

L.2.7
Clinical Results for Acoustic Neuromas

L.2.7.1
Proton Therapy

The clinical experience with protons for acoustic tumours is relatively limited. At the NAC in South Africa, about 37 such tumours have been treated up to January 1999. The follow-up period is still too short to make a meaningful comment. Protons may be especially useful if the nerve is centrally located in the tumour, as may happen with Type 2 neurofibromatosis, because of the dose homogeneity across the target. Homogeneity comes at a price, however, since a larger penumbra results if the dose is prescribed at 90% as opposed to, for example, 50%. Prescribing at the 90% isodose may cause excessive brain tissue to be irradiated. This is an area of practical proton therapy that needs investigation. (See Chapter L.1.2.14, Proton Beam Profiles and Appendix P.4)

L.2.7.2
Gamma Knife and Linear Accelerator

The recorded cumulative experience shows that acoustic neuromas can be controlled in up to 90% of cases. Table G2.1 shows the result.

Protons: No reported proton series could be found to date, although these tumours are being treated by protons, inter alia at NAC, RSA.

NB : The dose ranges quoted in Table L2.1 should not be used clinically, as the trend is strongly toward much lower single doses, with 15 Gy single dose as a probable ceiling.

The local control rate is superior for unilateral tumours: 88% *versus* 76% for the bilateral type associated with neurofibromatosis Type 2. Hearing was preserved in 77% of those with good hearing prior to treatment. Transient facial paresis was seen in 17%–29% and trigeminal neuropathy in 19%–33% (Mehta 1995)

Ogunrinde *et al.* (1994) reported on 20 patients with acoustic neuromas less than 30 mm in mean diameter. Tumour control was achieved in 95% and useful hearing was preserved in 45% at 2 years, facial nerve function was normal in 90% and trigeminal function in 75% of the patients.

Mendelhall *et al.* (1994) treated non-ideal patients by linear accelerator with a mean dose of 15.5 Gy. The tumours were relatively large (23 mm collimator mean size), yet no patient suffered progression.

The typical radiological response observed for the Gamma Knife series of Karolinska in 70% of the patients, was early loss of contrast enhancement on CT or MRI imaging.

Table L2.1 Clinical results with photon radiosurgery for acoustic neuroma (*GK* Gamma Knife, *SALA* Specially adapted linear accelerator)	Lesion	Institution	Unit	Dose (Gy)	Number	Local control (%)	Follow-up years
	Acoustic neuroma	Karolinska (Norén et al. 1992)	GK	10–35	182/227	85	4.5
		Florida (Mendenhall et al. 1994)	SALA	10–22	32/32	100	2.25
		Pittsburgh (Flickinger et al. 1993)	GK	12–20	121/136	89	2
	Total				335/395	84.8	4.1

Note: Maximum doses > 15 Gy not recommended

L.2.7.3
Risk Factors for Complications

Tumour volumes for these lesions may vary 150-fold from about 0.2 cm^3 to 30 cm^3. The large lesions are especially prone to lead to complications (Engenhart *et al.* 1990).

New facial- or trigeminal neuropathy may develop up to 2 years later in nearly 1/3 of the patients (Flickinger *et al.* 1993) Such neuropathies are usually mild and may resolve about a year later.

Total dose: The risk of other neuropathies is related to total dose and volume irradiated. Larger lesions imply that larger lengths of the relevant nerves (acoustic, facial or trigeminal) will be irradiated. The risks appear to vary about 30% between facial and trigeminal neuropathies.

Location: According to Kondziolka *et al.* (1993) location is important. For patients with pons-petrous tumours less than 20 mm in diameter, the risk of facial neuropathy is about 10%, and for patients with intracanalicular tumours, the risk is less than 5%.

Hydrocephalus has been reported in some patients treated with radiosurgery.

Radiation effects are likely to manifest in 6–18 months, and very few patients are likely to suffer additional effects after 2 years.

L.2.7.4
Recommended Doses for Acoustic Neuromas

There is a steady decrease in the recommended radiation doses as experience is gained with radiosurgery.

The Karolinska Group (Gamma Knife) first used a peripheral dose of from 25–35 Gy. In this group facial paralysis occurred in 38% of patients and useful hearing was preserved in 20% with a 71% local control.

The recommended dose range was then lowered to 18–20 Gy (a reduction of about 40% in the nominal dose) and most recently, *to between 10 Gy and 15 Gy* – a further reduction in the nominal dose of 33%–50% – with a dramatic reduction in the incidence of facial paralysis (17%) and hearing preservation in 77%.

What should be the dose for proton therapy? There may be no reason to go beyond 10–15 Gy single dose equivalent.

L.2.7.5
Radiological Changes After Radiosurgery

At 12 months, the typical radiographic change in 70% of the patients was early loss of contrast enhancement on both CT and MRI.

Recently, Mabanta *et al.* (1999) reported favourable results (100%) preliminary tumour control rates (18/18 patients) with schwannomas located in the jugular foramen region, trigeminal and facial nerve. Minimal tumour doses ranged from 10–15 Gy, (mean 13.1 Gy). Complications occurred in 3 patients, but did not require surgery or steroids.

L.2.8
Summary

Radiosurgery is becoming a strong contender as treatment of choice for acoustic neuromas. The trend is towards lower single doses, in the order of 10–15 Gy and controlled trials are necessary between the available modalities. Single doses as low as 10 Gy may suffice, and could possibly be repeated once if found not to be effective.

The equivalent photon doses for conventionally fractionated therapy are about 55–60 Gy, which should be well within tolerance for well-collimated small volumes.

Dose reductions from doses 20 Gy or larger to doses in the order of 10–15 Gy led to a very good reduction in complications.

Proton beams could offer a more homogeneous dose distribution than the Gamma Knife, and may be of use where the nerve bundles are likely to be entrapped in the nerve. Proton beams used at the Bragg peak have a penumbra that is not insignificant, and consideration should be given to prescribing with Bragg peak protons at a prescription isodose less than 90%. Although these tumours are less likely to cause complications than AVMs, the volume of normal brain irradiated, despite the apparently lower doses needed for control of these tumours, should always be kept as small as reasonably achievable.

L.3
Meningiomas

L.3.1
Incidence and Pathology

Meningiomas make up about 15% of all primary intracranial tumours. They are usually, but not always, slow growing and almost all, about 98%, are benign. The incidence is somewhat greater for women than for men. They may show great variability in their natural history and growth rate although they are generally slow growing and extra-axial. Because of the slow growth rate, patients should be followed up for a lifetime.

They cause symptoms by compression of the brain.

Meningiomas that are histologically benign, like osteoblastic, fibroblastic or meningotheliomatous types tend to have a more favourable prognosis than the highly vascular meningiomas. Calcified meningiomas tend to be more benign.

Cranial base meningiomas have a high recurrence rate after surgery and they are more dangerous than convexity meningiomas. The variability in behaviour makes the comparison of treatment modes difficult (Rosseau *et al.* 1995). Mehta (1995) stressed the possible importance of oestrogen receptors. Up to 33% if these tumours have hormone receptors, and in vitro results suggest that progestogens may be a therapeutic alternative. Lesions of the cerebellopontine angle commonly present with cranial neuropathies.

Parasagittal meningiomas may be especially prone to oedematous degeneration following radiosurgery (Ganz *et al.* 1996; Kalapurakal *et al.* 1997)

L.3.2
Treatment Options

Microsurgical complete resection is presently the treatment of choice. The location of basal meningiomas often precludes complete resection. Recurrence is a troublesome problem and Jääskeläinen *et al.* (1986) reported a median time to recurrence of 7 years with a risk still present at 25 years! New post operative cranial nerve deficits occur in 19%–86% of patients.

Radiosurgery: Rousseau and Cerullo (1995) observed that the prospect of 100% control with minimal morbidity with radiosurgery in patients who had previously undergone one to five craniotomies deserves serious further study for the exclusive use of radiosurgery for these lesions.

Duma *et al.* (1993) reported, with radiosurgery, tumour regression in 56% of 34 patients with 100% tumour growth control.

Indications for radiosurgery:
- Incomplete surgical resection
- Other medical conditions that would make conventional surgery unacceptable
- Patient rejection of surgery

Eligibility:
Lesions should be less than 40 mm in diameter, and should have no *en plaque* component, and should be situated away from cranial nerves. (Also see Fig. I6.2)

Meningiomas are suitable lesions for radiosurgical treatment, because they usually have well-defined margins, do not invade the brain parenchyma and are easily visualised by CT and MRI. They grow slowly and because they are reasonably vascular, radiotherapy can be expected to cause a vascular shutdown with time. They often arise in the elderly where surgery may be risky (Mehta 1995).

Because meningiomas are usually very well demarcated and very little normal brain needs to be irradiated, the superior conformation of the isodoses obtainable with proton therapy for lesions larger than 5 cm^3 (diameter > 2.1 cm) may offer an advantage over other types of radiosurgery, where the isodose conformation is much more difficult to obtain, especially for the larger and more irregularly shaped lesions where multiple isocentres are needed. Conformity indices for irregular lesions have been published (Verhey *et al.* 1998; Hamilton 1995).

The entire lesion with as little normal brain as possible should be irradiated. Inclusion of the dural blood supply to the meningioma may help as radiotherapy is likely to destroy the blood supply, This may contribute to the arrest of growth of the lesion provided that the critical volume of brain tissue irradiated is not exceeded. Long term disease free survival can be obtained with microsurgery, but delayed tumour recurrence may necessitate radiosurgery.

L.3.3
Results of Treatment

Control rate: The early data for radiosurgery for meningiomas are promising, but it will require several more years and many more patients to fully evaluate the efficacy of radiosurgery in comparison to surgery and conventional radiotherapy.

Loeffler *et al.* (1995) quoted the results of 97 patients treated with radiosurgery at the Joint Centre for Radiation Therapy in Boston. Of these 67% had failed previous surgery and were treated for recurrent tumour. The 2-year actuarial progression free rate was 96%.

Engenhart *et al.* (1990) had an excellent control rate of 84%.

Kondziolka *et al.* (1993) used radiosurgery in 103 patients with the Gamma Knife. Only lesions smaller than 35 mm in average diameter and more than 4 mm from the optic chiasm were accepted. Basal meningiomas occurred in 89% of the patients and 2/3 of the patients had undergone previous surgery. They found that cavernous sinus and para-cellar tumours tended to be very irregular in outline, because of a tendency to extend into multiple intracranial and extra-cranial compartments. In these patients the superior conformity of protons may be an advantage. The presence of major blood vessels in the tumour like the internal carotid or the anterior cerebral arteries did not prevent the application of a therapeutically effective dose. They managed to do follow-up MRI scans in 85 patients from 6–60 months after treatment. Of these 64% showed no progression in tumour size, 28% had a decrease in tumour size and 7% had an increase in tumour size. Reasons for failure in these were malignant gliomas in a third, and "geographical miss" with tumour outside the high dose zone in a third and a third had multiple prior craniotomies.

Clinically, 6–60 months after therapy, 72/89 of patients remained clinically stable, 10/89 improved and 2.2% worsened.

The results are summarised in Table L3.1. The doses are not the recommended doses. Evidence is accumulating that the doses in the 10–15 Gy range may suffice (see below). Controlled trials with protons *versus* the Gamma Knife and the linear accelerator are needed.

L.3.4
Recommended Doses

Conventional radiotherapy can give reasonable results postoperatively (Goldsmith *et al.* 1994). Conventional doses of 52 Gy will control 93% of meningiomas at 10 years, whereas the control rate is 65% for patients who received less than 52 Gy. A minimum of 53 Gy is recommended for malignant meningiomas. The single dose equivalent would be about 12.7 Gy. Conventional radiotherapy may be used for recurrences after

Table L3.1 Radiosurgical results for meningiomas (*ICP* = Intracranial pressure, *GK* = Gamma Knife, *Linac* = linear accelerator, *N/A* = not available). Note: No proton results could be found

Author	Radiation regime	Pt No	Control rate %	Complication rate
Goldsmith (1994) LA	27 # x 2 Gy adjuvant to resection	140	93	3.6% (sudden blindness or cerebral necrosis)
Hodes (1996) GK	1 # x 10–19 Gy	20	95	1 death
Ganz (1996) GK	1 # x 10–12 Gy (peripheral dose with 12 Gy max.)	34		Progression rate of 40% in patients receiving ≤ 10 Gy
Hudgins (1996) GK	1 # x 15 Gy	100	81	17% deteriorated
Duma (1993) GK	1 # x 16 Gy		100	4/34 (two with transient and two with permanent deficit
Engenhardt (1990) Linac	1 # x 29 Gy	17	100	12% mortality (4 pts) 24% significant oedema (8 pts)
Shafron (1999) GK	1 # x 10–20 Gy (median 12.7 Gy)	70	100	3% (in two pts who had higher doses than their present norm)
Valentino (1993) LA	1 # x 37 Gy	72	94	3/37 transient increase in ICP
Kondziolka (1991) GK	1 # x 10–25 Gy	97	95	N/A
Castro (1994) He^{++}	(~30 # x 2 GyE) 65 CgyE	27	85	~20% grade 3,4,5 (all skull base lesions

Note: Single doses > 15 Gy not recommended

surgery for large lesions, especially with the multileaf collimators or miniature multileaf collimators intensity modulation and 3-D planning presently available.

Radiosurgical doses: Hodes *et al.* (1996) used single doses of 10–19 Gy at the periphery with good control. Ganz *et al.* (1996) suggest a threshold dose of 10 Gy for control but no higher than 12 Gy for Gamma Knife radiosurgery in order to avoid radiation induced oedema.

Hudgins *et al.* (1996) for an average tumour diameter of 2.4 cm (about 7.3 cm^3) applied a minimal dose of 15 Gy using up to 5 isocentres. Duma *et al.* (1993) used a single fraction marginal dose of 10–20 Gy, with a maximal dose to the optic nerve of 9 Gy, with good results. Good conformation was obtained with skilful selective plugging of the gamma sources of the Gamma Unit, which may explain why they did not have many complications in patients receiving 20 Gy. The BED$_2$ = 242 Gy for 20 Gy single dose, which is probably excessive in any case.

Shafron *et al.* (1999) reported on 70 patients with 76 meningiomas. The mean dose to the periphery of the lesion (linear accelerator) was 12.7 Gy (range 10–20 Gy) which in most cases was delivered at the 80% isodose line. The control rate with a follow-up of at least 1 year was 100%. Only two patients developed complications – both received doses in excess of the presently recommended doses. One had a lesion of about 17 cm^3 and received a dose of 15 Gy at the periphery, the other had a lesion of about 12 cm^3 and received a dose of 17.5 Gy (values read off from the published dose-volume scattergram.

L.3.5
Complications of Radiosurgery for Meningioma

Complications due to the radiosurgery quoted in Loeffler *et al.* (1995) occurred in 14.43% of 97 patients. In five patients *(5.2%) cranial neuropathies* developed and in five more, *malignant oedema*, which necessitated re-operation in 2. Larger and deep-seated lesions were found to be more prone to complications.

Engenhart *et al.* (1990) had an excellent control rate of 84% for a complication rate for patients with large lesions of 42%. High doses were used: 29 Gy which is a dose with an astronomical biological effect (BED$_2$ = 449 Gy). The complications were high, as can be expected: *2/17 deaths from herniation*, with about *24% of patients developing significant oedema*. Less severe complications were reported in patients treated with lower doses – see under treatment results above.

Temporary neurological deficits occurred in 3/72 of the patients classified as stable (Kondziolka *et al.* 1993).

(See also Chapter M on Complications of Radiosurgery.)

L.3.6
Summary

Meningiomas are slow growing lesions, adequately treated by microsurgery where feasible.

Relatively low single doses of irradiation – in the 12 to 15 Gy range, seem to be sufficient, with the lower doses reserved for the larger lesions. Proton therapy is especially indicated for lesions of a complex outline, but the level of the prescription isodose may warrant careful consideration. Prescribing at a lower isodose may increase the inhomogeneity, but will result in a smaller penumbra with no loss of conformation and it will not affect the advantageous integral dose obtainable with protons.

Conventional radiotherapy, in the order of 52 Gy in 1.8–2 Gy fractions give good results, and may be used for recurrences after surgery for large lesions. Fractionation with radiosurgery is not considered essential, but may have benefits, e.g. to avoid acute oedema.

Non-skull base meningiomas, for example parasagittal meningiomas, are especially prone to develop symptomatic oedema and should be approached with extreme caution.

L.3.7
References

Andrews DW, Siverman CL, Glas J *et al.* (1995) Preservation of cranial nerve function of Acoustic Neurinomas with fractionated stereotactic radiotherapy. Stereotact Funct Neurosurg 64:165–182

Brackmann DE (1996) Commentary on Sekhar. Am J of Otol 17:683

Castro JR, Linstadt DE, Bahary J-P *et al.* (1994) Experience in charged particle irradiation of tumours of the skull base: 1997–1992. Int J Radiat Oncol Biol Phys 29:647-655

Duma CM , Lunsford LD, Kondziolka D, Harsch GR, Flickinger JC (1993) Stereotactic radiosurgery of cavernous sinus meningiomas as an addition or alternative to microsurgery. Neurosurgery 32:699–705

Ebershold M, Harner S, Beatty C *et al.* (1992) Current results of the retrosigmoid approach to acoustic neurinoma. J Neurosurg 76:901–909

Engenhart R, Kimming BN, Hover K *et al.* (1990) Stereotactic single high dose irradiation of benign intracranial meningiomas. Int J Radiat Onc Biol Phys 19:1021–1026

Flickinger JC, Lunsford LD, Linskey ME *et al.* (1993) Gamma Knife Radiosurgery for acoustic tumours: multivariate analysis of four year results. Radiother Oncol 27:91–98

Ganz JC, Schrottner O, Pendl G (1996) Radiation induced oedema after Gamma Knife treatment for meningiomas. Stereotact Funct Neurosurg 66 [Suppl II]:129–133

Goldsmith BJ, Wara WM, Wilson CB *et al.* (1994) Postoperative irradiation for subtotally resected meningiomas. J Neurosurg 80:195–201

Hamilton RJ, Kuchnir FT, Sweeney P, Rubin SJ *et al.* (l995) Comparison of static conformal field with multiple non-coplanar arc techniques for stereotactic radiotherapy. Int J Onc Biol Phys 33:1221–1228

Hodes JE, Sanders M, Patel P, Patchell RA (1996) Radiosurgical management of meningiomas. Stereotact Funct Neurosurg 66:1–3, 15–18

Hudgins WR, Barker JL, Schwartz DE, Nichols TD (1996) Gamma Knife treatment of 100 consecutive meningiomas. Stereotact Funct Neurosurg [Suppl] 1:121–128

Jääskeläinen J, Haltia M, Sevo A (1986) Atypical and anaplastic meningiomas: radiology surgery and outcome. J Surg Neurol 25:233–242

Kalapurakal, JA Silverman CL, Akhtar N *et al.* (1997) Intracranial meningiomas: factors that influence the development of cerebral oedema after stereotactic radiosurgery and radiation therapy. Radiology 204:461–465

Kondziolka D, Lunsford LD (1993) Stereotactic radiosurgery for brain tumours. In: Salcman M (ed) Current techniques in neurosurgery, 1st edn. Current Medicine, Philadelphia

Linskey ME, Lunsford LD, Flickinger JC (1992) Tumour control after stereotactic radiosurgery in neurofibromatosis patients with bilateral acoustic tumours. Neurosurgery 31:829–838

Linskey ME, Flickinger JC, Lunsford LD (1993) Cranial nerve length predicts the risk of delayed facial and trigeminal neuropathies after acoustic tumour stereotactic radiosurgery. Int J Radiat Oncol Biol Phys 25:227–233

Loeffler JS, DA, Shrieve DC *et al.* (1995) Radiosurgery for the treatment of intracranial lesions. In: DeVita VT, Hellman S, Rosenberg S (eds). Lippincott, Philadelphia pp 141–156

Mabanta SK, Buatti JM, Friedman WA *et al.* (1999) Linear accelerator radiosurgery for non-acoustic schwannomas. Int J Radiat Oncol Biol Phys 43:545-548

Mehta MP, Boyd TS, Sinha P (1998) The status of stereotactic radiosurgery for cerebral metastases in 1998. J Radiosurg 1:17–33

Mehta MP, Rozental JM, Levin AB *et al.* (1992) Defying the role of radiosurgery in the management of brain metastases. Int J Radiat Oncol Biol Phys 24:619–623

Mehta M (September/October 1995) The physical, biologic and clinical basis of radiosurgery. In: Kinsella T (ed) Current problems in cancer pp 269–329

Mendelhall WM, Friedman WA, Bova FJ (1994) Linear accelerator based stereotactic radiosurgery for acoustic schwannomas. Int J Radiat Oncol Biol Phys 28:803–810

Norén G (1996) Commentary on Sekhar. Am J Otol 17:685–686

Norén G, Greitz D, Hirsch A *et al.* (1992) Gamma Knife surgery in acoustic neurinoma. In: Steiner *et al.* (eds) Radiosurgery: baseline and trends. Raven Press, New York

Ogunrinde OK, Lunsford LD, Flickinger JC *et al.* (1995) Stereotactic radiosurgery for acoustic nerve tumours in patients with useful pre-operative hearing: results of a 2 year follow-up examination. J Neurosurg 80:1011–1017

Ogunrinde OK, Lunsford LD, Flickinger JC *et al.* (1995) Cranial nerve preservation after radiosurgery of intracanalicular acoustic tumours. Stereotact Funct Neurosurg 64 [Suppl 1]:87–97

Rosseau G, Cerullo L (1995) Current challenges in management of cranial base meningiomas. Am J Otol 16:1–3

Rowed DW, Nedzelski JM (1997) Hearing preservation in the removal of inracanalicular acoustic neu-
    romas via the retrosigmoid approach. J Neurosurg 86:456–461
Sekhar LN, Gormley WB , Wright DC (1996) The best treatment for vestibular schwannoma (acoustic
    neuroma): microsurgey or radiosurgery? Am J of Otol 17:676–682
Shafron DH, Friedman WA, Buatti JM et al. (1999) Linac radiosurgery for benign meningiomas. Int J
    Radiat Oncol Biol Phys 43:321–327
Steiner L (1996) Commentary on Sekhar. Am J of Otol 17:685–686
Thompsen J (1996) Commentary on Sekhar. Am J Otol 17:689
Valentino V, Schinaia G, Raimondi AJ (1993) The result of radiosurgical management of 72 middle fos-
    sa meningiomas. Acta Neurochir (Wien) 122:60–70
Verhey LJ, Smith V, Serago F (1998) Comparison of radiosurgery treatment modalities based on phys-
    ical dose distributions. Int J Radiat Oncol Biol Phys 40:497–505
Voges J, Treuer H, Sturm V, Buchner C, Lehrke R, Kocher M, Staar S, Kuchta J, Müller RP. Risk analysis
    of linear accelerator radiosurgery. Int J Radiat Oncol Biol Phys 36:1055–1063
Yoshida J (1996) Molecular neurosurgery using gene therapy to treat malignant glioma. Nagoya J Med
    Sci 59:97–105

L.4
Pituitary Tumours

L.4.1
Introduction

Microsurgical transsphenoidal techniques have superseded craniotomies, and even
these are undergoing continued refinement, for example endonasal transsphenoidal
endoscopic surgery, which enables magnification, illumination and excellent visualisation of the tiny structures.

Even so, recurrences after surgery or residuals left behind are not uncommon. Conventional radiation techniques as adjuvant therapy give good results, but for extension
into specific areas, example the cavernous sinus, cobalt 60 or linear accelerator based
radiosurgery offers a good therapeutic approach. Protons or other particle therapy has
been used, but the Bragg peak should probably not be used in these settings, as the lateral dose fall-off is a problem where sensitive structures like the optic nerve and tract
are only millimetres away. In these situations, multiple coplanar plateau beams may be
used for protons.

Since many pituitary tumours respond well to conventional radiotherapy, only
some potentially resistant or large odd-shaped pituitary tumours should be considered for proton therapy after careful consideration of several treatment plans for protons and photons.

The results with particle therapy in < 2000 patients with pituitary tumours have
been reviewed and have been judged excellent, (Mehta 1995). Some conditions are
presently of historical interest only and are discussed in Chapter F.1.1. For an excellent
overview of pituitary tumour pathology and treatment see Grigs by (1988, 1998).

In an academic hospital patients from the ear, nose and throat, endocrine, infertility (proloactinomas) and paediatric departments often have an interest in a contribution to make in these clinics.

Chapter I on Dose-Volume Relationships will illustrate some of the problems associated with proton therapy in this situation.

L.4.2
Anatomy

Anatomy: The pituitary gland is situated in the sella turcica in the body of the sphenoid bone. Superiorly the diaphragma sellae separates the pituitary gland from the chiasmatic cisterns and the floor of the anterior part of the third ventricle. *The optic chiasm* overlies the diaphragma sellae and the pituitary in most cases but is sometimes fixed over the tuberculum sellae (10%) and sometimes over the dorsum sellae, *but it is only millimetres away from the upper part of the pituitary gland.* The anterior cerebral arteries are superior and the cavernous sinuses laterally.

The cavernous sinuses contain the internal carotid arteries, the abducens, oculomotor, trochlear and branches of the trigeminal nerve in the lateral wall of each sinus. The sphenoid sinus is inferior to the gland, which normally has a mass of only 0.6 grams.

Pathology: Tumours of the pituitary gland are complex with regard to secretory products, growth patterns and response to therapy. The heterogeneity of these tumours is shown by immunological staining methods of tumour tissue and by current serologic tests. Contemporary studies show that many pituitary adenomas thought to be non-functioning are in fact secreting hormonal products. Careful evaluation has also revealed the presence of mixed tumours (Grigsby 1988). In this regard, Kovacs *et al.* (1996) proposed a 5-tier system of classification based on endocrine profile, imaging, operative findings, histology, immunocytochemistry and ultrastucture, based on 8000 surgically removed human pituitary tumours.

L.4.3
Classification

The old classification into basophilic (ACTH) acidophylic (GH) and chromophobic (inactive) is of no use, and is in fact misleading. In addition, a significant proportion of pituitary adenomas produces more than one hormone.

Hardy (1973), and Hardy and Vezine (1976) developed a classification system that has gained partial acceptance with neurosurgeons (Grigsby 1988). They classified pituitary tumours into four grades:

I.   Normal sized sella with asymmetry of the floor
II. Enlarged sella with intact floor
III. Localised erosion or destruction of the sellar floor
IV. Diffusely eroded floor

Suprasellar extension is qualified as:

A. Tumour bulges into chiasmatic cistern
B. Tumour reaches the floor of the third ventricle
C. As B but larger with extension to the Foramen of Monro
D. Tumour extends into the temporal or frontal fossa.

For radiosurgery, extension into the cavernous sinus, optic apparatus and brain has important implications for therapy.

The proposed 5-tier classification system of Kovacs *et al.* (1996) is very informative and emphasises the fact that the management of these lesions should be a team effort involving the ophthalmologist, neurosurgeon, endocrinologist neuroradiologist, radiation oncologist and endocrine laboratory.

L.4.4
The Aims of Therapy

The aims of therapy are to define the extent of the tumour, evaluate the hormonal status, remove, shrink, or render non-functional tumour masses, control hypersecretion and give supplementary hormones where necessary (Leavens *et al.* 1992).

L.4.5
Signs and Symptoms

Pituitary adenomas are mostly benign tumours originating from the adenohypophysial cells. They represent the most common neoplasm of the sellar region – about 15% of all intracranial tumours.

Mass effects produced by pituitary adenomas can include headache and visual field or visual acuity problems. Pressure effects may lead to blindness or even death (Kovacs 1996)

Hormonal effects due to prolactinoma include hypertension, amenorrhoea, galactorrhoea, decreased libido, impotence and infertility. Cardiomyopathy occurs in acromegaly in adults or gigantism in young people before the epiphysis close, due to an excess of growth hormone secreted.

Increased secretion of adrenocorticotrophic hormone (ACTH) leads to Cushing's disease, thyrotropin (TSH) hypersecretion to hyperthyroidism. Increase in follicle stimulating and luteinising hormone (FSH/LH) hypersecretion leads to hypogonadism or no discernible endocrine effect.

Pituitary tumours may secrete the α-subunit, the biologically inactive chain of glycoprotein hormones which causes no clinical signs suggesting an endocrine abnormality, but it can be used as a *marker* for monitoring disease progress.

Hypopituitarism: Pituitary tumours may damage the hypothalamus or the pituitary stalk resulting in reduced synthesis or transport of hypothalamic releasing or inhibitory hormones causing varying degrees of hypopituitarism.

L.4.6
Diagnosis

The presence of such a tumour must be suspected in patients with headache and the often associated visual disturbances, sometimes with the stigmata of hormone over or under-secretion.

Radiologically, plain skull films, computed tomography (CT) magnetic resonance scanning and angiography all have their place.

All patients with a suspected pituitary tumour should have a thorough clinical, endocrinological and neurological examination as well as an assessment of visual acuity and visual field defects before therapy is commenced, to enable proper assessment afterwards and to avoid later possible litigation.

Full endocrinological examination includes gonadal, thyroid and adrenal function, growth hormone and prolactin levels (Rush *et al.* 1989).

L.4.7
Treatment

Microadenomas need a multidisciplinary approach: medical/endocrinological, microsurgical plus or minus external beam radiotherapy, and sometimes radiosurgery.

Medical management: Useful drugs include bromocriptine, cyproheptadine, mitotane and somatostatin.

Surgery: Transsphenoidal surgery is a safe and effective treatment for microadenomas, and the techniques are being refined continually. Jho *et al.* (1997) developed and described a minimally invasive approach by endoscopic endonasal transsphenoidal technique for the treatment of pituitary tumours, including micro- and macroadenomas and even some invading the cavernous sinus. Endoscopic surgery offers an excellent view of the sellar and suprasellar structures and provides the potential for more complete tumour resection as well as offering faster postoperative recovery.

Surgery plus radiosurgery: A combined approach of transsphenoidal resection and radiosurgery for adenomas invading the cavernous sinus has been described by Ikeda *et al.* (1998). Radiation doses varied from 25–60 Gy centrally with marginal doses of 12.5 Gy to 30 Gy delivered by Gamma Knife. All 13 patients treated showed an excellent response. The combined approach can preserve normal pituitary function and eradicate adenoma invading the cavernous sinus. The dose limiting factor for such treatment is the distance between the tumour and the optic pathway. They recommend the combined approach as the optimal therapy for adenomas invading the cavernous sinus.

Macroadenomas: The treatment for macroadenomas is less clear-cut because of a high recurrence rate after surgery, the inability of bromocriptine to shrink tumours and to normalise prolactin in about 1/3 of the patients. The results with postoperative conventional radiotherapy in such cases seem to be good.

L.4.7.1
Conventional Radiation Therapy

In macroadenomas there is paucity in the literature regarding the value of radiotherapy especially with regard to visual improvement, hypersecretion and tumour reduction.

Conventional linear accelerator therapy is possible in the majority of patients, preferably postoperatively.

Commenting on radiotherapy as the sole treatment, Rush and Newall (1989) retrospectively analysed the results in 29 patients treated by radiotherapy alone. Twenty-eight patients received a dose of 45 Gy in 4–5 weeks. *The tumours were controlled in 26 out of 28 patients for an observed period of 3–14 years.* Seventeen of 21 patients experienced normalisation or improved vision, and 7/10 patients who had raised prolactin levels reverted to normal levels. They used a 1 cm margin at the 90% isodose and gave 3-field therapy: two lateral fields and one coronal field. Doses employed were 45–46 Gy in 1.8–2 Gy fractions. Field sizes ranged from 4–8 cm^2.

The dose recommended by Grigsby *et al.* (1988) is about 45–50 Gy in 1.8 Gy fractions.

Patients with visual field defects who have inoperable disease or who refuse surgery should be given 54 Gy.

It appears that Cushing's disease can be controlled with relatively low doses: about 30–45 Gy.

Acromegaly, amenorrhoea/galactorrhoea and non-functioning tumours all do better on 45 Gy and more.

External conventional radiotherapy can control 80% of patients with acromegaly, 50%–80% of those with Cushing's disease and about 33% of those with prolactinomas (Grigsby 1988). The return to normal levels of the hormone may take months to years. Movsas et al. (1995) conclude that postoperative conventionally fractionated radiotherapy for incompletely resected, recurrent or persistent hormone elevation levels can be curative by treating to a median dose of 50 Gy, with a median field size of 6 × 6 cm by linear accelerator. This resulted in control of recurrences with no deterioration in visual fields or recurrences in 95% of the patients. Six out of 21 patients had neurologic symptoms in follow-up, most of which appeared vascular in nature. Four patients complained of atypical migraine-like headaches beginning 1.5–3 years following treatment. Most of the complications occurred in patients receiving doses more than 50 Gy.

McCord et al. (1997) found that pituitary adenomas are well-controlled by external beam radiotherapy, that visual symptoms often improve after radiotherapy and that hormonal problems usually require medical intervention. Combined surgery/conventional radiotherapy resulted in 95% of control at 10 years, which was not statistically significantly different from patients treated with radiotherapy alone (90% at 5 years).

Younger patients, patients with recurrent tumours, prolactinomas and ACTH secreting tumours did worse.

Individualised portals are necessary to cover the tumour with a 1.5–2 cm margin and the field sizes are typically 5–6 cm^2.

L.4.7.2
Radiosurgery for Pituitary Tumours

Gamma Knife and Linear Accelerator: The experience with radiosurgery is not very large this includes proton therapy. The first Gamma Knife treatment for a pituitary adenoma was done in 1967. Thoren et al. (1991) reported on the use of radiosurgery with the Gamma Knife for growth hormone producing pituitary tumours with favourable results.

Of 21 patients with growth hormone producing macroadenomas with parasellar growth extension and acromegaly, 7 patients had radiosurgery alone and 14 patients had previous surgery of which 8 had conventional radiotherapy. Two patients had a remission with normalisation of growth hormone levels, 8 obtained a significant reduction of hormone levels with clinical improvement. Eleven of the 21 patients had minor or no therapy-related effects. For large invasive lesions these results can be considered good.

Pituitary adenomas comprise, surprisingly, only 7.8% of the 27,000 patients treated by Gamma Knife treated world-wide to 1996 (Motti et al. 1996). These authors feel that radiosurgery has a definite role following failed pituitary surgery and for tumours extending into the cavernous sinus. The extreme sensitivity of the optic tract (maximal dose tolerable 8–9 Gy) and the extremely close proximity of these structures to the pituitary gland explains why radiosurgery is not often used for pituitary lesions.

Voges *et al.* (1996) reported on 32 consecutive patients treated with linear accelerator radiosurgery for recurrent pituitary macroadenomas after neurosurgery or conventional radiotherapy. They used single doses ranging from 8–20 Gy with a median of 14.5 Gy. They treated 14 patients with acromegaly, 5 with Cushing's disease, 4 with Nelson's syndrome, 5 with prolactinomas and 4 with non-functioning adenomas. Analysis of 26 patients with more than 6 months follow-up revealed no significant endocrinologic response in patients with Cushing's disease, Nelson's syndrome or prolactinoma. In contrast, in 12 patients with acromegaly the median growth hormone value decreased significantly, and in 3 non-functioning tumours a reduction in the size of the tumour was observed. They concluded that relatively low radiosurgical doses may be safe and effective for acromegaly or non-functioning tumours resistant to conventional therapy. In Cushing's disease, Nelson's tumours or prolactinomas higher doses may be required.

Rocher *et al.* (1995) reported on 135 patients treated by stereotactic radiosurgery plus or minus external beam radiotherapy, of which 42 were pituitary adenomas. The biological and radiological results were good, but they *had a high visual complication rate (12/42 = 28.6%), eight of which were classed as grade 3 complications. This led them to abandon radiosurgery for pituitary tumours, except those less than 2 cm and at "some distance" from the optic nerves.* The visual complications correlated with the tumour volume, the distance between the adenoma and the visual tract, and with pre-existing visual disturbances.

In an analysis of 77 patients treated at the Karolinska Institute by Gamma Knife 42 of 51 patients with Cushing's disease were cured (Rahn *et al.* 1991)

Valentino (1991) described 52 patients with pituitary adenoma treated by linear accelerator radiosurgery postoperatively for incompletely removed lesions or for recurrent lesions. Symptomatic improvement was observed in 67% of the patients and of 33 endocrine-active tumours only 2 remained active. Follow-up CT scans revealed measurable tumour reduction in 40 of the 52 patients.

L.4.7.3
Dose Response and Dose-Volume Relationships

Conventional radiotherapy: Sheline and Wara (1975) found that in 56% of patients the tumour *recurred after 30 Gy versus 11.1% after 30–40 Gy.* Doses between 45–50 Gy appear to be safe, whereas doses in excess of 50 Gy conventional therapy carry a fair amount of risk, as discussed.

Radiosurgery: Kjellberg and Abe (1988) published a nomogram for the dose determination for pituitary adenomas according to the tumour type, tumour diameter, and the total dose.

L.4.7.4
Clinical Results

Proton radiosurgery for pituitary adenomas: The penumbra or lateral fall-off of proton beams can vary considerably, depending on the beam characteristics. Bragg peak therapy may in fact not be optimal because of the relatively large penumbra of small diameter proton beams. (See Chapter G.1.2.14). Another factor is that the Bragg peak is poorly developed in narrow proton beams. (See section on physics.) The certainty of dose delivery is suspect for protons where there is bone and adjacent air cavities, as the margin must be made larger to take care of the uncertainties introduced in the position of the Bragg peak under such conditions. The use of the Bragg peak for a pituitary lesion should be very carefully considered, due to the sensitivity of the nearby optic chiasm and tract. With coplanar plateau region therapy the penumbra is very steep and plateau plans may miss the chiasm where Bragg peak therapy may not.

Large doses per fraction are particularly hazardous for the optic nerve and chiasm, and single doses of > 8 Gy should be avoided.

The experience with proton beams: Kjellberg *et al.* (1968) reported on 80% remission rate by 4 years for acromegaly. Minakova *et al.* (1983) had similar results with a 90% remission rate at 4 years in 145 patients.

Kjellberg *et al.* (1968) showed for 175 patients with Cushing's disease, complete remission in laboratory and clinical parameters in over 60% of patients. Minakova's result (1983) for Cushing's disease in 224 patients is simular.

Table L4.1 gives the available results with particle therapy.

Table L4.1 Results with particle therapy for pituitary tumours. Doses are stated at the periphery of the lesions. Data from Levy et al. (1992), Kjellberg (1988, 1991) and Loeffler *et al.* (1995). The very large doses should be given only with very great caution. A dose of 150 Gy prescribed at the 50% isodose will deliver 10 Gy at the 3.3% isodose. The 3.3% isodose may inscribe a very large volume of surrounding brain tissue (See Chapter I)

Tumour	Institute	Modality	dose (Gy)	Patients'	response (%)
Acromegaly	Harvard	Protons	30–150	511–581	88
	Berkeley	Helium/ protons	30–50	302/318	95
Total				813/899	90.4
Cushing's disease	Harvard	Proton	30–150	153/180	89
	Berkeley	Helium/ proton	50–150	73/82	
Total				226/262	86.25

NB: The dose ranges quoted in Table L4.1 are of historical interest only and should not be used clinically. For a guide to clinically safe doses, refer to Chapter I on Dose-Volume Relationships and the guidelines of Kjellberg and Abe (1988). Fractionated proton therapy may improve this gross discrepancy. Four fractions of 6 Gy each will do virtually as much damage (BED_2 = 96 Gy as 25 fractions of 2 Gy each; BED_2 = 100 Gy). The doses quoted in Table L4.1 have BED_2 values of 480 Gy up to 11,400 Gy, which should have an almost unlimited potential for causing late damage, especially if this is contrasted with fractionated conventional radiation i.e. 1.8–2 Gy to 45–50 Gy, (BED_2 = 85.5 Gy to 100 Gy, respectively). For a discussion of the BED see Chapter H.3.

L.4.7.5
Complications

After conventional radiotherapy: Complications for conventional irradiation include *epilation, scalp swelling, and otitis.* Late reactions include *panhypopituitarism* that may occur within months or years, and these patients will need thyroid hormone replacement and corticosteroids, which may be needed from 6 months to a year following treatment. Patients evaluated after 3–20 years: 54/65 patients showed evidence of hypothalamic-pituitary impairment. Growth hormone deficiency may occur but is of little clinical relevance in adults. ACTH and TSH deficiencies develop rarely, if at all. *Damage to the optic nerves* is more frequent in patients receiving conventional doses greater than 50 Gy and by patients treated by fractions larger than 2 Gy or both (Grigsby 1998).

In this regard, long term visual changes were noticed by Movsas *et al.* (1995) who reported on the late changes in vision in 21 evaluable patients. Of 38 sighted eyes in the 21 patients 27 had normal visual fields that remained normal after irradiation, 7 showed improvement and 4 eyes had a stable defect mostly in the superior temporal region. No patient suffered deterioration in visual fields or acuity. Six out of the 21 patients developed neurological symptoms: 4 of *migraine-like headaches* that developed 1.5 to 3 years after treatment.

One patient developed *vertical diploplia* and one patient had a *stroke* 7 years after treatment.

In 11 patients who had 50 Gy or less only 1 patient developed symptoms, as against 5/10 of those receiving > 50 Gy. The daily fractions were 1.8–2.0 Gy per fraction on a 10 MV linear accelerator. The authors conclude that postoperative radiotherapy delivered in 1.8–2.0 Gy fractions to total doses of 50 Gy is effective and safe.

There is a small risk of < 2% of cerebral necrosis at doses > 54 Gy.

Persistent but non-symptomatic space occupying residual lesions was observed in 9 of 17 patients despite clinical improvement. The authors conclude that radiation therapy alone is an effective treatment for these tumours, that doses need not exceed 45 Gy in 25 fractions (1.8 Gy per fraction), that radiation can normalise hyperprolactinaemia and that tumour regression is variable and unrelated to the observed symptom regression.

After radiosurgery: See Chapter M on Complications.

L.4.8
Summary

Proton therapy for selected problem cases following pituitary surgery may have a place. The relatively large penumbra of small Bragg peak beams may render protons unsuitable for the treatment of pituitary lesions, especially if the lesion is close to the optic apparatus.

A re-examination of the role of the prescription isodose for protons may be needed. There is a trend to prescribe at the 90% isodose. It may be more advantageous to prescribe at, for example, the 50% isodose. Comparative plans with the plateau beam and alternative photon options should be carefully evaluated.

It may be better to use coplanar plateau region proton therapy for these tumours, because of the proximity of the optic chiasm, and due to the fact that the Bragg peak is poorly developed in narrow proton beams.

Alternatives to protons include stereotactic radiosurgery by other means, or even conformally planned conventionally fractionated radiotherapy in conjunction with microsurgery or endocrinological management.

The results of conventional radiotherapy are good, with few complications.

The response for particle therapy reported in the literature is good, but extreme caution is necessary with radiosurgery for patients with non-malignant, non-life threatening conditions because of the close proximity of the optic nerve.

L.4.9
References

Grigsby PW, Stokes S, Marks JE *et al.* (1988) Prognostic factors and results of radiotherapy alone in the management of pituitary adenomas. Int J Radiat Oncol Biol Phys 15:1103–1110

Grigsby PW (1998) Pituitary. In: Carlos Perez and Luther Brady (eds) Principles and practice of radiation oncology, 3rd edn. Lippincott-Raven, pp 829–848

Hardy J (1973) Transsphenoidal surgery of hypersecreting pituitary tumours. In: Koyler P, Ross ST (eds) Diagnosis and treatment of pituitary tumours. Excerpta Medica, New York, p 179

Hardy J, Vezina JL (1976) Transsphenoidal neurosurgery of intracranial neoplasm. Adv Neurol 15:261–273

Ikeda H, Jokuru H, Yoshimoto T (1998) Gamma Knife Radiosurgery for pituitary adenomas: usefulness of combined transsphenoidal and Gamma Knife radiosurgery for adenomas invading the cavernous sinus. Radiat Oncol Invest 6:26–34

Jho *et al.* (1997) Endoscopic pituitary surgery: an early experience. Surg Neurol 47:213–222; discussion 222–223

Kjellberg RN, Shintani A, Franzt AG (1968) Proton beam therapy for acromegaly. N Engl J Med 278:689–695

Kjellberg RN (1991) Proton beam (PB) therapy of pituitary tumours. Proceedings of the International Stereotactic Radiosurgery Symposium, Pittsburgh

Kovacs K, Scheithauer BW, Horvath E *et al.* (1996) The World Health Organisation Classification of Adenohypophysial Neoplasms. Cancer 78:502–510

Leavens ME, McCutcheon IF, Samaan NA (1992) Management of pituitary adenomas. Oncology 6:69

Levy RP, Fabrikant JI, Lyman JT *et al.* (1992) Clinical results of stereotactic heavy-charged particle radiosurgery of the pituitary gland. In: Steiner *et al.* (ed). Radiosurgery: baseline and trends. Raven Press, New York

Loeffler JS, Larson DA, Shrieve DC *et al.* (1995) Radiosurgery for the treatment of intracranial lesions. In: De Vita V, Hellman S, Rosenberg A (eds) Important advances in oncology. Lippincott, Philadelphia pp 141–156

McCord MW, Buatti J, Fennel EM *et al.* (1997) Radiotherapy for pituitary adenoma: long-term outcome and sequelae. Int J Radiat Oncol Biol Phys 39:437–444

Minakova Y, Kerpatorskaya LY, Lyass FM (1983)Proton beam therapy for pituitary tumours. Med Radial (Mosk) 28:7–13

Motti ED, Losa M, Pieralli S *et al.* (1996) Stereotactic radiosurgery of pituitary adenomas. Metabolism 45 [Suppl 1]:111–114

Movsas B, Movsas TZ, Steinberg S *et al.* (1993) Long-term visual changes following pituitary irradiation. Int J Radiat Oncol Biol Phys 33:599–605

Rahn T, Thoren M, Warner S (1991) In: Faglia G, Peck-Peuoz P, Ambrosi B (eds) Pituitary adenomas new trends in basic and clinical research. Excerpta Medica, New York, pp 303–212

Rocher FP, Sentenac I, Berger *et al.* (1995) Stereotactic radiosurgery: the Lyon experience. Acta Neurochir Suppl (Wien) 63:109–114

Rush SC, Newall J (1989) Pituitary adenoma: the efficacy of radiotherapy as the sole treatment. Int J Radiat Oncol Biol Phys 17:165–169

Sheline GE, Wara WM (1975) Radiation therapy of acromegaly and nonsecretory chromophobe adenomas of the pituitary. In: HG Seydel HH (ed) Tumours of the nervous system. Wiley, New York, pp 117–131

Thoren M, Rahn T, Guo WY *et al.* (1991) Stereotactic radiosurgery with cobalt-60 gamma unit in the treatment of growth hormone producing pituitary tumours. Neurosurgery 29:663

Valentino V (1991) Postoperative radiosurgery of pituitary adenomas. J Neurosurg Sci 35:207–211

Voges J, Sturm V, Deuss U (1996) Linac radiosurgery (linac RS) in pituitary adenomas: preliminary results. Acta Neurochir Suppl (Wien) 65:41–43

L.5
Proton and Stereotactic Radiotherapy for Primary and Secondary Brain Tumours

L.5.1
Introduction

The current results of radiotherapy for primary brain tumours are not good, but stereotactic treatment holds some promise for improvement, possibly combined with surgery or chemotherapy.

Proton therapy should have the edge on other forms of radiosurgery for the treatment of brain tumours, especially for lesions > 5 cm^3 because the dose distribution with protons is more homogeneous, the integral dose to the brain is lower, especially for larger lesions, and conformation is superior. There may be a distinct advantage for a homogeneous dose distribution for malignant tumours, best achievable with protons, but which is not necessarily important for benign lesions.

Re-locatable immobilisation systems allowing fractionated stereotactic proton therapy have been developed, which satisfies the need. High single doses have no biological benefit for malignant lesions; fractionated therapy should give much better results.

For metastatic lesions, however, a single large dose may offer good palliation for normally otherwise incurable patients and stereotactic therapy has been found to be very efficient and economical since radiosurgery requires minimal hospitalisation (reduced costs) and avoids the risk of haemorrhage, infection and tumour seeding. Some authors are of the opinion that it may displace surgery as the optimal method of management because of minimal morbidity and because radiosurgery is non-invasive. Surgery has the advantage of an immediate resolution of mass effect. Response rates of up to 80% are typically reported Loeffler *et al.* (1995).

L.5.2
The Importance of Fractionation

Fractionation is a key ingredient for the successful therapy of primary malignant tumours. (See Chapter H.1.6 on Radiobiology.) Fractionation may be easier to achieve with particle beams like protons for technical reasons. An example of a system that allows easy fractionation is the stereophotogrammetric (SPG) system of the National Accelerator Centre (NAC) in South Africa (Jones *et al.* 1995; Levin 1993). (See Chapter F.1.6.)

Fractionated therapy is gentle on the late reacting tissues like the brain and blood vessels and it reduces the late complication rate (Chapter H.1.6).

However, the results for single fraction boosts with modalities other than protons appear to be good where the tumours were pre-treated with conventionally fractionated photon beam radiotherapy.

Re-locatable frames used with the Gamma Knife or specially adapted linear accelerators have also been described. (Delannes *et al.* 1991; Mehta 1995).

Brenner *et al.* (1991) suggested a table for fractionated radiosurgery (up to 9 fractions) for recurrent malignant brain tumours. (See Chapter H.2.6 and Appendix P.5)

The importance of (hypo)fractionation is emphasised by Hudes *et al.* (1999) for persistent or recurrent malignant glioma.

L.5.3
Clinical Results Obtained with Primary Malignant Brain Tumours with Radiosurgery

Conventional radiotherapy: As a benchmark, the Brain Tumour Co-operative Study Group (BTCSG) showed a median survival of 3.5 months (14 weeks) for conventional therapy for patients who received 45 Gy or less, *versus 10.5 months* (42 weeks) median survival at *60 Gy*, and a dose response between 50 Gy and 60 Gy conventionally fractionated radiotherapy (Walker *et al.* 1979).

Wara *et al.* (1998) is of the opinion that the available data suggest that a total dose of 60–64 Gy in daily fractions of 1.8–2 Gy is adequate to treat most patients with malignant gliomas, and that higher doses will probably be of no benefit.

Radiosurgery: Loeffler *et al.* (1992) gave 59 Gy in 33 fractions external radiotherapy, encompassing the lesion with a 3–4 cm margin, followed by a radiosurgical boost of 12 Gy to the contrast enhancing volume 4 weeks after completion of the external therapy. Twenty three patients had glioblastoma multiforme and 14 anaplastic astrocytomas. Nine of the 37 patients were dead after a median follow-up of 19 months, 6 of these from recurrent tumour, 2 died of treatment related complications and 1 died of intercurrent disease. This means that *75% of the patients survived at a median follow-up time of 19 months*, almost a doubling of conventional therapy.

Seven patients needed re-operation at a median time of 5 months post treatment.

Brachytherapy boosts improves survival in patients with brain tumours, but radiosurgery has the additional advantage that it is less invasive and inherently less risky than brachytherapy (Mehta 1995). The data to date suggest that a central, highly localised (radiosurgical) "boost" is beneficial.

Radiosurgery for low grade astrocytomas have been reported on by Pozzo and Colombo (1989) in a small study. They noted improvement in 10 out of 14 patients with only one patient dying of the disease at 38 months. Further clinical trials are required to corroborate these findings.

Williams *et al.* (1998) found that low grade gliomas fared better than high grade gliomas. They used single doses of 16.5 ± 1.9 Gy and 19.32 ± 1.82 Gy, respectively, for low and high grade lesions.

A mean survival in *recurrent* high grade tumours of 11.6 ± 1.5 months is recorded. In recurrent low grade tumours, five of out of nine patients died 31.6 ± 6 months after SRS. They conclude tentatively that for patients with recurrent gliomas, stereotactic radiosurgery (SRS) offers a precise local administration of radiotherapy that may result in both tumour control and prolongation of survival, but that randomised studies are needed to verify the findings.

Recurrent malignant gliomas in 103 patients from two centres achieved good palliation with a median survival of just over 10 months, and a median follow-up time of 17.5 months. (Selch at al 1993; Shrieve *et al.* 1995).

Hudes *et al.* (1999) obtained a median survival in 20 patients (with 25 lesions) after completion of hypofractionated radiosurgery, of 10.5 months with a 1 year survival of 20%.

Woo *et al.* (1997) reported on a radiosurgical boost for medulloblastomas in four patients (age 7–42 years).

All patients had debulking surgery followed by external radiotherapy and a stereotactic boost with doses ranging from 4.0 to 10 Gy and volumes 1.1–8.1 cm^3. All four patients were alive without evidence of recurrence at 8 to 35 months. They concluded that the results merit inclusion of a stereotactic boost in future clinical trials for medulloblastoma.

Larson *et al.* (1996) analysed 189 patients who were treated by Gamma Knife radiosurgery for gliomas, WHO grade 1–4.

The median single tumour dose was 16 Gy (8–30 Gy). This dose was delivered *0–2 mm beyond the radiological enhancing volume* and the median volume was 5.9 cm^3 (1.3–52 cm^3). The median survival was 21.5 months (86 weeks) if brachytherapy criteria were satisfied and the survival was reduced to 10 months (40 weeks) if they were not (p = 0.01) which indicated that selection factors (see below) strongly influenced survival.

Buatti *et al.* (1995) reported on the first carefully selected 11 patients treated at the University of Florida. External beam radiotherapy was delivered as a mean dose of 60 Gy. A stereotactic boost was added to the enhancing tumour without margin. The median treatment volume was 14 cm^3 (sphere radius of 15 mm), and the maximum volume was 22.5 cm^3 (radius 17.5 mm) The median stereotactic boost dose was 12.5 Gy at the 80% prescription isodose shell.

Despite rigorous selection and aggressive stereotactic boost irradiation, this patient cohort had a median actuarial survival of only 17 months. All patients had progression of intracranial disease within a year of radiosurgery and only 3 out of 11 remain alive within a follow-up of 13 months.

These results differed significantly from others reported, and the authors advocate *stringent clinical trials.*

L.5.4
Selection Factors for Glioma Patients and the Hazard Ratio Model for Radiosurgey

A multivariate analysis identified low pathologic grade, younger age, good performance status, small volume and unifocal tumour as favourable factors (Larson *et al.* 1993).

Survival was not found to be significantly related to the technical parameters of the radiosurgery like total dose, prescription isodose and number of isocentres.

Their hazard ratio (HR) model may help to predict the outcome in any specific patient. The Hazards ratio model. The Hazards Ratio took into account the performance status, pathology, age, tumour volume and number of lesions. (Larson *et al.* 1996)

Patients with a HR < 3 had about a 70% 3-year survival, an HR between 3 and 12 about 35% 3-year survival and patients with an HR > 12 had only about a 50% survival at 1 year.

Figure L5.1 shows the survival curves stratified according to the Hazard Ratio Model.

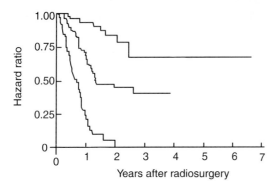

Fig. L5.1 Selection factors and survival: hazard ratio model of Larson *et al.* (1996) determining survival of patients with malignant glioma. Kaplan-Meier survival curves are shown according to Hazard Ratio model with p < 0.001 (log rank test). (Redrawn from DA Larson *et al.*, 1996, Int J Radiat Oncol Biol Phys 36:1045–1053)

While this model cannot be directly extrapolated to proton therapy, it may serve as a useful basis for analysing the results of proton radiosurgery for brain tumours.

In conclusion, there is evidence that radiosurgical boosts for malignant gliomas are beneficial, but radiosurgery for these tumours should probably be done within controlled multicentre co-operative trials. Fractionated boosts may improve the results further and should probably be investigated.

L.5.5
Dose Response for Brain Tumours

Of the malignant gliomas, glioblastoma multiforme accounts for about 80% of the tumours. The expected median survival for the latter subgroup is 9 to 10 months, and the 5-year survival only about 5%. (Mehta 1995)

More than 80% of these tumours fail in regions less than 2 cm away from the apparent edge of the primary tumour.

The Brain Tumour Co-operative Study Group showed a median survival of 3.5 months (14 weeks) for conventional therapy for patients who received 45 Gy or less, *versus* 10.5 months (42 weeks) median survival at 60 Gy (Walker *et al.* 1979).

A trial by the Brain Tumour Co-operative Group showed that a dose of 60.2 Gy to the tumour plus a 3 cm margin plus BCNU at 200 mg/M^2 every 8 weeks plus or minus a brachytherapy boost of 60 Gy over 150 hours (about 1 week) at the tumour periphery, resulted in a statistically significant advantage for the group receiving the brachytherapy (Green *et al.* 1994).

Radiosurgery is however less invasive than brachytherapy and radiosurgical boosts should be tested in a trial against brachytherapy.

For a discussion and a table of radiotherapy regimens presenting brain tolerance see Chapter H.3 on the BED.

Further answers to the question of acceptable dose levels comes from the RTOG phase I study in patients with *previously irradiated primary and metastatic brain tumours* (Shaw *et al.* 1994). This study established maximum tolerable doses (MTDs) for tumour diameters in 10 mm increments from less than 20 mm to 40 mm.

Hudes *et al.* (1999) found that hypofractionated radiosurgery in patients previously irradiated by conventional fractionation to a median dose of 60 Gy (44–72 Gy) benefited from the addition of a hypofractionated stereotactic boost. None of six lesions treated with 21 Gy or 24 Gy hypofractionated radiosurgery responded, whereas there was a 79% response rate among the 19 lesions treated to 30 or 35 Gy.

The values obtained are tabulated in adapted form (Table L5.1)

Table L5.1 Maximally tolerated radiosurgical doses (*MTDs*) for previously irradiated primary and secondary brain tumours. Data from Shaw *et al.* (1994)

Tumour diameter (cm)	MTD (Gy)
> 2	27
2.1–3.0	21
3.1–4.0	15

These values may be in order for patients with a limited prognosis, since the doses are higher than the 1% brain necrosis risk line of Kjellberg (1983). As indicated above, doses of 16–20 Gy may be prudent for patients with a good performance status and good prognosis. Here again, the total volume of brain that gets more than 10–12 Gy may be the determining factor. The reader is referred to Chapter I on Dose-Volume Relationships.

Finally, the acceptable dose for brain tumours is a function of the tumour size, the tumour type, previous surgery or radiotherapy concomitant disease like hypertension and diabetis mellitus, and very importantly, the fraction sizes used.

L.5.6
Brain Tolerance

See Chapter D.

L.6
Secondary Malignant Brain Tumours

About 10 to 20 percent of all patients with cancer will develop brain metastases.

L.6.1
Conventional Radiotherapy (Whole Brain)

Conventional radiotherapy (whole brain) improves the survival to about 4–5 months. Thirty Gy in ten fractions yield near optimal results. Patients with three or fewer lesions achieve better survival times.

More recent RTOG studies reported accelerated fractionation using 1.6 Gy twice daily to total doses of 48–70.4 Gy; the optimally tolerated dose was found to be 54.4 Gy (Curran *et al.* 1991).

Local control of metastatic tumours obtained by surgery followed by whole brain irradiation improved survival and quality of life (Patchell *et al.* 1990).

L.6.2
Radiosurgery

The rationale for radiosurgery in patients with metastatic brain tumours has been enunciated by Mehta (1995). Metastatic lesions are usually almost spherical and thus ideal in shape, the grey/white junction is relatively "quiet", i.e. not very prone to cause radiation induced symptoms and metastatic lesions are usually detected before they are large (< 0.3 cm). The near spherical shapes, usually well circumscribed, allow tight planning and margins and therefore a diminished risk of complications, provided that the lateral fall-off of the beams is steep, e.g. 15% per millimetre.

The median survival time of these patients, if untreated, may be as little as 1 month

Reports on over 1000 patients support response rates in excess of 80%, with few complications.

A sharp decline in the control rate occurs in patients with lesions > 6 cm in diameter.

Lymphomas give a 100% response rate, 50% for non-small cell lung cancer, 33% for breast cancer and only 11% for renal cell carcinoma. For melanomas and sarcomas a surprising response rate of 67% was achieved by radiosurgery.

Doses varied from 18 Gy to 29 Gy median peripheral dose, the vast majority of the reported cases are from Gamma Knife or Linear Accelerator centres.

The dose level should be considered in terms of the patient's overall prognosis. Lower doses in the 16–20 Gy range may be prudent in patients with a good performance status and no other major metastatic disease process, to avoid the catastrophe of serious late complications in an otherwise well patient.

Mehta *et al.* (1998) reviewed the data of 1250 patients with 2100 metastatic lesions. Untreated, a survival of only 1 month can be expected. *Stereotactic radiosurgery (SRS) offered an 83% local control rate and a median survival of 9.6 months, which is comparable to recent surgical reports.* A dose of 18 Gy or more may be needed. Again a plea is made for randomised trials by the author.

Nausea was reported in 11.2% of patients who had more than 2.75 Gy to the area postrema, seizures in 6.1% within 24 h and transient motor weakness in 2% of patients within 36 hours in patients with motor cortex lesions. All patients receiving > 3.75 Gy to the area postrema should receive anti-emetic therapy prior to treatment.

Since 1990 the Boston group recommends anti-convulsant therapy for all patients with cortical lesions before radiosurgery

The major chronic complications were radiation necrosis in 8% of patients from 2–22 months after therapy, all of which eventually required resection. The risk of necrosis was a function of tumour volume and prior or concurrent whole brain irradiation.

Chronic steroid dependence (use longer than 6/12) is a consequence of persistent cerebral oedema after radiosurgery, with all its accompanying complications, and this may occur in about 8% of patients at 12 months.

L.6.3
Radiosurgery for Metastases *versus* Surgery

Surgical resection requires a hospital stay of about 7 days, versus 1.3 days for radio-surgery. The total surgical cost may amount to 3.4 times more than that for radio-surgery (Mehta 1995). Even with fractionated therapy, the hospital stay is short, since the patients will come in on an outpatient basis. There is evidence that stereotactic radiosurgery is as efficient as surgical resection, has a lower morbidity, better quality of life and better maintenance of function than resection for solitary brain metastases. There may also be a survival advantage and in patients with good neurological status, 2–4 lesions may be treated (Callaghan 1997).

Mehta *et al.* (1992) concludes that stereotactic radiosurgery (by linear accelerator) can be used effectively for patients with brain metastases, with a high tumour response rates associated with improved quality of life. The minimal tumour doses ranged from 12 Gy to 37 Gy with a mean of 18.3 Gy and the dose varied inversely with the collimator size. The tumour volumes ranged from 0.2 cm^3 to 30.6 cm^3, with a mean of 5.2 cm^3. An overall tumour control rate of 82% was realised and a complete response rate of 43%.

Breneman *et al.* (1997) found that the treatment of brain metastases by radio-surgery (linear accelerator) gave comparable results to that of surgery. Radiosurgical (single) doses employed were 10–20 Gy with a median minimal dose of 16 Gy. The results were superior to that of whole brain radiotherapy alone. Survival was best for patients with three or fewer lesions, and local control the best in patients who received more than 18 Gy.

Kocher *et al.* (1998) found that patients with brain metastases have a high risk of cancer related death due to extra- or intracranial tumour manifestations. Their retro-spective analysis demonstrates the ability of linear accelerator based radiosurgery to control intracranial disease and to prolong survival in patients with one to three metastases and with various approaches an overall median survival of 8 months was achieved. Prognostic factors included Karnofsky performance status, presence of extracranial tumour, and the volume of the largest lesions. They conclude that linear accelerator based radiosurgery in patients with up to three cerebral metastases results in survival rates approaching those of patients with resected single brain metastases.

Whether brain metastases should be managed by radiosurgery, has been ques-tioned by Sperduto *et al.* (1995). They state that patients with brain metastases with uncontrolled primary malignant tumours should receive whole brain radiotherapy in the conventional manner plus steroids, patients with local control of their disease could be considered for whole brain irradiation plus a radiosurgical boost, and patients with a mass effect should be managed surgically followed by whole brain irra-diation.

A trial involving Gamma Knife, linear accelerator and proton radiosurgery for metastatic brain lesions seems to be called for.

L.6.4
Complications of Radiosurgery for Brain Tumours

Within the dose ranges mentioned, Breneman (1997) found that out of 82 patients, 7 acute and 2 chronic complications developed for a total complication rate of 11%.

Three patients experienced grand mal seizures for lesions in the motor cortex. Two patients developed worsening neurological symptoms associated with increasing mass effect after radiosurgery, which required surgical decompression.

The sharpness of the beam (steep dose fall-off) will help to reduce the radiation dose to the normal brain, and thus to reduce complications. (See also Chapters M on Complications and I on Dose-Volume Relationships)

L.7
Summary

There is evidence for a dose-response for primary malignant tumours of the brain within a narrow band of 54–64 Gy in 1.8 Gy fractions, for conventional therapy. The data on radiosurgical boosts or interstitial brachytherapy favours boost doses of about 10 Gy, added to reduced volumes after previous external therapy of about 60 Gy conventionally fractionated.

For primary malignant lesions, fractionated radiosurgery may have a key role to play in order to optimise damage to the tumour, whilst sparing the normal tissues. In general terms, the smaller the dose per fraction, the bigger the probability of a cure.

Surgical debulking prior to radiotherapy (where possible) plus fractionated localised external beam therapy followed by a radiosurgical boost, which should probably be fractionated as well, may be the best course of action from a radiobiological point of view.

Radiosurgery without prior external therapy for metastatic brain lesions seems to compete with surgery both with respect to cost and efficacy, and where life expectancy is normally not good, single radiosurgical doses may be useful and will not cause the patient to spend a large percentage of his or her remaining life span in hospital.

A newcomer in the radiosurgical arena is the "photon radiosurgical (PRS) system". This device is discussed further in Chapter N on Alternatives to Proton Beams.

L.8
References

Breneman JC, Warnick RE, Albright RE (JR) et al. (1997) Stereotactic radiosurgery for the treatment of brain metastases results of a single institution. Cancer 79:551–557

Brenner DJ, Martel MK, Hall EJ (1991) Fractionated regimens for stereotactic radiotherapy of recurrent tumours in the brain. Int J Radiat Oncol Biol Phys 21:819–824

Buatti JM, Friedman WA, Bova FJ, Mendelhall WM (1995) Linac radiosurgery for high-grade gliomas: the University of Florida experience. Int J Radiat Oncol Biol Phys 32:205–210

Callaghan RM (1997) Stereotactic radiosurgery – a novel treatment for brain lesions. Hosp Supplies 38–46

Curran W, Scott C, Nelson D et al. (1991) Results from the RTOG Phase I/II twice daily RT dose escalation trials for malignant glioma (83-02) and brain metastases (85-28). Ninth International Conference on Brain Tumour Research and Therapy, Asilomar, California

Delannes M, Daly N, Bonnet J, Tremoulet M (1991) Fractionated radiotherapy of small inoperable lesions of the brain using a non-invasive stereotactic frame. Int J Radiat Oncol Biol Phys 21:749–755

Flickinger JC, Fulton DS, Artisan RC, Scott-Brown I et al. (1992) Increasing radiation dose intensity in patients with malignant glioma: final report of prospective Phase I–II dose-response study. J Neurol Oncol 14:63–72

Green SD, Shapiro WR, Burger RC et al. (1994) A randomised trial of interstitial brachytherapy (RT) boost for newly diagnosed malignant glioma. Brain Tumour Co-operative Group (BTCG) trial 8701. American Society of Clinical Oncology

Hall E, Brenner DJ (1993) Radiobiology of radiosurgery: rationale for different treatment regimes for AVMs and malignancies. Int J Radiat Oncol Biol Phys 25:381–385

Hudes RS, Corn BW, Werner-Wasik M et al. (1999) A phase I dose escalation study of hypofractionated stereotactic radiotherapy as salvage therapy for persistent or recurrent malignant gliomas. Int J Radiat Oncol Biol Phys 43:293–298

Jones DTL, Schreuder AN, Symons JE Rüther, Van der Vlugt G, Bennett KF, Yates ADB (1995) Use of stereophotogrammetry in proton radiation therapy. Proceedings FIG Commission 6. International FIG Symposium February, Cape Town

Kjellberg RN, Hanamura T, Davis KR, Lyons SL, Adams RN, Adams R (1983) Bragg-peak proton-beam therapy for arteriovenous malformations of the brain. N Engl J Med 309:269–273

Kocher M, Voges J, Muller RP et al. (1998) Linac radiosurgery for patients with a limited number of brain metastases. J Radiosurg 1:9–15

Larson DA, Flickinger JC, Loeffler JS (1993) The radiobiology of radiosurgery. Int J Radiat Oncol Biol Phys 25:557–561

Larson DA, Gutin PH, McDermott M et al. (1996) Gamma Knife for glioma: selection factors and survival. Int J Radiat Oncol Biol Phys 36:1045–1053

Levin CV, Hough J, Adams LP, Boonzaaier D, Rüther H, Wynchank S (1993) Determining locations of intracerebral lesions for proton radiotherapy. Phys Med Biol 38:1393–1401

Loeffler JS, Alexander E (1990) The role of stereotactic radiosurgery in the management of intracranial tumours. Oncology 4:21–31

Loeffler JS, DA, Shrieve DC et al. (1995) Radiosurgery for the treatment of intracranial lesions. In: De Vita VT, Hellman S, Rosenberg S (eds). Lippincott, Philadelphia, pp 141–156

Marks JE, Baglan RJ, Prassad SC et al. (1981) Cerebral radionecrosis: incidence and risk in relation to dose time and fractionation. Int J Radiat Oncol Biol Phys 7:243–252

Mehta MP, Rozental JM, Levin AB et al. (1992) Defying the role of radiosurgery in the management of brain metastases. In J Radiat Oncol Biol Phys 24:619–623

Mehta M (September/October 1995) The physical, biologic and clinical basis of radiosurgery. In: Kinsella T (ed) Current problems in cancer pp 269–329

Patchell RA, Tibbs PA, Walsh JW et al. (1990) A randomised trial of surgery in the treatment of single metastases to the brain. N Engl J Med 322:494–500

Penar PL (1996) Cost and outcome analysis (in the management of cerebral metastases). Neurosurg Clin North Am 7:547–558

Pozzo F, Colombo F (1989) Low grade astrocytomas: Treatment with unconventionally fractionated external beam stereotactic radiation therapy. Radiology 171:565–569

Sakarja JN, Mehta MP, Loeffler JS et al. (1994) Stereotactic radiosurgery improves survival in malignant gliomas compared with the RTOG recursive partitioning analysis. Int J Radiat Oncol Biol Phys 30:164–165

Selch MT, Ciacci JD, DeSalles AA et al. (1993) Radiosurgery for primary malignant brain tumours. In: DeSalles AF, Goetsch SJ (eds) Stereotactic surgery and radiosurgery. Medical Physics, Madison, pp 335–352

Shaw E, Scott C, Souhami L et al. (1996) Radiosurgery for the treatment of previously irradiated recurrent primary brain tumours and brain metastases: initial report of the Radiation Therapy Oncology Group Protocol (90-05) Int J Radiat Oncol Biol Phys 34:647–654

Shrieve DC, Loeffler JS (1995) Advances in radiation therapy for brain tumours. Neurol Clin 13:773–93

Sperduto P, Hall WA (1996) Radiosurgery: cost effectiveness, gold standards, the scientific method, cavalier cowboys, and the cost of hope. (editorial) Int J Radiat Oncol Biol Phys 36:511–513

Voges J, Treuer H, Sturm V, Buchner C, Lehrke R, Kocher M, Staar S, Kuchta J, Müller RP (1996) Risk analysis of linear accelerator radiosurgery. Int J Radiat Oncol Biol Phys 36:1055–1063

Walker MD, Strike TA, Sheline GE (1979) An analysis of dose effect relationship in the radiotherapy of malignant gliomas. Int J Radiat Oncol Biol Phys 5:1725–1731

Wara WM, Baumann GS, Sneed PK et al. (1998) Brain, brainstem and cerebellum. In: Perez CA, Brady (eds) Principles and practice of radiation oncology, 3rdedn. Lippincott-Raven, pp 777–828

Williams J, Zakhary AB, Watts MD et al. (1998) Stereotactic radiosurgery for human glioma: treatment parameters and outcome for low versus high grade. J Radiosurg 1:3–7

Woo C, Stea B, Lulu B, Hamilton MD, Cassady JB (1997) The use of stereotactic boost in the treatment of medulloblastomas. Int J Radiat Oncol Biol Phys 37:761–764

M The Complications of Single Large Intracranial Doses of Radiation and Their Management

M.1
Introduction

Some complications have been discussed under the individual clinical conditions. This chapter is intended to give a more comprehensive overview of the causes, mechanisms, contributing factors, prevention and management of complications should they occur.

Although radiosurgery is regarded as reasonably safe, complication rates are high at the largest doses and volumes treated and complications of up to 60% for some dose-volume situations have been reported. It is therefore important to be aware of the minimal doses required to get the desired effect. Immediate side effects (ISEs) occur in about one third of patients following radiosurgery.

Multidisciplinary clinics with all the relevant members of a team are imperative to minimise the risks. The likely effects of damage to any brain area should be discussed with the neurosurgeon, or neurologist, then with the patient. An atlas of functional neuro-anatomy, like that of Orrison (1995) relating structure to brain function is very useful in this regard. The complications of large-field fractionated proton therapy have been discussed in Chapters K.3 and K.4.

M.2
Classification of Radiation Effects

M.2.1
Acute Effects

The adverse effects of radiation on the brain and spinal cord are classified according to the time of appearance. Acute reactions occur during or immediately after a course of radiation therapy. Acute reactions are likely to be due to swelling and oedema.

Cerebral oedema can occur within days to weeks after therapy. The oedema is reversible and is usually ameliorated by steroids. The acute effects are dose- and volume-dependent.

Whenever a large single dose of radiation is intended, it is wise to give prophylactic steroids. The recommendations vary, but 10–20 mg of dexamethasone 2 hours before each radiosurgical dose and 8 hours afterwards is indicated (Engenhart 1995). The effects of radiosurgery and radiotherapy are likely to vary depending on the single dose equivalent, the volume of the lesion irradiated and the sensitivity of the area irradiated. For example, the brain stem is much more liable to injury than the brain parenchyma in silent areas. If the area postrema is included in the radiation field, acute nausea and vomiting may ensue. Premedication is essential where this area is expected to receive a radiation dose larger than a few Gray, since doses as low as 2–3 Gy may trigger serious nausea and vomiting.

Seizures can be expected in about 3% of patients, especially in those with a pre-treatment history of seizures. Seizures may be due to acute oedema, but it is more frequently seen in patients who had a previous history of seizures as part of their symptomatology. Steroids should be combined with a continuation of existing suitable anti-convulsants.

Headaches have been reported, and some patients who presented with headache before treatment had more severe headache for a few days following treatment. These headaches are usually controlled by simple analgesics.

Headaches could also be a consequence of vasogenic oedema, and if so, suitable analgesics like paracetamol should be combined with steroids. If there is no evidence of cerebral oedema on CT or MRI, then non-steroidal anti-inflammatory agents or simple analgesics may suffice.

Haemorrhage is not directly related to radiosurgical procedures, although some haemodynamic disturbances in AVMs may follow radiosurgery within weeks or months. If haemorrhage occurs it is obviously a dire neurosurgical emergency and should be handled as such. The patient or his family should be alerted to this possibility at the time of treatment and consultation and the necessary communication channels should be established well in advance, and a plan of action/options established.

The risk of haemorrhage with AVMs fortunately diminishes with time after treatment. The cumulative risk of haemorrhage in the first 2 years after treatment is 6%–8%. (Steiner *et al.* 1992; Livingstone and Hopkins 1992).

Partially obliterated AVMs do not offer a reduced risk of haemorrhage after 2 years, emphasising the need for good planning and lesion coverage, yet avoiding the irradiation of normal brain as far as possible. Fabrikant *et al.*, with helium ions, reported in 10/86 cases incidence of haemorrhage in patients with AVMs, of which 7/86 patients bled in the first year, and 3 patients later than 1 year. In their experience serious early sequelae of treatment were negligible. They used dexamethasone immediately prior to therapy, and tapered the dose off over 2 weeks. Seizures occurred in only a few patients who had a history of seizures. Helium ions have very sharp (steep) distal and lateral dose fall-offs, which may partially explain the low complication rate.

Immediate side effects (any side effects occurring during the course of therapy or up to 2 weeks later) following radiosurgery by linear accelerator have been reported by Werner-Wasik *et al.* (1999). They analysed the ISEs in 78 patients, which included 13 gliomas, 2 ependymomas, 19 metastatic tumours, 15 meningiomas, 12 acoustic neuromas, 1 optic neuroma, 1 chondrosarcoma and 11 AVMs. Stereotactic radiation therapy (STR) was used in 51 and stereotactic fractionated radiosurgery (SRS) in 27 patients. The mean target volume was 9 cm^3. Of these, 28/78 patients experienced ISEs of which 87% were mild (nausea and vomiting in 5, dizziness vertigo in 5, seizures in 6 and new persistent headaches in 17). Moderate ISEs: Two patients experienced worsening neurological deficit and two orbital pain.

Severe: Two required hospitalisation, one for seizure and one for worsening neurological deficit. ISE in six cases prompted CT of the brain, which revealed perilesional oedema in six patients.

ISE occurred in 50% of acoustic neuromas and in 36% of AVMs, approximately the same in the other lesion types. Higher radiotherapy doses to the lesion margins and higher maximum radiotherapy doses were associated with a higher incidence of ISE.

ISEs occurred in 26% of patients taking corticosteroids before SRT/SRS and in 42% of patients not taking them (p = 0.15), not statistically significant. Dizziness/vertigo are common and unique for patients with acoustic neuromas and are not associated with higher brainstem doses.

Doses employed: SRS for brain metastases 13–21 Gy. Pituitary and optic neuroma patients received 46–50 Gy in 2 Gy fractions using the Gill-Thomas Cosman frame. AVMs received 14–20 Gy with the largest diameter not exceeding 2 cm and 6 fractions of 7 Gy each for lesions larger than 2 cm in diameter.

Patients or their families should be briefed on what symptoms to be on the look-out for and what action to take.

M.2.2
Late Effects

Delayed reactions are sub-classified into "early delayed", appearing a few weeks to a few months after radiotherapy, or "late delayed" appearing months to years later (Sheline 1986).

The early delayed reaction in the brain is partially due to transient demyelination because of temporary depletion of the oligodendroglia; damage to the blood-brain barrier with radiosurgery causes the leakage of protein-rich, hygroscopic fluid into the brain, especially into the white matter, which is loosely woven compared to the cortex. The resultant oedema may be a contributing cause of early delayed phenomena.

Late delayed damage results from the combination of oligodendroglial loss and endothelial damage, leading to demyelination and necrosis (Brada and Thomas 1995; Mehta 1995). Brain tolerance has been discussed in Chapter H.3.10. Cerebral necrosis, usually a serious and undesirable complication, should be avoided as far as possible. Young patients are at greater risk of complications and special caution should be exercised with them.

Vasogenic oedema: Late effects include asymptomatic and symptomatic vasogenic oedema, occlusion of functional arteries or veins, and radionecrosis.

The manifestations and incidence of the complications depend in part on the region of the brain involved, the volume of normal and abnormal brain affected, the radiation dose, the presence of prior tissue injury as a result of haemorrhage or interventional procedures, the timing and the nature of the therapeutic efforts and concomitant medical conditions like diabetes mellitus and hypertensive disease. Flickinger *et al.* (1999) found a lower than 41% rate of symptom resolution in patients who had a history of prior haemorrhage than those who had no such history 66%. They suggested that steroid therapy may hasten the resolution of symptoms without changing whether or not a deficit ulltimately resolves. Cyst formation occurred in 5 out of 102 patients with complications.

Mehta (1995) suggested a "unifying model" to explain radiation damage to the brain, see Fig. M2.1.

M.2.2.1
Cerebral Oedema

Asymptomatic vasogenic oedema: It is somewhat artificial to divide radiation effects into "early" and "late" as different types of lesions are being recognised with overlap-

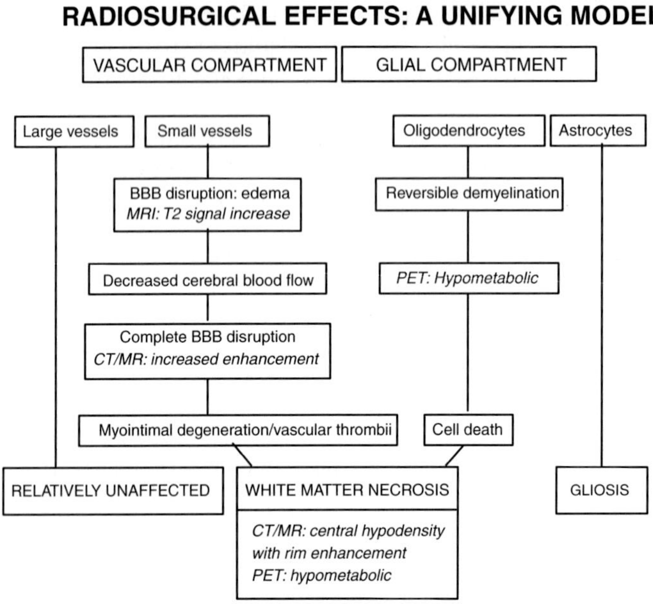

RADIOSURGICAL EFFECTS: A UNIFYING MODEL ?

Fig. M2.1 A unifying concept that explains the radiosurgery effect as an outcome resulting from the effect on multiple cell populations, resulting in varying clinical and radiographic manifestations. (Redrawn from MP Mehta, 1995, In: Current Problems in Cancer)

ping time distributions. The use of CT and MRI allows earlier recognition and potential discrimination between the transient and more severe progressive injuries. This contributes to removing the boundaries between early and delayed reactions. Within the "early delayed" category, changes ranging from a mild form of transient cerebral oedema without CT contrast enhancement to pronounced oedema with contrast enhancement or even frank radiation necrosis have been described (Van der Kogel et al. 1995; Watne et al. 1990).

Fabrikant et al. (1992) found that vasogenic oedema is usually asymptomatic and is usually discovered by chance on MRI on routine follow-up. Radiographically, the oedema is seen in the immediate region of AVMs as a high intensity signal on T_2 weighted MR images or as a region of low attenuation on CT images. These changes were observed in almost 50% of patients irradiated to more than 25 GyE (helium ions) for lesions in the deep white matter. This is ascribed to the relatively loose cellular packing in the white matter that permits diffusion of fluid into the surrounding tissues, and may be due to local breakdown of the blood-brain barrier (BBB). The process may be limited to the immediate 2–3 mm rim around the irradiated volume. The process is limited to the irradiated hemisphere. Even extensive regions of white matter oedema may be present without symptoms and it is usually observed 12–24 months after therapy and may regress to normal at about 36 months without intervention.

The oedema may suddenly appear and may coincide with thrombotic changes in the AVM or AOVM (angiographically occult venous malformation) vessels about

6 months after treatment, as a result of thrombus formation with haemodynamic changes, and it may become symptomatic very suddenly.

If the patient has any symptom possibly related to vasogenic oedema, it is wise to start sooner rather than later on steroids like dexamethasone, 4–10 mg 8-hourly and to institute the neurological or neurosurgical investigations immediately.

"Steroid dependence" is a term where the patients redevelop symptoms as soon as the steroids are withdrawn and it should be classed as a serious and undesirable side effect.

Symptomatic vasogenic oedema

Symptomatic vasogenic oedema seems to occur between 8 and 27 months after treatment and it is probably an indication that too large a volume of brain received too large a dose of radiation. In principle it should be avoidable, but the dose and volume must be weighed against the risks associated with the patients condition, and the risk *versus* possible benefit should be discussed with him or her.

The symptoms include headache, nausea, vomiting like other mass lesions.

Cortisone may have to be administered intravenously initially, and then orally for months, plus analgesics where indicated for headaches, anti-nauseants where nausea is a problem. A drug to protect the stomach and duodenum, like a proton pump inhibitor, keeping in mind that the latter may interfere with the uptake of anti-convulsants should be discussed with a gastroenterologist. Close liaison between family doctor, physician, radiosurgeon, neurosurgeon and family is essential.

As usual, the possibility of aggravating other conditions or infections by cortisone administration must be kept in mind.

In the experience of Fabrikant *et al.* (1992), no case of symptomatic vasogenic oedema has occurred below a dose of 25 GyE, but it occurred in 12%–14% of their patients, all treated with higher doses than 25 GyE, usually 35–45 GyE. However, the high doses applied with impunity may be misleading, because the fall-off of the helium beams used is very steep; about 14% dose fall-off per millimetre (Appendix P.4 and chapter G). Other radiosurgical modalities do not necessarily have these very sharp penumbras; if a beam is used for "radiosurgery" it may be a semantic trap and extreme caution is needed in evaluating any beam or system for real suitability for radiosurgery. Recent evidence suggests that the above quoted doses may be too large in any case; single doses of the order of 13–15 Gy may be sufficient for meningiomas and 18 Gy for acoustic neuromas and AVMs.

The patient, family and family doctor should be instructed verbally and per pro forma of possible symptoms, follow-up procedures and actions to be taken in case of persistent headache or other symptoms as a matter of routine. A high "index of suspicion" after radiosurgery is advisable.

M.2.2.2
Cerebral Radionecrosis

Fabrikant (1992) reported this complication in 2%–3% of their patients who received doses from 25 CGyE to 45 GyE, delivered in 1–2 sessions. The timing and the extent of the necrosis appear to depend on the radiation dose and the volume of brain treated. Again, these doses are probably too high and are not recommended, as the desired effects could probably have been reached with lower single doses, in the order of 18 GyE.

Non particle therapy groups reported that for AVMs, for a given target volume, there is a strict relationship between the applied dose, the obliteration rate, and the side effects (Flickinger *et al.* 1990; Marks and Spencer 1991).

Engenhart *et al.* (1994) reported a 10% necrosis rate in patients with Spetzler and Martin Grade 5 lesions – and a 4% incidence of necrosis for Grade 4 AVMs. This high complication rate may be due to the large lesion sizes in these categories or the sensitivity of the areas concerned.

The volume of brain irradiated to 10 Gy (Voges 1996) or 12 Gy (Flickinger 1997) may be the critical factor. (See Chapter I on Dose-Volume Relationships)

Figure M2.2a, b shows an area of cerebral radionecrosis in a 16-year-old with an AOVM. The treatment plan shows that the 10 Gy isodose surface enclosed a volume of about 10 cm^3.

Very small areas of cerebral necrosis may respond to steroid therapy, but often the associated mass effect will mandate neurosurgical intervention. It is therefore essential to take every precaution to avoid the occurrence of radionecrosis.

M.2.2.3
Vascular Occlusion and Aneurysms

Arterial Occlusion: Functional arteries can be occluded within or adjacent to for example, an AVM. This can cause infarction, which is a more serious problem than sympto-

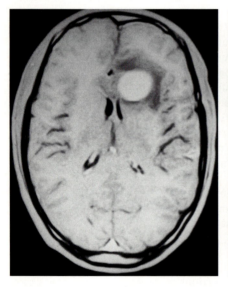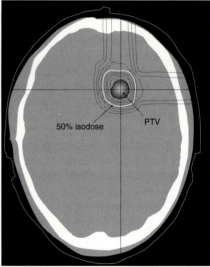

Fig. M2.2 *(a)* CT scan 6 months post post radiosurgery for a symptomatic AOVM in a 16-year old boy which shows an area of central necrosis with peri-lesional oedema and mass effect. Surgical intervention showed a thrombosed lesion that could be removed easily with some necrotic tissue. The eventual outcome was a completely functional patient. *(b)* The treatment plan shows that the 50% isodose corresponds well to the outline of the necrotic lesion, which has an approximate volume of 10.2 cm^3. The patient received a single dose equivalent of 18.7 CgyE, and the 10 Gy isodose line corresponds to the 10/18.7 x prescription isodose = 48% isodose. This corresponds well to the observations that the volume of brain tissue receiving 10 Gy minimum may be critical. (See Chapter I)

matic vasogenic oedema. Serious consequences have been observed as a result of vascular occlusion in 2%–3% of patients (Fabrikant *et al.* 1992).

Venous thrombosis: Veins are less sensitive to radiation than arteries. The veins constituting the pathologic shunts of AVMs can all be occluded without problems, but obstruction of the venous outflow tract may be undesirable because of the risk of venous infarction (Fabrikant 1992).

Treatment planning should take into account the initial venous phase on angiography and the plan should be such that as far as possible, the larger outflow venous structures will not be irradiated. Patients with thrombosed veins are often asymptomatic, however.

Aneurysms: Haemodynamic changes can cause pressure effects and aneurysms may rarely arise after the successful occlusion of an AVM, and cause bleeding.

Clinical complications are most often seen in patients with AVMs of the brain stem (Flickinger *et al.* 1997), thalamus or basal ganglia. Lesions in the brain stem have about twice the incidence of parenchymal lesions with regard to symptomatic post radiosurgical imaging changes.

M.2.2.4
Other Reported Complications

Minor: About 20% (17/86) of patients irradiated with helium ions had complications between 3 and 38 months after therapy (mean, 13.4 months). Seven of the 17 had minor complications like *diploplia, visual field defects, unilateral hearing impairment, slight ataxia or mild paresis.* Three of these recovered quickly, and completely; four partially.

Major: Ten patients (12%) had major complications including *hemiparesis, ataxia, cranial nerve palsies, partial aphasia or hypothalamic syndrome* (Fabrikant *et al.* 1992).

Significantly, and in line with the findings of Voges *et al.* (1996), Fabrikant *et al.* (1992) found that of 20 patients who received doses above 25 CGyE and whose angiographic volumes of treated tissue were more than 13 cm³, 10 experienced complications of major or minor nature, but they represented almost 60% of all the complications.

None of the 40 patients in the series treated with lower doses to lower volumes (< 25 CGyE to < 13 cm³) experienced any complications.

M.2.2.5
Cranial Nerve Complications

Acoustic neuromas: Flickinger *et al.* (1996) reviewed changing techniques and lower doses to curb the complication rate in acoustic neuromas. Lower doses lead to fewer complications but to no decrease in the control rate.

Lower doses were associated with the more discrete planning associated with MRI imaging and MRI based planning.

They reported an actuarial 7-year control rate, with no need for surgical intervention, of 96±2.3%. Smaller tumours and those planned with MRI rather than CT had significantly *fewer facial, trigeminal and auditory nerve* complications.

The mean minimum dose for MRI planned patients was 14 Gy and that of CT planned patients 17 Gy, with corresponding maximum doses of 28 Gy and 34 Gy, respectively (due to 100% inhomogeneity of dose across the target).

The lower doses were associated with fewer complications.

Wu *et al.* (1996) emphasise the importance of MRI scanning, smaller doses, the use of conformal isodoses by using multiple isocentres for the Gamma Knife, and earlier, smaller tumour identification for reducing complications in the treatment of vestibular schwannomas.

Miller *et al.* (1999) reported on the results of 42 consecutive patients with acoustic neuromas treated prospectively, examining the effects of 16, 18, and 20 Gy (prescribed at the 50% isodose for tumour diameters of 3.1–4 cm, 2.1–3 and < 2 cm, respectively. The next 40 patients were treated with 12, 14, and 16 Gy for tumour volumes of 14.1 cm^3, 4.2–14.1 cm^3, and (4.2cm^3 respectively.

They found that at a median follow-up of 2.3 years, the actuarial incidence of facial neuropathy was 38% for the standard dose protocol and 8% for the reduced dose protocol (p = 0.006). The only factor associated with increased risk of facial neuropathy was a tumour margin dose of > 18 Gy. The incidence of trigeminal neuropathy at 2 years was 29% for the standard dose protocol and 15% for the reduced dose protocol. The results suggest that marginal tumour dose of > 18 Gy is the most significant risk factor for facial nerve complications after acoustic neuroma radiosurgery by Gamma Knife. Patients receiving a minimum tumour dose of < 16 Gy are at significantly lower risk. The control rate seems to be good at the reduced doses, but longer follow-up is needed. Patients with the larger diameter tumours are at greater risk for trigeminal neuropathy.

Facial neuropathy developed in 36/260 evaluable patients for an actuarial incidence of 17.2±2.7% at 3 years, of which MRI planned patients only developed 7.6±4.3% *versus* 27.1±4.3% of CT planned patients.

Trigemnial neuropathy is defined as any temporary or permanent subjective change in sensation in the ipsilateral trigeminal nerve distribution. Flickinger *et al.* (1996, Gamma Knife) reported trigeminal neuralgia in 35.6±4.6% in patients planned with CT scans, *versus* only 7.6±2.5% actuarially at 3 years in patients planned with MRI and who also received lower doses as a result.

Acoustic nerve and hearing: With CT planning, a drop of 60.6±6.6% *versus* a drop of 32.3±6.7% in MRI planning occurred in patients with pre-operative Gardner Robertson hearing class I–IV.

Loss of any testable speech discrimination (deterioration to Class V hearing) developed in 50.9±6.7% patients planned with CT, versus 14.1±4.5% of MRI planned patients actuarially at 3 years; these differences are statistically significant.

Loss of serviceable hearing (deterioration from Class I–II to Class III–V) developed in 60.1±12.3% of the CT planned group, *versus* 44.2±8.5% in the MRI planned patients. Flickinger *et al.* (1996) is consequently reducing the minimum (peripheral) tumour doses to only 13–15 Gy, a dose at which no trigeminal or facial neuropathy was observed.

Cranial neuropathies also correlate with the length of the nerve irradiated, represented by the extracanalicular transverse tumour diameter for the trigeminal nerve and the combined extracanalicular plus intracanalicular midporus transverse tumour diameter for the facial and auditory nerves, rather than the volume of the acoustic neuroma per se (Linskey *et al.* 1990, 1993)

Andrews *et al.* (1995) reported a further conservation of cranial nerve function for acoustic nerve tumours if the stereotactic treatment was fractionated.

Image fusion with planning will reduce the uncertainties of lesion localisation and extent, and ensures the use of minimal irradiated volumes.

M.2.2.6
Radiation Induced Complications from Pituitary Lesions, Skull Base Tumours, Uveal Melanoma, Nasopharyngeal Carcinomas and Sarcomas of the Skull Base

The complication rate for *surgery* at the skull base is high. New cranial nerve deficits have been reported by experienced surgeons in 19%–86% and cerebrospinal fluid leaks in 20% of cases (Rosseau *et al.* 1995).

Results with *radiosurgery* have been good. Duma *et al.* (1993) reported 100% control with only 2/34 patients developing lasting *cranial nerve deficits.*

Subtotal resection followed by ordinary teletherapy gave very good control rates and only a 3.6% morbidity (Lunsford *et al.* 1994). Further information will be found under the relevant chapters wherein the above conditions are discussed.

M.2.2.7
Cavernous Sinus Meningiomas

Duma *et al.* (1993) obtained excellent results (100% progression free survival) with a 9% incidence of clinical complications of which 4.5% were temporary, in these patients with peripheral (Gamma Knife) doses of 10–20 Gy; the dose to the optic nerve was limited to 9 Gy.

M.2.2.8
Parasagittal meningiomas

These are much more prone to develop oedema than the skull base meningiomas. (See Chapter L.3.5)

Neuropsychological changes: Wentz *et al.* (1998) studied the neuropsychological changes following radiosurgery for AVMs, with special focus on attention and memory. Radiosurgery was given by linear accelerator and minimum doses to the target were 15–22 Gy, median 20 Gy. Estimated whole brain dose was 0.5–2 Gy. The pretherapeutic evaluation revealed marked deviations from the normal population, with a significant improvement ($p = 0.05$) in the test scores in 3 of 4 subtests of attention functions. The data indicated a tendency to slight improvement in the overall neuropsychological performance of AVM patients in the chronic phase after radiosurgery.

M.3
Summary

Irrespective of the radiosurgical modality, and generalised statements that the complication rate with radiosurgery is low, including proton therapy, the brain is very susceptible to injury by radiation, and extreme caution is necessary in the selection of patients with detailed attention to dose, lesion localisation and volume.

For all benign intracranial tumours it seems that the complication rate can be kept to a minimum if the irradiated brain volume is kept as small as possible by ensuring adequate conformation of the tumour shapes and the isodoses. The dose should be kept as low as is commensurate with a reasonable probability of cure and a low probability of complications.

There seems to be a steeply increasing risk of complications if more than 10 cm^3 of brain or brain-containing tissue receives more than 10 Gy.

A wide variety of complications are associated with radiosurgery. These include minor complications like headaches and seizures. More serious complications like symptomatic and asymptomatic vasogenic oedema, brain necrosis and optic nerve, acoustic trigeminal and facial nerve damage may be induced.

Arteries and veins may be occluded, aneurysms may develop, the brain stem may be damaged with serious consequences.

Much lower dose levels than initially used by radiosurgical pioneers fortunately seem to be equally effective achieving the therapeutic goals and will undoubtedly reduce the complication rates.

MRI planning is essential in reducing uncertainties, which allows smaller volumes and doses to be irradiated, leading to both a reduction in dose and in the complication rate.

Meticulous attention to dose-volume relationships, accurate planning and all technical parameters may help to reduce the complication rate.

Image fusion technique in planning will reduce the uncertainties of lesion localisation and extent, and ensures the use of minimal irradiated volumes.

Multidisciplinary team discussions are essential prior to therapy, and good liaison between radiosurgeon, neurosurgeon, patient and family is essential before and after radiosurgery.

M.4
References

Andrews DW, Siverman CL, Glas J et al. (1995) Preservation of cranial nerve function of acoustic neurinomas with fractionated stereotactic radiotherapy. Stereotact Funct Neurosurg 64:165–182

Brada M, Thomas GT (1995) Tumours of the brain and spinal cord in adults. In: Oxford Textbook of Oncology, vol 2. Oxford University Press,

Duma CM , Lunsford LD, Kondziolka D, Harsch GR, Flickinger JC (1993) Stereotactic radiosurgery of cavernous sinus meningiomas as an addition or alternative to microsurgery. Neurosurgery 32:699–705

Edwards MS, Wilson CB (1980) Treatment of radiation necrosis. In: Gilbert H, Cag R (eds) Radiation damage to the nervous system: a delayed therapeutic hazard. Raven Press, New York, pp 129–144

Engenhart R, Wowra B, Debus J, Kimmig B, Hover KH, Lorenz W, Wannenmacher M (1994) The role of high dose single-fraction irradiation in small and large intracranial arteriovenous malformations. Int J Radiat Oncol Biol Phys 30:521–529

Fabrikant JI, Levy RP, Steinberg GK, Phillips MH, Frankel KA, Lyman JT, Marks MP, Silverberg GD (1992) Charged particle radiosurgery for intracranial vascular malformations. Neurosurg Clin North Am 3:99–139

Flickinger JC, Schell M, Larson DA (1990) Estimation of complications for linear accelerator radiosurgery with the integrated logistic formula. Int J Radiat Oncol Biol Phys 19:143–148

Flickinger JC, Kondziolka D, Pollock BE, Lunsford LD (1996) Evolution in technique for vestibular schwannoma radiosurgery and effect on outcome. Int J Radiat Oncol Biol Phys 36:275–280

Flickinger JC, Kondziolka D, Pollock BE et al. (1997) Complications from arteriovenous malformation radiosurgery: multivariate analysis and risk modelling. Int J Radiat Oncol Biol Phys 38:485–490

Flickinger JC, Kondziolka D, Lunsford, LD et al. (1999) A Multi-institutional analysis of complication outcomes after arteriovenous malformation radiosurgery. Int J Radiat Oncol Biol Phys 44:67–74

Grigsby PW, Stokes S, Marks JE, Simpson JR (1988) Prognostic factors and results of radiotherapy alone in the management of pituitary adenomas. Int J Radiat Oncol Biol Phys 15:1103–1110

Linskey ME, Lunsford LD, Flickinger JC (1990) Stereotactic radiosurgery for acoustic neurinomas: early experience. Neurosurgery 26:933–938

Linskey ME, Flickinger JC, Lunsford LD(1993) The relationship of cranial nerve length to the development of delayed facial and trigeminal neuropathies after stereotactic radiosurgery for acoustic tumours. Int J Radiat Oncol Biol Phys 15:227–234

Livingston K, Hopkins LN (1992) Endovascular treatment of intracerebral arteriovenous malformations. Clin Neurosurg 39:331–347

Lunsford LD. Contemporary management of meningiomas: radiation therapy as an adjuvant and radiosurgery as an alternative to surgical removal? J Neurosurg 80:187–190

Marks LB, Spencer PD (1991) The influence of volume on the tolerance of the brain to radiosurgery. J Neurosurg 75:177–180

Matula C, Czech T, Kitz K, Roessler K, Koos W (1995) The intra-operative markings of neuroanatomical details – helpful for radiosurgery? Acta Neurochir Suppl 63:5–8

Mehta M (1995) The physical, biological and clinical basis of radiosurgery. In: Current problems in cancer, vol XIX. Mosby Yearsbook, St Louis, pp 267–328

Miller RC, Foote RL, Coffey RJ et al. (1999) Decrease in cranial nerve complications after radiosurgery for acoustic neuromas: a prospective study of dose-volume. Int J Radiat Oncol Biol Phys 43:305–311

Motti ED, Losa M, Pieralli et al. (1996) Metabolism 45 [Suppl 1]:111–114

Movsas B, Movsas TZ, Steinberg SM, Okunieff P (1995) Long-term visual changes following pituitary irradiation. Int J Radiat Oncol Biol Phys 33:599–605

Orrison WW (1995) Atlas of brain function. Thieme, New York

Rocher FP, Sentenac I, Berger C, Marquis I, Romestaing P, Gerard JP (1995) Acta Neurochir Suppl (Wien) 63:109–114

Rosseau G, Cerullo L (1995) Current challenges in management of cranial base meningiomas. Am J Otol 16:1–3

Sekhar LN, Gormley WB, Wright DC (1996) The best treatment for vestibular schwannoma (acoustic neuroma): microsurgery or radiosurgery? Am J Otol 17:676–682

Sheline GE (1986) Normal tissue tolerance and radiotherapy of the brain. In: Bleehen MN (ed) Tumours of the brain. Springer, Berlin Heidelberg New York, pp 141–160

Shiu AS, Kooy HM, Ewton JR, Tung SS, Wong J, Antes K, Maor MH (1997) Comparison of miniature multileaf collimation (MMLC) with circular collimation for stereotactic treatment. Int J Radiat Oncol Biol Phys 37:679–688

Steiner L, Lindquist C, Adler JR et al. (1992) Clinical outcome of radiosurgery for cerebral arteriovenous malformations. J Neurosurg 77:1–8

Suit H, Urie M (1992) Proton beams in radiotherapy. J Natl Cancer Inst 84:155–164

Urie MM, Fullerton B, Tatsuzaki H, Birnbaum S, Suit HD, Convery K, Skates S, Goitein M (1992) A dose-response analysis of injury to the cranial nerves and/or nuclei following proton beam irradiation. Int J Radiat Oncol Biol Phys 23:27–39

Van der Kogel AJ, Ang KK (1995) Complications related to radiotherapy. In: Pecham M, Pinedo, HM, Veronesi U (eds) Oxford textbook of oncology, vol 2. Oxford Medical Publications

Voges J, Sturm V, Deuss U, Traud C, Treuer H, Schlegel W, Einkelmann W, Muller RP (1996) Linac radiosurgery (linac RS) in pituitary adenomas: preliminary results. Acta Neurochir Suppl (Wien) 65:41–43

Voges J, Treuer H, Sturm V, Buchner C, Lehrke R, Kocher M, Staar S, Kuchta J, Müller RP (1996) Risk analysis of linear accelerator radiosurgery. Int J Radiat Oncol Biol Phys 36:1055–1063

Watne K, Hager B, Heier M, Hirschberg H (1990) Reversible oedema and necrosis after irradiation of the brain. Acta Oncol 29:891–895

Wener-Wasik M, Rudoler S, Preston PE et al. (1999) Immediate side effects of stereotactic radiosurgery and radiosurgery. Int J Radiat Oncol Biol Phys 43:299–304

Wentz F, Steinvorth S, Wildermuth S et al. (1998) Assessment of neuropsychological changes in patients with arteriovenous malformation (AVM) after radiosurgery. Int J Radiat Oncol Biol Phys 42:995–999

Woo SY, Grant WH 3rd, Belezza D, Grossman R, Gildenberg P, Carpentar LS, Carol M, Butler EB (1996) A comparison of intensity modulated conformal therapy with a conventional external beam stereotactic radiosurgery system for the treatment of single and multiple intracranial lesions. Int J Radiat Oncol Biol Phys 35:593–597

Wu A, Kalnick S, Schell MC (1996) MRI: an important factor for decreasing the morbidities of treating vestibular schwannoma with radiosurgery. Int J Radiat Oncol Biol Phys 36:1283–1284

N Alternatives to Proton Therapy for Radiosurgery

N.1
Introduction

It is apparent that specially adapted linear accelerators have the benefit of a rapidly developing technology.

Sophisticated computerised planning systems and conformal therapy possibilities for the linear accelerator and the Gamma Knife have rapidly evolved in the last decade and are cheaper by a considerable margin compared to protons.

Simple hand held devices like the photon radiosurgery system (PRS) must be regarded as experimental, but may prove to be a very useful and cheap additional device for some intracranial tumours. Another promising newcomer is the Cyber Knife.

N.1.1
The Linear Accelerator

According to a pessimistic view by Podgorsak *et al.* (1989) protons and heavier ions will *never* be used widely in radiosurgery because of the costs involved! These authors favoured the specially adapted linear accelerator.

Larsson *et al.* (1958) used protons as a radiosurgical tool. Betti and Derichinsky (1983) made one of the first reports about special adaptation for a linear accelerator for stereotactic radiosurgery. The linear accelerator quickly gained acceptance and popularity for the reasons listed in the following sections.

N.1.1.1
Ease of Conversion

To transform a linear accelerator (LA) to a radiosurgical tool only a few additions are needed:
• Stabilisation of head movement during scanning and therapy (**see below**)
• Improving mechanical rigidity
• Acquiring special computing equipment
• Special collimators

Since the majority of radiation oncology departments already have linear accelerators that can be adapted, they are becoming the most widely used apparatus for radiosurgery.

N.1.1.2
Versatility and Flexibility

With LA based radiosurgery, absorbed dose (beam weight), degrees of arc and collimator size may be selected separately for each arc for arc therapy. This permits great flexibility in treatment planning and execution. The energy of the beam, from 4 MV upwards, has little influence on the dosimetry in the multi-arc mode. An often-used energy is 6 MV.

Dynamic stereotactic radiosurgery is a further refinement, which in principle utilises simultaneous rather than sequential movement of the couch and gantry. The dynamic technique also saves time, as it is a continuous process, not interrupted as in multiple arc therapy, where time is needed to set up each sequential arc (Luxton *et al.* 1993).

The utility of the linear accelerator is improved further by miniature multileaf collimation (MMLC), (Shiu *et al.* 1997). (Also, see Chapter N.1.1.7 below)

Dose-Volume histograms showed that single isocentre MMLC treatment is superior to both single and multiple isocentre circular collimator treatment because it provides a more uniform dose distribution to an irregularly shaped target volume and reduces the dose to surrounding brain tissue.

Hamilton *et al.* (1995) compared static conformal fields to multiple non-coplanar arcs for an irregularly shaped lesion and found that multiple arcs treated 1.6 times more normal tissue than that treated by 4 static conformal fields, and the volume of normal tissue is further reduced by increasing the number of static fields from 4 to 8. Despite this, they found that the volume receiving the prescription isodose is more than 3.5 times larger than the target volume for all six treatment plans for the irregular target of 3.5 cm^3 examined.

This means that for all the plans for a lesion of 3.5 cm^3 at least 8.75 cm^3 of the surrounding brain would have received the full prescription isodose of 80%.

The dose to the target is more uniform with static fields. Close conformation with static fields, however, was only possible with target shapes with an axis of rotational symmetry or a plane of mirror symmetry. With modern proton therapy delivered by Gantry, all of the above benefits can be realised or improved upon for lesions > 5 cm^3. (See Chapter F.1.1.2)

N.1.1.3
Relocatable Frames

A notable advance for linear accelerator radiosurgery was, *inter alia*, the relocatable head-frame described by Thomson *et al.* (1990). These frames can be precisely relocated more than once and this makes fractionated treatment possible, which was impossible with the older types of head-frame, which were fixed to the head by steel screws. Once removed these frames could not be replaced with sufficient accuracy.

N.1.1.4
Thermoplastic Masks

Uematsu *et al.* (1996) utilises a linear accelerator at one end and a CT scanner at the other end of a common table, which can be swung through 180°. Immobilisation of the patient is achieved by a simple thermoplastic mask, and the accuracy needed (< 1 mm) is achieved by careful checking of the alignment for each treatment session by a scanning check. With this system three to ten fractions can be administered with ease, thus bringing the linear accelerator into the realm of accurate, fractionated stereotactic radiotherapy without using stereotactic head-frames.

Jones et al. (1995) described a removable mask for proton therapy, which is a noninvasive, comfortable and accurate system. It is the stereophotogrammetric (SPG) system used at NAC in the RSA and may well be a trend setter for linear accelerator based radiosurgery as well. (See Appendix P.7 for a description)

N.1.1.5
Good Beam Delivery and Planning

Intensity modulation for linear accelerators with the "Peacock System" (Woo et al. 1995) contributes to improved conformal delivery of the beam and encroaches on the ability of protons to deliver good conformal plans. The "Peacock" system has the capability of handling intensity modulation, back projection and the simulated annealing optimisation technique. This methodology enhances the scope of the linear accelerator based radiosurgery to generate plans superior to conventional collimated plans for lesions larger than 4 cm^3 and irregularly shaped, thus intruding directly into the advantage zone of protons. An excellent expose of this system is given by Carol and associates (1996).

Spot scanning techniques may restore the advantage of protons relative to photons despite these advances for the linear accelerator. The problem remains the penumbra for small lesions with Bragg peak therapy and spot scanning for protons. (See Chapter I on Dose-Volume Relationships)

N.1.1.6
Extracranial Radiosurgery

A spinal stereotactic frame for use with a linear accelerator for spinal radiosurgery has been described by Hamilton et al. (1995). This is in the form of a 3-dimensional orthogonal frame of reference used in conjunction with two arcades for skeletal fixation. CT imaging is performed between the arcades to carry out 3-dimensional reconstruction and dosimetric planning. New systems utilise infrared detectors.

N.1.1.7
Miniature Multileaf Collimators

The linear accelerator is available with miniature multileaf collimators, which make conformal static field radiosurgery possible. It eliminates multiple arcs, reduces the integral dose to the brain and shortens set-up times. The transmission through these collimators is about 6%. Selected arcs (with the multi-arc technique) can be arranged to avoid sensitive structures like the optic nerve. This problem is not usually significant with multiple non-coplanar fields with the MMLC.

Kubo et al. (1999) showed that for most lesions treated with radiosurgery the use of a micro-multileaf collimator (MMLC) with a leaf width of 1.7–3.0 mm at isocentre and

3–5 static fields, allows one to meet the Radiation Therapy Oncology Group guidelines for treatment planning. Both planning and treatment are relatively straight forward with MMLC.

N.1.2
The Leksell Gamma Knife

Presently Gamma Knives are mainly found in neurosurgical institutions, whereas linear accelerators are found more frequently in radiation oncology departments.

Drawbacks associated with the GK include the large quantity of radioactive material (6000 Ci); the high price and weighty installation problems with the associated special re-loading problems. Reloading of the GK every 5–10 years is necessary, because the ^{60}Co pellets have a half-life of about 5 years and the sources need to be replaced when the dose rate is too low. An example of the GK is the Gamma Knife model U (Elekta Instruments Atlanta) which consists of a permanent 18,000 kg shield surrounding a primary hemispheric array of 201 ^{60}Co sources. The central beam of radiation is fixed at an angle of 55° to the horizontal plane with the other beams arranged in an arc, all reaching a focal point 403 mm from the sources. The original Leksell unit (1968) irradiated a discoid volume, which has been changed to a roughly spherical volume at isocentre in 1974.

Goetsch et al. (1999) described a rotating gamma system for stereotactic radiosurgery. This novel unit has been distributed to fifteen hospitals in China. Instead of 201 ^{60}Co sources, it has only 30, with 200 Ci total initial activity. The sources are placed in a gantry and rotate as a group in an axis orthogonal to the patient's body. The unit can produce well collimated beams similar to the "Model U" Gamma Knife® unit. It has less leakage radiation than the Leksell GK and 1/3 of the initial radioactivity. It can give 3 Gy per minute at isocentre.

N.1.2.1
Limited Choice of Collimators

A secondary collimator helmet with beam channel diameters of 4, 8, 14 or 18 mm is used to vary the volume of the prescribed radiation. The 18 mm collimators can inscribe a volume of 3.1 cm^3 for a single isocentre.

Local anaesthesia supplemented with mild intravenous sedation is used for the GK. Children under the age of 14 years need general endotracheal anaesthesia.

These interventions, except for very small children, are not usually needed for proton therapy or for linear accelerator based radiosurgery using relocatable frames.

Multiple isocentres are used for larger lesions of irregular shape, but it causes significant dose inhomogeneity across the lesion. Selected collimators can be blocked to avoid sensitive structures like the optic nerve.

N.1.2.2
Fractionated Treatment

Even with the Gamma Knife, technical improvements expanded its scope. Simonova et al. (1995) showed that fractionated therapy is also possible with the GK.

N.1.3
The Photon Radiosurgery System

This may become a supplemental tool in radiosurgery and neurosurgery departments. This device may be seen as an alternative to stereotactic ^{125}I source implants, or high dose rate brachytherapy. The device is a battery driven miniature X-ray machine. It comprises a metallic probe, 3 mm in diameter and 100 mm long, that produces low energy X-rays with an effective energy of 10–20 keV emanating from the tip of the probe. The X-rays emerge from a virtual point and give a radiation field uniform in all directions. A full description of the device is given by Beatty *et al.* (1995). It can be used within minutes after a stereotactic biopsy has been taken. This probe is suitable for human tumours, which are smaller than **3 cm** in diameter (Douglas *et al.* 1996).

The dosimetry is at least as good as that obtained using a 6 MV LA or 160 MeV protons and the authors feel that PRS treatment is safe and effective as tested in 14 patients. Further more, the PRS device also appears to offer a modest sparing of normal tissues compared to protons or linear accelerator based radiosurgery for brain tumours, at a fraction of the cost of proton therapy. They used doses of 10–20 Gy (median 12.5 Gy) for spherical intracranial metastases of 10 to 35 mm in diameter, for treatment volumes ranging from 0.52 cm³ to 22.5 cm³ (median = 4.2 cm³)

The probe tip should be placed in the middle of the lesion and the dose should be prescribed at the periphery of the tumour plus 2 mm. Dose volume histograms for a 20 mm diameter spherical lesion were made for the PRS device, a 6 MV linear accelerator with four circular beam portals and a proton beam using three circular beam portals. The results are shown in Fig N1.1.

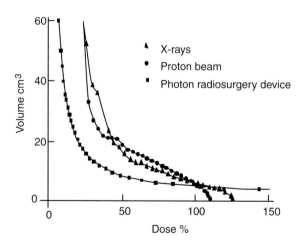

Fig. N1.1 Dose-volume histogram comparing brain irradiated during treatment of a lesion with proton beam radiosurgery, X-ray radiosurgery and with the PRS device. Each technique treated to the same prescribed dose. PRS treatment may offer some normal tissue sparing beyond that achievable with the other techniques under certain clinical conditions. (Redrawn from RM Douglas *et al.*, 1996, Int J Radiat Oncol Biol Phys 36:443–450)

The Cyber Knife

The Cyber Knife is an image-guided robotic system fitted with a miniature 6 MV linear accelerator, designed for stereotactic radiosurgery. The device meets typical accuracy required for radiosurgery, and the first 14 patients have been treated. The device can accomplish precisely localised irradiation of focal lesions *anywhere in the body*.

The image-guided robotic system includes treatment planning imaging and delivers components, all of which are integrated by a powerful computer workstation. The Cyber Knife does not depend on stereotactic frames attached to the head, but relies instead on internal registration of CT robot and imaging co-ordinate systems to provide automatic registration of the clinical target to the beam.

The image guidance system is composed of two diagnostic X-ray units controlled by computer. Thirteen circular collimators from 5–80 mm are available. The reference system for the Cyber Knife is the patient's cranium itself instead of a frame with fiducial markers. Thermoplastic masks are used, however, as in conventional radiotherapy (Chenery *et al.* 1998)

N.1.4
A Comparison of the Fall-off in Dose

The dose fall-off is a measure of the normal tissue sparing capacity of each device, and may be of paramount importance in avoiding complications.

There is little to choose between the linear accelerator and the Gamma Knife in terms of the penumbra; the average dose fall-off is about 9%–10% per mm from the 90% to 20% isodoses, or about 7.6 mm. For particle beams the situation is more complex. The lateral dose fall-off is quite sharp in the plateau region and distal to the Bragg peak, but the fall off is shallowing considerably towards the end of the Bragg peak laterally.

In order to assess whether a particular proton therapy plan will be superior to a Gamma Knife or linear accelerator plan, comparative dose-volume histograms should ideally be carefully assessed. (Also see Section I.3)

This aspect is further discussed in Chapter I on Dose-Volume Relationships. For a summary of penumbral characteristics, see Appendix P.4.

N.1.5
Comparative Clinical Results

Direct comparison of clinical results in radiosurgically treated patients is difficult because of lack of standardisation in published reports regarding the size and location of the target and details of the prescribed dose.

The use of stereotactic radiosurgery outside of carefully controlled trials is still not warranted (Luxton *et al.* 1993) because treatment methodology requires multidisciplinary effort and treatment prescription conventions are not yet widely accepted.

N.2
Large Field Therapy and Alternatives to Protons

Proton therapy offers advantages for the treatment of many sites with large fields. This includes irradiation of the para-aortic nodes (Levin *et al.* 1992) in the uterine cervix, where up to 60% of the volume of a conventional 4-field "box" could be spared (Smit 1991). Many other examples can be quoted. However, since these assembled contributions became available, 3-D planning systems, which could accommodate 3-D lead block shielding for photon therapy became commonplace. With intensity modulation, reverse planning and other refinements available, new comparative treatment plans are needed since the older comparisons were largely with obsolete photon techniques. (See also Chapters G, J and K.)

N.3
Eye Lesions and Protons

Please refer to Chapter J for a brief discussion of alternative to proton therapy. Proton therapy seems to give the best results.

N.4
Reliability of Equipment

Reliability of beam availability is an extremely important factor in the practical execution of radiotherapeutic programs of any kind. It is extremely frustrating to radiation oncologist/radiosurgeon and patient alike to have long gaps or long delays in the appointed times for therapy.

The Gamma Knife is, like any ^{60}Co radiation unit, intrinsically extremely reliable since there are no significant moving parts or complicated electrical circuitry involved. It is simple to operate.

The modern linear accelerator has a satisfactory reliability, yet it is a complex piece of equipment and a certain amount of time for maintenance and repair is to be expected. It can be classed as a very reliable treatment unit of great flexibility, usually surrounded by an adequate complement of very competent staff members with good institutional support.

The cyclotron or synchrocyclotron: These are very complicated machines and where frequent energy changes are needed, reliability is bound to suffer. This may be the one aspect of proton therapy that may offset its benefits in non-hospital-based facilities, since it is axiomatic that delays for most malignant tumours allow cell repopulation, and treatment gaps are bound to compromise the prospects of cure for the majority of such patients. Delays for non-malignant lesions have less serious consequences, but are no less frustrating. Reliability and availability of beam, more than any other factor, may determine the future of proton therapy.

N.5
Summary

There are several devices, which can do many of the radiosurgical tasks that a proton beam can do, but not all equally well.

Dosimetrically, there is little to choose between the Gamma Knife and the linear accelerator.

Proton therapy results in a very much smaller integral dose to the brain for any given dose, it's dose distribution is uniform over the target in contrast to a quite non-uniform target dose with the GK. However, this apparent advantage needs to be carefully evaluated against what is in fact a larger penumbra with some proton beams in the Bragg peak zone, than the penumbra of the photon modalities, especially for small fields.

Proton isodoses can conform better to the shapes of irregular targets, and are especially advantageous for lesions so large that adequate treatment with the Gamma Knife or linear accelerator becomes problematical. For example, with more than six isocentres with the Gamma Knife, the integral dose becomes very large and the inhomogeneity of dose may become a problem.

The cost factor remains the main inhibition to the rapid proliferation of proton facilities. This is discussed in Chapter O.

Protons remain superior in dose distribution for the treatment of eye lesions, as well as wide field irradiation to other anatomical areas in the body.

Reliability is a very important factor, and here the Gamma Knife and modern linear accelerator seem to have the advantage over cyclotrons and synchrocyclotrons. Good comparative studies on the reliability of units and the clinical consequences thereof will be interesting. (Also see Section B.2.1a)

N.6
References

Beatty J, Biggs PJ, Gall K, Okunieff P, Pardo FS (1996) A new miniature device for interstitial radiosurgery. Med Phys 23:53–62

Becker G, Kortmann R, Kaulich TW, Duffner F, Bamberg M (1996) Gamma Knife *versus* stereotactic linear accelerator utilisation, clinical results and cost-benefit relations Radiology 36:345–353

Betti O, Derichinsky VE (1983) Irradiation stereotacxique multifaisceau. Neurochirurgie 29:295–298

Carol M, Grant WH, Pavord D et al. (1996) Initial clinical experience with the Peacock intensity modulation of a 3-D Conformal Radiation Therapy System. Proceedings of the American Society for Stereotactic and Functional Neurosurgery, Marina del Rey, California 1995, Part II. Stereotact Funct Neurosurg 66:1–9

Chenery SG, Chehabi HH, Davis DM et al. (1998) The Cyber Knife: beta system descriptions and initial clinical results. J Radiosurg 1:241–249

Douglas RM, Beatty J, Gall K, Valenzuela RF, Biggs P, Okunieff P, Pardo FS (1996) Dosimetric results from a feasibility study of a novel radiological source for irradiation of intracranial metastases. Int J Radiat Oncol Biol Phys 36:443–50

Gademan G (1994) Hadrontherapy in Oncology. Ugo Amaldi and Borje Larsson (eds) Excerpta Medica Int Congr Ser 1077:59–66

Goetsch SJ, Murphy BD, Schmidt R et al. (1999) Physics of rotating gamma systems for stereotactic radiosurgery. Int J Radiat Oncol Biol Phys 43:689–697

Flickinger JC, Kondziolka D, Pollock BE, Maitz A, Lunsford LD (1997) Complications from arteriovenous malformation radiosurgery: multivariate analysis and risk modelling. Int J Radiat Oncol Biol Phys 38:485–490

Hamilton RJ, Kuchnir FT, Sweeney P, Rubin SJ et al. (1995) Comparison of static conformal field with multiple non-coplanar arc techniques for stereotactic radiotherapy. Int J Radiat Oncol Biol Phys 33:1221–1228

Jones DTL, Schreuder AN, Symons JE, Rüther, Van der Vlugt G, Bennett KF, Yates ADB (1995) Use of stereophotogrammetry in proton radiation therapy. Proceedings FIG Commission 6. International FIG Symposium, Cape Town

Kubo HD, Wilder RB, Pappas CTE (1999) Impact of collimator leaf width on stereotactic radiosurgery an 3-D conformal radiotherapy treatment plans. Int J Radiat Oncol Biol Phys 44:937–945

Larsson B, Leksell L, Rexed B, Sourandar P, Mair W, Andersson B (1958) The high energy proton beam as a neurosurgical tool. Nature 182:1222–1223

LeMay DR, Chen THC, Petrovich Z, Luxton G, Zelman V, Zee CS, Green J, Apuzzu MLJ (1996) Gamma unit facility: concept and genesis, architectural design and practical realisation. Stereotact Funct Neurosurg 66:41–49

Levin CV (1992) Potential for gain in the use of proton beam boost to the para-aortic lymph nods in carcinoma of the cervix. Int J Radiat Oncol Biol Phys 22:355–361

Luxton G, Petrovich Z, Jozsef G, Nedzi L, Apuzzo M (1993) Stereotactic radiosurgery: principles and comparisons of treatment methods. Neurosurgery 32:242–259

Phillips MH, Steltzer KJ, Griffin TW *et al.* (1994) Stereotactic radiosurgery: a review and comparison of methods. J Clin Oncol 12:1085–1099

Podgorsak EB, Pike GB, Olivier A, Pla M, Souhami L (1989) Radiosurgery with high energy photon beams: a comparison among techniques. Int J Radiat Oncol Biol Phys 16:857–865

Simonova G, Novotny J, Novotny J Jr, Vladyka V, Liscak R (1995) Fractionated stereotactic radiotherapy with the Leksell Gamma Knife: a feasibility study. Radiother Oncol 37:108–116

Shiu AS, Kooy HM, Ewton JR, Tung SS, Wong J, Antes K, Maor MH (1997) Comparison of miniature multileaf collimation with circular collimation for stereotactic treatment (with a linear accelerator) Int J Radiat Oncol Biol Phys 17:679–688

Smit BJ (1992) Prospects for proton therapy in carcinoma of the cervix. Int J Radiat Oncol Biol Phys 22:349–355

Smith A, Goitein M, Durlacher S, Flanz J, Levine A, Reardon P, Woods S (1994) The Massachusetts General Hospital Northeast Proton Therapy Centre. In: Amaldi U, Larsson B (eds) Hadrontherapy in oncology. Excerpta Medica Int Congr Ser 1077

Thomson ES, Gill SS, Doughty D (1990) Stereotactic multiple arc radiotherapy. BJR 63:745–751

Uematsu M, Fukui T, Tokimitsu H, Kojima T, Asai Y, Kusano S (1996) A dual computed tomography linear accelerator unit for stereotactic radiation therapy: a new approach without cranially fixated frames. Int J Radiat Oncol Biol Phys 35:587–592

Woo S, Butler BB, Grant W, King D, Nizin P, Grossman R (1995) Initial clinical experience of Peacock intensity conformal radiotherapy. Proceedings of the American Radium Society 78th Annual Meeting, Paris, 29 April, p 36

Zehetmayer M, Menapace R, Kitz K, Ertl A (1995) Experience with a suction fixation system for stereotactic radiosurgery of intra-ocular malignancies. Stereotact Funct Neurosurg 64 [Suppl 1]:80–86

O Costs of Proton Therapy and Radiosurgery

O.1
Introduction

Proton therapy mandates expensive specially developed apparatus for beam delivery, planning computers, dedicated highly trained staff, and often labour intensive adjunctive activities like the manufacturing of sophisticated collimators, immobilisation devices, compensators etc. Planning can take many hours for complex plans. Adequate staff and workstations are needed to leave the radiosurgical team sufficient time to evaluate several alternative plans unhurriedly.

The pre-therapy investigations for all modalities (protons, Gamma Knife etc.) are expensive, and include MRI, CT, stereotactic angiography, and sometimes PET scanning.

Gamma units are expensive to purchase and maintain for dedicated radiosurgery.

Linear accelerators are common and the costs for conversion to a radiosurgical facility is not very high.

Because of rapidly fluctuating exchange rates especially in 1998, all the figures quoted are rough approximations, and any reader should verify costs at each institution. There are various ways of looking at cost and some reference will be made to more sophisticated cost analysis.

Cost definitions and categories
Eisenberg (1989), Weinstein (1990) and Rutigliano (1995) analysed the principles of medical cost analysis. Penar (1996) summarised the available literature and identified cost as:
1. Direct health care costs (or savings) like costs related to the program technology, costs related to tests or treatments avoided, treatment of side effects and complications, savings due to avoidance of treatment of morbidity and treatment of conditions during added years of life.
2. Direct personal costs or savings.
3. Direct non-health related costs or savings.
4. Indirect costs or savings, e.g. productivity gains or losses.

Since the clinical factors for proton radiosurgery and proton radiotherapy are not vastly different, we have chosen to make simple cost comparisons based on available information on fees charged. (Also see Table B1.)

O.2
Patient Fees for Stereotactic Treatment

O.2.1
Linear Accelerator

In the USA:
Ancillary fees: fees for treatment planning, physicist, radiologist and follow-up services (excluding magnetic resonance imaging or MRI fees) varies between *$18,000 and $22,150* (Becker *et al.* 1996).

Accelerator fees: Becker *et al.* (1996) found that the most cost effective option is the special modification of an existing linear accelerator resulting in treatment costs per patient of DM 9,201 (about *$5331*). They could find no methodological, physical or cost reasons for using a Gamma Knife especially because the trend is towards fractionated conformal therapy and away from the application of high single doses.

Alleyne *et al.* (1997) reported a possibly still cheaper delivery system for radiosurgery by linear accelerator by rotating the patient instead of the gantry.

O.2.2
Gamma Knife

Ancillary fees plus treatment fees: The available information on charges for treatment with work-up varied between *$26,000 to $34,000* including three days in hospital. Other Gamma Knife units charged from $9,800 to $11,800, hospital stay not specified.

O.2.3
Proton Therapy

South Africa:
• Machine fee: $5675.00 including fees for planning, physicists and radiographers as well as for artefacts like collimators etc.
• "Clinician's fee" is about $900.00.
• The host hospital charges a nominal fee for CT scanning for planning, and some artefacts; *total cost therefore about $7000.00 in 1998.*
  Germany (Estimate)
  The estimated costs (Gademann *et al.* 1993) of a curative *conventional* radiotherapy course in Germany amounts to about DM 7,000 (about $4,055), curative oncological surgery to 15,000 DM (about $8,690) and chemotherapy to DM 62,000 (about $36,000).

Gademann (1993) estimates that a "course of proton therapy" in Germany may cost 15,000 DM *($8,690).*
  USA neurosurgical fees:
  The radiosurgical fees should be compared to neurosurgery charges in the USA including 8–11 days in hospital, of *$28,000 to $36,000.*
  USA radiosurgical fees:
  Suit and Urie (1992) estimate the cost of proton therapy to be "two to three times" as much as photon therapy. This cost comparison is not for radiosurgery, but for general radiotherapy.

A few representative listed fees for proton therapy for stereotactic proton therapy are as follows: For an AVM for the total procedure, about *$25,000–$35000*, excluding radiological and neurosurgical charges.

A total proton fee for astrocytoma: *$38,630,* and the fee for a choroidal melanoma would be in the order of *$21,500.* Treating an acoustic neuroma would cost about *$38,000.*

O.3
Installation Costs

Linear accelerator: To retrofit an existing accelerator may cost $300,000 and a planning system, if needed, may require an additional $300,000, about *$600,000.*

Gamma Knife: Needs to be specially bought and housed at a cost of about *$4 million.* Gamma knives are available in two models with different source configurations and the cost range from $2.5–$3.5 million.

A proton therapy facility will cost upwards of *$26 million.* (Gademann *et al.* 1993) and may supply several rooms.

The installation of a proton beam is a prodigious undertaking (Luxton *et al.* 1992) and will require the construction of a large well-shielded building $25 \times 60 \times 10$ m^3 (15,000 m^3) in size or larger.

O.4
Maintenance Costs

Linear accelerator: The maintenance costs *are usually absorbed by the radiation oncology department.* Some cost must be added to ensure that the required quality control with respect to mechanical rigidity and accuracy is maintained. According to Alleyne *et al.* (1997) the cost is *$249,000* for a dedicated linear accelerator and $123,000 for the patient rotator.

Gamma Knife: A gamma unit can be operated with a small staff because it is a relatively uncomplicated single purpose facility. According to Alleyne *et al.* (1997), the annual maintenance cost for the Gamma Knife is about *$442,000*

Proton therapy: Particle therapy units are comparatively expensive to maintain, and need a big staff of physicists and engineers to run it. If maintenance is assumed to cost about 10% of the purchase price, it could cost *$2,600,000* per annum, Gademann estimated $5.5 million (Table O6.2).

O.5
Life Span of Treatment Units

Table O5.1 gives an estimate of the life span of treatment units.

O.6
Cost Comparison: Surgery *versus* Radiosurgery

Table O6.1 shows the estimated radiosurgical costs for particle therapy *versus* photon therapy.

Table O5.1 Estimate of life span of radiosurgical units. Estimates: Epstein and Linguist (1993)

Unit	Years
Gamma Knife	20
Linear accelerator	10
Proton accelerator	18 (Gademann 1993)

Table O6.1 Radiosurgical costs for the treatment of metastatic brain tumours have been compared to neurosurgical costs by Rutigliano *et al.* (1995)

Uncomplicated procedure cost	
Radiosurgery	$20,209
Neurosurgery	$27,587

Average complication cost per case	
Radiosurgery	$2,534
Neurosurgery	$2,874

Total cost per procedure	
Radiosurgery	$22,743
Neurosurgery	$30,461

Table O6.2 summarises some comparative data on costs.

Table O6.2 Comparison of approximate radiosurgical costs

	Linear accelerator	Gamma Knife	Proton facility
Capital cost	$2.0	$4	$21–$40 (× 1 million)
Radio-surgical fees	$ 5,331 to $22,000	$ 9,800 to $34,000	$6,720 (NAC 1998) to $8,690 (estimate to $20,000 upwards)
Maintenance	$123,000 to $249,000	$442,000	$5.5 million (Gademann 1993)

O.7
Summary

The Linear accelerator for <u>radiosurgical</u> work seems to be the least costly. This versatile unit is suitable for radiosurgical and general oncological work. A proton facility could probably treat lesions > 5 cm^3 do the same or better, but at greater cost in terms of maintenance, installation and costs per case. On the other hand, the life expectancy of a proton installation may be about twice that of a linear accelerator.

The Gamma Knife is a dedicated facility with high initial installation costs, small staff requirements, fairly expensive source replacements every 5 years or so, and limited general utility outside of the radiosurgical arena.

The linear accelerator and the isocentric proton facility are both very versatile general radiotherapy units, whereas the Gamma Knife is a dedicated mostly single purpose unit for neuroradiosurgery. The high cost of a proton facility may be partially offset by its relatively long life expectancy. Gamma Knives are only suitable for intracranial lesions, whereas the linear accelerator and proton units are suitable for treatment of lesions at all body sites.

O.8
References

Alleyne CH, Fox TH, Olsen JJ et al. (1997) Stereotactic radiosurgery of malignant and benign lesions using a patient rotator. Radiat Oncol Invest 5:20–30

Becker G, Kortmann R, Kaulich TW et al. (1996) Gamma Knife *versus* stereotactic linear accelerator. Utilisation, clinical results and cost benefit relations. (in German) Radiologie 36:345–353

Eisenberg JM (1989) Clinical economics. A guide to the economic analysis of clinical practices. JAMA 262:2879

Epstein ME, Linquist C (1993) Cost accounting the Gamma Knife. Stereotact Funct Neurosurg 61 Suppl 1:6–10

Gademann G (1994) In: Amaldi, Larsson (eds) Hadrontherapy in oncology. Proceedings of the First International Symposium on Hadrontherapy, Como, Italy, October 1993. Elsevier, Amsterdam, pp 59–67

Luxton G, Petrovich Z, Jozsef G et al. (1993) Stereotactic radiosurgery: principles and comparisons of treatment methods. Neurosurgery 32:241–259

Penar PL (1996) Cost and outcome analysis (of the management of cerebral metastases). Neurosurg Clin North Am 7:547–558

Rutigliano MJ, Lunsford LD, Kondziolka D, Strauss MJ, Khanna V, Green M (1995) The cost effectiveness of stereotactic radiosurgery of solitary metastatic brain tumours. Neurosurgery 37:445–353

Rutigliano MJ (1995) Cost effectiveness analysis: a review. Neurosurgery 37:436

Suit H, Urie M (1992) Proton beams in radiotherapy. J Natl Cancer Inst 84:155–164

Weinstein MC (1990) Principles of cost-effective resource allocation in health care organisation. Int J Technol Assess Health Care 6:93

P Appendix

P.1
The Spetzler Martin Grading System (with Some Remarks)

1. Size

The AVM is regarded as:
- Small if the greatest *diameter* of the nidus is < 3 cm (radius < 1.5 cm, volume < 14 cm^3). (This is already "large" for radiosurgery.)
- Medium if the greatest diameter of the lesion is between 3–6 cm (radius 1.5–3 cm, volume 15–102 cm^3).
- Large, if the AVM diameter is > 6 cm (> 102 cm^3).

The size of the AVM is usually closely related to the number of feeding arteries, the amount of flow, and the degree of "steal".

2. Pattern of venous drainage

- Drainage is considered to be superficial if all the drainage is through the cortical venous system, as determined by the angiogram.
- The drainage is considered to be deep if any or all of the drainage is through deep veins such as the internal cerebral veins, basal veins or pre-central cerebellar vein.

The deep veins are difficult and dangerous for the surgeon to manage and AVMs with deep drainage are likely to be referred for radiosurgery.

3. Eloquence of the adjacent brain

Eloquent brain regions are defined as those when damaged will have debilitating effects.

Eloquent areas:
- The sensorimotor, language and visual cortex
- The hypothalamus and the thalamus
- The internal capsule and the brain stem.
- The cerebellar peduncles and the deep cerebellar nuclei.

Areas such as the anterior frontal and temporal lobes and the cerebellar cortex are considered to be "non-eloquent".

Spetzler-Martin Grade 1, 2 and 3 are basically small superficial nidi in non-critical brain areas, and Grade 4 and 5 are large, deep seated lesions, or lesions in critical brain areas.

Table P1.1 Determination of AVM grade according to the Spetzler-Martin system. Grade = size + elo-quence + drainage: maximum score = 5. A Grade 5 lesion is associated with a significant risk of surgi-cal morbidity and mortality. Some lesions are so large as to be obviously "inoperable" and are referred to as "Grade 6" inoperable lesions due to size, or location, and lesions of the midbrain, pons or the thal-amus fall into this class.

Graded feature	Points assigned
Size of AVM	
Small < 3 cm	1 (< 14 cc)
Medium 3–6 cm	2 (15–102 cc)
Large > 6 cm	3 (> 102 cc)
Eloquence	
Non-eloquent	0
Eloquent	1
Pattern of venous drainage	
Superficial	0
Deep	1

As far as radiosurgery is concerned, the radiation oncologist is likely to be asked to treat patients who are medically unfit for surgery, for whatever reason, and patients who are considered inoperable by the neurosurgeon.

All the parameters of interest do not carry the same weight for the radiation oncol-ogist as for the neurosurgeon, therefore a grading system that may be of more use to the radiation oncologist is proposed in P.2.

In general, the lesion sizes of the Spetzler-Martin system (1986) are considered too large to be of much use for radiosurgical work.

Reference and Acknowledgement

Spetzler RF, Martin NA (1986) A proposed grading system for arteriovenous mal-formations. J Neurosurg 65:476–483

P.2
A Proposed Grading System for AVMs for Radiosurgery

Examples:

Grade 1. Low risk: (Score 2–4)

A lesion of < 1.8 cm (3 cm^3) (1) non-eloquent, low sensitivity (1) points = 2 has a low risk and can be assumed to have a good chance of complication free control. The factors that should be carefully weighed are the fall-off ("penumbra") of the treatment plan, the total dose and the number of beams, three or more entry points should be used with protons wherever possible. (See chapter I.)

Grade 2. Medium risk: (Score 4–5)

A medium sized lesion (2) located in a medium sensitive area (3) score 5, should have a reasonable prognosis and fair complication risk, as would have patients with a very small lesion (1) in a sensitive area (3), score 4.

Grade 3. High risk: (Score 6–7)

Table P2.1 Graded features

Size of AVM (Diameter and volume)	Points assigned and comments
Lesion sizes suitable for treatment by:	
Small < 1.8 cm diam, 3 cm^3	1 Gamma Knife, LA and plateau prtons, maximum GK collimator 18 mm, 3.1 cm^3
Medium 1.9 cm diam, 3.6 cm^3 2.1 cm diam, 5.1 cm^3	2 LA, protons, multiple isocentre GK
Large > 2.2 cm diam, > 5.1 cm^3*	3 Protons or other heavy charged particles multiple isocentre LA or GK
Eloquence	
Non-eloquent	1 Frontal lobe
Eloquent a) Not very sensitive	2 Motor and speech = Cerebellum, temporal parietal lobes
b) Medium sensitivity	3 Optical cortex = basal ganglia
c) Highly sensitive	4 Brainstem, midbrain, pons thalamus and corpuscallosum

* Over 5.1 cm^3 the integral dose with the linear accelerator becomes too large and over 5.1 cm^3 the risk of complication increases rapidly. (See Chapter I on Dose-Volume Relationships) The pattern of venous drainage has been excluded from this classification. See PIE score (Flickinger *et al.* 1999).

A large lesion of more than 5 cm^3 (3) in a highly sensitive area, e.g. pons (4), will have a score of 7 and a high risk of radiation induced complications. In the final analysis it may be the volume of normal brain irradiated that is the critical factor and doses of > 10 Gy (Voges 1996) or 12 Gy (Flickinger 1997) of normal brain (including the lesion for AVMs may be a cut-off point). See chapter I.

References and Acknowledgement

Flickinger JC, Kondziolka D, Maitz A *et al.* (1997) Analysis of neurological sequelae from radiosurgery of arteriovenous malformation. How location affects outcome. Int J Radiat Oncol Biol Phys 40:273-278

Flickinger JC, Kondziolka D, Pollock BE, Maitz A, Lunsford LD (1997) Complications from arteriovenous malformation radiosurgery: multivariate analysis and risk modelling. Int J Radiat Oncol Biol Phys 38:485-490

Spetzler RF, Martin NA (1986) A proposed grading system for arteriovenous malformations. J Neurosurg 65:476-483

Voges J, Treuer H, Sturm V, Buchner C, Lehrke R, Kocher M, Staar S, Kuchta J, Müller RP (1996) Risk analysis of linear accelerator radiosurgery. Int J Radiat Oncol Biol Phys 36:1055-1063

P.3
Planning Target Volumes

Table P3.1 Planning target volumes (PTVs) in cm^3 for penumbral widths of 3, 2, 1.6, 1.3, 0.8, 0.5 cm – for the [10 Gy 10 cm^3] constraint

90% PI

Radiosurgical dose (Gy)	PTVs (cm^3)						
	3.00	2.00	1.60	1.30	1.00	0.08	0.05
25			0.07	0.40	1.21	2.11	4.17
22.5			0.15	0.60	1.50	2.45	4.49
20		0.03	0.35	0.92	1.93	2.91	4.91
17.5		0.22	0.75	1.49	2.60	3.59	5.50
15		0.84	1.67	2.55	3.71	4.65	6.34
12.5	1.2	2.91	3.89	4.76	5.74	6.47	7.67
12	1.9	3.71	4.66	5.46	6.34	6.99	8.03
10	10.0	10.00	10.00	10.00	10.00	10.00	10.00

80% PI

Radiosurgical dose (Gy)	PTVs (cm^3)						
	3.00	2.00	1.60	1.30	1.00	0.08	0.05
25		0.01	0.22	0.72	1.67	2.63	4.65
22.5		0.05	0.37	0.96	1.99	2.97	4.96
20		0.16	0.65	1.35	2.44	3.27	5.36
17.5		0.46	1.15	1.89	3.13	4.10	5.47
15	0.16	1.26	2.17	3.08	5.29	5.12	6.70
12.5	1.67	3.43	4.39	5.22	6.14	6.81	7.91
12	2.45	4.22	5.12	5.87	6.70	7.29	8.23
10	10.00	10.00	10.00	10.00	10.00	10.00	10.00

65% PI

Radiosurgical dose (Gy)	PTVs (cm^3)						
	3.00	2.00	1.60	1.30	1.00	0.08	0.05
25		0.19	0.72	1.45	2.55	3.54	5.46
22.5		0.34	0.96	1.76	2.90	3.88	5.73
20		0.60	1.35	2.20	3.36	4.33	6.09
17.5	0.10	1.09	1.97	2.88	4.03	4.95	6.57
15	0.60	2.10	3.08	3.99	5.06	5.87	7.25
12.5	2.55	4.33	5.22	5.96	6.77	7.35	8.27
12	3.37	5.06	5.87	6.54	7.25	7.75	8.54
10	10.00	10.00	10.00	10.00	10.00	10.00	10.00

50% PI

Radiosurgical dose (Gy)	PTVs (cm^3)						
	3.00	2.00	1.60	1.30	1.00	0.08	0.05
25	0.04	0.84	1.67	2.27	3.71	4.65	6.34
22.5	0.11	1.10	1.99	2.90	4.05	4.96	6.58
20	0.26	1.56	2.44	3.83	4.49	5.36	6.88
17.5	0.63	2.14	3.13	4.03	5.10	5.91	7.27
15	1.50	3.25	4.22	5.06	6.00	6.70	7.83
12.5	4.33	5.36	6.14	6.77	7.44	7.91	8.65
12	4.09	6.00	6.70	7.25	7.83	8.23	8.86
10	10.00	10.00	10.00	10.00	10.00	10.00	10.00

Table P3.2 Skull base lesions - calculation of safe doses for the constraint of 10 Gy administered to the lesion volume plus an additional volume of 10^3. The maximum dose has been limited to 20 Gy for safety reasons. Special caution is needed for parasagittal meningiomas. Note that the PTV (planning treatment volume) will be somewhat larger than the actual volume of the meningiomas or similar lesion type.

Lesion volume (cm³)	90% Prescription isodose Dose fall-off per millimetre (%)					80% Prescription isodose Dose fall-off per millimetre (%)				
	2.7	4	6	8	10	2.7	4	6	8	10
	Penumbral width (cm)					Penumbral width (cm)				
	3.0	2.0	1.6	1.0	0.8	3.0	2.0	1.6	1.0	0.8
0.1	14.6	18.8				15.5	21.1			
0.5	13.5	16.3	19.3			14.1	17.6	21.8		
1	12.9	15.1	17.3			13.4	16.1	19		
1.5	12.6	14.4	16.2			13	15.3	17.6		
2	12.4	14	15.5			12.7	14.7	16.6		
3	12	13.3	14.5	20.1		12.4	13.9	15.4		
4	11.8	12.9	14	18.3		12.1	13.4	14.7	20.4	
5	11.6	12.6	13.5	17.2	20.9	11.9	13.1	14.1	18.8	
6	11.5	12.4	13.2	16.3	19.4	11.7	12.8	13.7	17.7	
7	11.4	12.2	12.9	15.7	18.3	11.6	12.6	13.4	16.9	20.4
8	11.3	12.1	12.7	15.2	17.5	11.5	12.4	13.2	16.3	19.3
10	11.2	11.8	12.4	14.5	16.3	11.3	12.1	12.8	15.3	17.7
15	10.9	11.4	11.9	13.4	14.6	11.1	11.7	12.2	14	15.5
20	10.8	11.2	11.6	12.8	13.7	10.9	11.4	11.8	13.2	14.4
25	10.7	11.1	11.4	12.4	13.1	10.8	11.2	11.6	12.7	13.7
30	10.6	10.9	11.2	12.1	12.7	10.7	11.1	11.4	12.4	13.2

Lesion volume (cm³)	65% Prescription isodose Dose fall-off per millimetre (%)					50% Prescription isodose Dose fall-off per millimetre (%)				
	2.7	4	6	8	10	2.7	4	6	8	10
	Penumbral width (cm)					Penumbral width (cm)				
	3.0	2.0	1.6	1.0	0.8	3.0	2.0	1.6	1.0	0.8
0.1	17.8					23.2				
0.5	15.6					18.8				
1	14.6	18.8				16.9				
1.5	14	17.4	21.3			15.9				
2	13.6	16.5	19.7			15.3	20.4			
3	13.1	15.3	17.7			14.4	18.2			
4	12.7	14.6	16.5			13.8	16.9	20.4		
5	12.4	14.1	15.6			13.4	16	18.8		
6	12.2	13.7	15	21.6		13.1	15.4	17.7		
7	12	13.4	14.6	20.1		12.8	14.9	16.9		
8	11.9	13.1	14.2	19		12.6	14.5	16.3		
10	11.7	12.7	13.6	17.5	21.5	12.3	13.8	15.3	22.5	
15	11.3	12.1	12.8	15.4	17.8	11.8	12.9	14	18.3	23.1
20	11.1	11.8	12.3	14.3	16	11.5	12.4	13.2	16.4	19.5
25	11	11.5	12	13.6	15	11.3	12.1	12.7	15.3	17.6
30	10.9	11.4	11.8	13.1	14.3	11.2	11.8	12.4	14.5	16.3

The influence of the prescription isodose on the dose distribution for a 2 cm diameter lesion for an 8 mm penumbra (90%-10% dose fall-off), for a single dose of 20 Gy prescribed at 80% or 50%.

To calculate the isodose for any given dose, the following formula is used:

$$\frac{\text{dose at isodose}}{\text{prescription dose}} \times \text{prescription isodose}$$

Volume at 10 Gy = 14.14 cm^3

10 Gy, 40%	80%, 20 Gy
5 Gy, 20 %	100%, 25 Gy
	120%, 30 Gy

Volume at 10 Gy = 9.21 cm^3

	50%, 20 Gy
10 Gy, 25 %	75%, 30 Gy
5 Gy, 12.5%	100%, 40 Gy

a.) Example illustrating graphically the effect of the prescription isodose on the dose distribution within a 4 cm^3 lesion. The penumbra is assumed to fall 1 mm per 10% dose fall-off. It is clear that the volume of brain irradiated to equivalent doses will be smaller for doses prescribed at the 50% isodose compared to the 80% isodose, for a single isocentre.

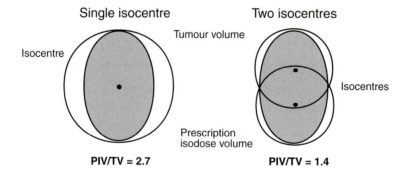

Single isocentre   **Two isocentres**

Isocentre   Tumour volume   Isocentres

Prescription isodose volume

PIV/TV = 2.7   **PIV/TV = 1.4**

b.) Example illustrating the concepts of PIV/TV. The same principle as in (a) above applies for a dose prescribed with multiple isocentres. The prescription isodose volume (PIV) devided by the tumour volume (TV) is a measure of dose conformity.
(Redrawn from Shaw et al. 1996, Int J Radiat Oncol Biol Phys 34:647-654)

P.4
Lateral Dose Fall-off of Various Stationary Radiation Beams

Table P4.1 Lateral dose fall-off of various stationary radiation beams, adapted and expanded from Luxton *et al.* (1993). Lee *et al.* 1993 mathematically modelled a 250 MeV proton beam and found that the lateral fall-off should be, for a 10 cm SOBP from 80% to 20% 2.7 mm at 100 mm deep and 7.8 mm at 200 mm depth in water (22.2%/mm and 7.6% per mm, respectively). The helium beams were scanned across the centre of the SOBP region at various depths (Smith *et al.* 1994). The figures *in* parentheses give the per cent lateral dose fall-off of dose in per cent per millimetre

Beam	Collimator diameter (mm)	Depth (cm)	Dose fall-off (mm) 90%–10%	Dose fall-off (mm) 80%–20%
He^{++}SOBP[b]				
27 mm SOBP	12.7 mm		12.5 (6.4)	4.4 (18.2)
27 mm SOBP	12.7 mm		8.0 (*10*)	2.7 (22.2)
			6.0 (*13.3*)	1.9 (31.5)
20 mm SOBP	20.0 mm		17.0 (4.7)	4.5 (17.7)
			9.0 (8.8)	3.5 (17.1)
			6.0 (*13.3*)	2.5 (24.0)
Protons	100 mm	10	4.1 (*19.5*)	2.7 (22.2)[a]
		20	10.2 (7.8)	7.8 (7.6)[a]
NAC	100 mm?	24	15.7 (5.33)	9.4 (6.3)
Linear acc. 6 MV	15 mm		7.5 (10.7)	3.9 (20.5)
Gamma Knife	15 mm		8.0 (10.0)	13.5 (4.4)
				3.0 (21.1)[c]

[a] Lee *et al.* (1993);
[b] *SOBP* Spread Out Bragg Peak;
[c] Corrected for stray irradiation

P.5
Expanded Tables Based on the Tables of Brenner, Martell and Hall (1991) for Fractionated Therapy for Recurrent Malignant Brain Tumours

Table P5.1 Tables for fractionated therapy for recurrent malignant brain tumours. The α/β assumed for brain tumours is 7, treatment to be completed in 4 days. Expanded and adapted from Brenner *et al.* (1991) and Hall and Brenner (1993)

Single fraction radiosurgical dose	Total fractionated dose							
	Fx=2	Fx=3	Fx=4	Fx=5	Fx=6	Fx=7	Fx=8	Fx=9
9	11.3	12.7	13.7	14.6	15.2	15.7	16.2	16.6
10	12.7	14.3	15.4	16.5	17.3	18.0	18.5	18.9
11	14.3	15.9	17.2	18.4	19.3	20.1	20.8	21.3
12	15.4	17.6	19.0	20.4	21.4	22.3	23.0	23.7
13	16.8	19.2	20.8	22.4	23.6	24.5	25.4	26.2
14	18.1	20.8	22.4	24.4	25.8	27.1	28.2	28.7
15	19.5	22.5	24.3	26.5	28.0	29.1	30.2	31.2

Table P5.1 (Continued)

Single fraction radiosurgical dose	Total fractionated dose							
16	20.9	24.1	25.6	28.5	31.1	31.6	32.8	33.8
17	22.3	25.8	28.2	30.6	32.4	34.0	35.5	36.4
18	23.6	27.4	30.2	32.6	34.6	36.3	37.8	39.0
19	25.0	29.1	31.9	34.7	36.8	38.7	40.6	41.6
20	*26.4*	*30.8*	*33.8*	*36.8*	*39.2*	*41.2*	*43.0*	*44.3*
21	27.8	32.5	35.7	38.9	41.5	43.7	45.5	47.0
22	29.2	34.1	37.6	41.0	43.7	46.0	47.9	49.7
23	30.6	35.5	39.4	43.2	46.1	48.6	50.7	52.4
24	32.0	37.5	41.4	45.3	48.4	51.1	53.3	55.1
25	33.4	39.2	43.3	47.4	50.7	53.5	55.9	57.8

References

Brenner DJ, Martell MK, Hall EJ (1991) Fractionated regimes for stereotactic radiotherapy of recurrent tumours in the brain. Int J Radiat Oncol Biol Phys 21:819–824

Hall EJ, Brenner DJ (1993) The radiobiology of radiosurgery: rationale for different treatment regimes for AVMs and malignancies. Int J Radiat Oncol Biol Phys 25:381–385

P.6.
Fractionated Treatment for AVMs

Table P6.1 shows the equivalent fractionated doses to replace a single large doses for late reacting tissues like AVMs and other related conditions with an assumed α/β ratio of 2, using the BED_2 formalism.

Table P6.1 Equivalent fractionated doses for single large doses for late reacting tissues like AVMs and other related conditions with an α/β ratio of 2

Single fraction radiosurgical dose	Total fractionated dose for $\alpha/\beta = 2$							
	Fx=2	Fx=3	Fx=4	Fx=5	Fx=6	Fx=7	Fx=8	Fx=9
9	12.2	14.5	16.2	17.7	18.9	20.2	21.3	22.0
10	13.8	16.2	18.3	20.0	21.8	22.6	24.0	25.4
11	15.0	17.8	20.2	22.2	23.9	25.4	26.7	28.0
12	16.4	19.6	22.2	24.4	26.2	28.2	29.6	31.0
13	17.8	21.4	24.4	26.6	28.7	30.6	32.2	33.7
14	19.3	23.1	26.3	28.8	31.1	33.2	34.1	36.8
15	20.6	24.7	28.2	31.5	33.3	35.7	37.7	39.8
16	22.0	26.6	30.1	33.3	36.0	38.4	40.6	42.7
17	23.5	28.3	32.2	35.5	38.4	41.1	43.5	45.6
18	24.9	30.0	34.2	37.7	40.8	43.7	46.2	48.5
19	26.3	31.7	36.1	39.9	43.4	46.3	49.1	51.6
20	27.8	33.4	38.2	42.25	45.7	48.9	51.8	54.5

Experience with fractionated radiosurgery is very limited.

Caution: This table indicates that an under-dosage for AVMs can result by from 2%–3% for two fractions and up to 21% for nine fractions for α/β values = 2 if Brenner's.

Doses of 20 Gy should only be used for very small lesions, provided the beam parameters are good. (See Chapter I on Dose-Volume Relationships) Table P6.2 shows the probable under-dosage for fractionated therapy if Brenner's tables should be used for AVMs.

Table P6.2 The fractionated equivalent doses for a single dose of 20 Gy for malignant tumours is compared for the required equivalent fractionated doses for AVMs

	Fx=2	Fx=3	Fx=4	Fx=5	Fx=6	Fx=7	Fx=8	Fx=9
Brenner	26.4	30.8	33.8	36.8	39.2	41.2	43.0	44.3
$\alpha/\beta = 2$	27.8	33.4	38.2	42.25	45.7	48.9	51.8	54.5

It should be clear that Brenner's tables cannot be applied for fractionated treatments for AVMs – the dose must be escalated from 5% to 23% depending on the number of fractions. It needs to be stressed that a single dose of 19 Gy will inflict as much damage to the late tissues as a conventionally fractionated dose of 100 fractions of 2 Gy each! It should seldom be necessary to give such large doses, and the trend is toward smaller volumes and smaller doses to ensure complication free therapy. (See also Chapter I on Dose-Volume Relationships and Chapter M on Complications)

P.7
The Stereophotogrammetric System of Patient Positioning and Immobilisation

The basic components of the system are a computer monitored motorised chair, eight digital video cameras and two computers. The chair has five degrees of freedom: three translations, rotation around the vertical axis, and backrest swing. The head rest can also be adjusted, aiding patient comfort and fine tuning of the position.

The immobilisation mask is a vacuum drawn thermoplastic mask, of very accurate fit, cast in two sections: a front facial section as is customary for standard radiotherapy practice in many centres, and a sturdy section of thicker plastic around the occipital part of the head.

The two parts can be drawn together by specially fitted Velcro straps. The back section also has two Plexiglas arcs glued on to enable fixation to the headrest/backrest of the chair (Jones *et al.* 1995).

Onto the mask (facial section) is fitted fiducial markers. These are retroflective, easily "seen" by the digital video cameras. The markers are drilled out with 1 mm central holes, which can be identified on CT, or MRI and serve as very accurate reference points. The reflective surface of the markers is 8 mm in diameter. The patient is CT scanned with the mask in place in the supine position, from the top of the head to well below the target area.

From the scan the 3-D co-ordinates for the target and other areas of interest are determined relative to a reference point in the target volume. This reference point is usually taken as the treatment isocentre.

The SPG system operates in two modes: The first for positioning and the second for monitoring the patient for movement once the set-up position has been verified.

During the positioning phase, the TV cameras capture video images of the marker positions from several angles through a "frame grabber". The images are then processed by the first computer according to an SPG algorithm.

The positions of the cameras and of the proton beam in space are accurately known, therefore it is possible to compute the position of the reference point (isocentre).

The co-ordinates from the entry points, marked on the mask, are also fed into the computer.

The computed data are then relayed to the second computer controlling the chair movements, executed by stepper motors.

The X,Y and Z translational accuracy is within 0.1 mm and the vertical and rotational movement is within 0.1 deg of arc.

The first computer also computes collimator rotation for each individual field.

Once the patient's treatment position has been determined by computer, the position is checked with front and back pointer lasers as an additional control. The set-up is then simulated. In this process, use is made of co-axial roentgenography. A first exposure is taken without the collimator in position, a second with the collimator in position, which shows up the collimators outline and position as a well-defined darker shadow.

This can be compared to the digitally reconstructed radiograph from the planning computer to verify that the location and orientation is as planned.

The system is accurate: Jones et al. (1995) quotes an accuracy of 1 mm. (The registration between the reference points on the masks and anatomical landmarks varies by less than 1 mm during the course of a treatment.)

The second function of the SPG system is to monitor the patient for movement during the time the beam is switched on. The sensitivity for this function can be adjusted, and the beam will switch off when patient movement exceeds the pre-set limits. A high level of sensitivity is chosen for very small targets, or targets near vital structures.

However, some problems of patient movement, the cameras and the software have been experienced and the National Accelerator Centre is presently investigating the possibility of a relocatable stereotactic frame with bite blocks.

Reference

Jones DTL, Schreuder AN, Symons JE Rüther, Van der Vlugt G, Bennett KF, Yates ADB (1995) Use of stereophotogrammetry in proton radiation therapy. Proceedings FIG Commission, 6th International FIG Symposium, February, Cape Town

Subject Index

Printing: Mercedes-Druck, Berlin
Binding: Buchbinderei Lüderitz & Bauer, Berlin